Negotiated Breastfeeding

Based on an ethnography of postpartum consultations by independent midwives in Switzerland, this book produces unique insights into home birth parents' breastfeeding journey from the first hours after birth to weaning. Considered the "natural" continuity of childbirth without intervention, breastfeeding is a fundamental component of the holistic, continuous, and individualised care independent midwives provide as they engage with parents in a shared construction of meaning around breastfeeding.

This book offers new perspectives on the conceptualisation of breastfeeding as a shared process. Parents, in collaboration with their midwife and baby, are jointly constructing "negotiated breastfeeding". As the child grows and develops, questions arise regarding the management of risks, the construction of the lactating body, the body work required, and the perception of breastfeeding as a means of communication with the child, consistent with a "child-centred" approach to parenting. Fostering a reflection on the contrasts and similarities between the marginal model of holistic care and the dominant biomedical model, this book sheds light on issues of a broader scope: the relationship to health risks and health promotion, gender inequalities regarding parental roles and responsibilities, the concept of the child as a "project", and the consequential "intensification" of parenthood. The book also explores transversal themes by outlining how reproduction and parenting are undertaken in Switzerland, framed by the local cultural, political, and economic context, including the gender system and resulting power relationships.

Caroline Chautems is a Swiss National Science Foundation research fellow at the Institute of Social Sciences, University of Lausanne, Switzerland. She is also a lecturer at the Geneva School of Health Sciences. A social and medical anthropologist, Dr Chautems is currently working on Swiss caesarean culture, including the emergence of new obstetrical and therapeutic practices. Her research interests focus on reproduction and parenthood, with particular attention given to gender and bodies in regard to parenting and health policy.

Social Science Perspectives on Childbirth and Reproduction

Series editor: Robbie Davis-Floyd (Rice University, Houston, Texas)

This series focuses on issues relating to childbirth and reproduction from social science perspectives. It includes single-authored, co-authored, or edited books concerned both with people's reproductive experiences and with birth practitioners such as midwives (both professional and traditional), obstetricians, nurses, doulas, and others. It seeks to provide new viewpoints on functional and sustainable birth models and the challenges to their creation and maintenance, as well as on obstetric violence, disrespect, and abuse and their root causes. Single-case or comparative ethnographies on birth and other reproductive issues are featured, from high-tech conceptions to normal pregnancy and birth, including reproductive politics and human-rights issues in reproduction worldwide.

Birthing Models on the Human Rights Frontier
Speaking Truth to Power
Edited by Betty-Anne Daviss and Robbie Davis-Floyd

Midwives in Mexico
Situated Politics, Politically Situated
Hanna Laako and Georgina Sánchez-Ramírez

Birthing Techno-Sapiens
Human-Technology Co-Evolution and the Future of Reproduction
Edited by Robbie Davis-Floyd

Negotiated Breastfeeding
Holistic Postpartum Care and Embodied Parenting
Caroline Chautems

https://www.routledge.com/Social-Science-Perspectives-on-Childbirth-and-Reproduction/book-series/SSPCR

Negotiated Breastfeeding

Holistic Postpartum Care and Embodied Parenting

Caroline Chautems

Routledge
Taylor & Francis Group

LONDON AND NEW YORK

First published 2022
by Routledge
2 Park Square, Milton Park, Abingdon, Oxon OX14 4RN

and by Routledge
605 Third Avenue, New York, NY 10158

Routledge is an imprint of the Taylor & Francis Group, an informa business

British Library Cataloguing-in-Publication Data
A catalogue record for this book is available from the British Library

Library of Congress Cataloging-in-Publication Data
A catalog record has been requested for this book

ISBN: 9780367643522 (hbk)
ISBN: 9780367643546 (pbk)
ISBN: 9781003124108 (ebk)

DOI: 10.4324/9781003124108

Typeset in Sabon
by Deanta Global Publishing Services, Chennai, India

To my mother, my grandmother, and all the women who were told by misinformed health professionals that they were not able to breastfeed their babies.

Contents

Foreword   viii
Acknowledgements   xi

Introduction   1

1 Holistic care in Switzerland and my ethnographic study   16

2 Reinventing parenthood through breastfeeding: Risk-
   centric society and embodied parenting   50

3 Feeding to thrive   84

4 Building the lactating body   124

5 The communicating feed   162

Conclusion   208

Bibliography   225
Index   245

Foreword

This book is based on an extensive ethnography by Dr Caroline Chautems into the experiences of breastfeeding in home birth parents and their postpartum consultations with independent midwives in Switzerland. It is truly an honour to be invited to write the foreword for this excellent piece of scholarship by a social and medical anthropologist who has, through rigorous and time-consuming ethnographic study, vividly illuminated an anthropological perspective on the lived, embodied practice of breastfeeding by mothers in collaboration with their babies, partners, and independent midwives.

As a midwife whose research training and expertise are in ethnography, I have observed that the fields of medical anthropology and midwifery have many interconnections. The anthropologist spends extensive hours conducting ethnographic fieldwork, quietly observing, listening, asking questions, and analysing. The skilled midwife, likewise, observes the mother as she labours, gives birth, feeds, and cares for her new baby, intervening only when necessary. Both, the anthropologist and the midwife, over time, come to know and understand the participants. The participants, in turn, develop a growing trust in the person accompanying them on their journeys. Both anthropologist and midwife reflexively attune to explicit and tacit knowledges through participating in people's lives, ideally over a considerable period of time. Both have complex ethical issues and dilemmas to consider; indeed, as Spradley (1980) argues, the ethnographer is required to actually protect the sensitivities, rights, and interests of participants. This is also the case for midwives when supporting women, their partners, and their babies during a very important time of their lives.

Dr Chautems firstly provides a socio-cultural, political, and economic context of how reproduction and parenting are undertaken in Switzerland. As in many other industrialised countries, home births are marginal and contrast with the institutionalised, medicalised settings within which most women give birth. The author describes an in-depth ethnography having attended one hundred and 18 postnatal postpartum visits by 11 independent midwives, observing between one and eight midwife–family consultations per family. She also conducted two to six interviews with each mother or couple during the period of breastfeeding. She adopts an anti-essentialist stance and a critical gender perspective in describing the breastfeeding "project" and associated embodied parenting styles of the home birth parents who were participants in the study.

The research offers new perspectives on the conceptualisation of breastfeeding as a collective and highly complex social process involving parents, the child, the wider family, and health professionals. It challenges the persistence of the public health promotion, informed-choice ideal, and individual-based paradigm that tends to place intense responsibility upon the mother. The concept of "negotiated breastfeeding" is introduced with negotiations at play between midwives and parents, parents and babies, and the embodied project of breastfeeding. This co-production of meanings develops and changes as the child grows, bringing with it tensions and conflicts and diverging meanings of breastfeeding.

Dr Chautems identifies the significant body and emotional work that mothers engage in to sustain breastfeeding and the nurture of their child through breastfeeding. This links to an ideological view of motherhood that requires sacrifice, tenacity, and in some cases, persevering through pain. The intensified approach to parenthood involved self-denial and time-consuming parenting practices to include demand feeding and long-term breastfeeding. The fathers invested considerably in the facilitation of the child-centred and demanding aspects of intensive parenting, although this was not specifically acknowledged by the essentially matricentric approaches of midwives.

I published my first monograph in 2006 (Dykes 2006), along with associated articles based on my own doctoral thesis (Dykes 2005a, 2005b). My research focused on the working conditions of hospital midwives and the early postpartum period of new mothers, whom I did not meet again after their hospital stay. The settings were highly medicalised hospitals with industrial concepts of time and production identified and explored as central to the experiences of both mothers and midwives. Women spoke about the temporal dilemmas they experienced with breastfeeding and the challenges in relating to midwives and in establishing a relationship with their infant in these settings (Dykes 2009a). Midwives expressed the constant tyranny of linear time upon them affording them little time to "care" within these hospital settings (Dykes 2009b).

This book by Dr Chautems, written 15 years later, fills a gap in the existing corpus of social sciences literature between the experience and practice of breastfeeding mothers, pregnancy, birth, and postpartum care. Focusing on breastfeeding, the originality of this work lies in exploring the postpartum period, understood in the light of the overall birth process, and taking into account the interaction between midwife and parents at the centre of its analyses. Since the author continued meeting with parents until their children were weaned, she had the opportunity to document the development of parents' feelings and practices over the longer term.

The home settings are in striking contrast to the hospitals referred to in my book (Dykes 2006); however, as Dr Chautems highlights, the holistic model of care, sought by parents and offered by midwives, did not surpass the pressure upon the independent midwives to adhere to aspects of the bio-medical model when required. Indeed, as she emphasises, the midwives had been educated within this paradigm bringing associated tensions for them-selves and parents. Parents also engaged in aspects of the risk-based, bio-medical paradigm where it was felt to be appropriate. Weighing the baby as a means of health monitoring is one example. Thus, there are both striking divergences between the settings of my research and that of Dr Chautems, but also some convergences with regard to the pervasive influence of the dominant biomedical model.

I wholeheartedly recommend this monograph to anthropologists and the wider social sciences community, as well as midwives and related health practitioners working in the fields of parenting and child health.

Fiona Dykes PhD, MA, RM, FHEA,
Professor Emeritus of Maternal and Infant Health,
Maternal and Infant Nutrition and Nurture Unit (MAINN), School of
Community Health and Midwifery, University of Central Lancashire,
Preston, UK.

Dykes Fiona. 2005a. "'Supply' and 'Demand': Breastfeeding as Labour". *Social Science and Medicine* 60, 2283–2293.

Dykes Fiona. 2005b. "A critical ethnographic study of encounters between midwives and breastfeeding women on postnatal wards in England". *Midwifery* 21, 241–252.

Dykes Fiona. 2006. *Breastfeeding in Hospital: Mothers, Midwives and the Production Line.* London: Routledge.

Dykes Fiona. 2009a. "'Feeding all the time': Women's temporal dilemmas around breastfeeding in hospital". In Mccourt Christine (ed.). *Childbirth, Midwifery and Concepts of Time.* London: Berghahn Books, 202–221.

Dykes Fiona. 2009b. "'No time to care': Midwifery work on postnatal wards in England". In Hunter Billie & Deery Ruth (eds.). *Emotions in Midwifery and Reproduction.* Basingstoke: Palgrave Macmillan, 90–104.

Spradley James P. 1980. *Participant Observation.* New York: Holt, Rinehart & Winston.

Acknowledgements

During my research, I witnessed breastfeeding journeys starting from the very first moments after birth. I am incredibly grateful to all the parents who welcomed me in their homes at such an intimate time of their existence and who shared their feelings, doubts, sad, and joyful moments—sometimes over years. I am equally thankful to all the midwives who warmly accepted to integrate me into their busy schedules and allowed me to attend their consultations. I am deeply impressed by your boundless commitment towards the families you care for and your ability to question your own practices, constantly adjusting to your clients' needs and aspirations. To parents and midwives, thank you for your generosity and your open-mindedness to my anthropological gaze. I had anticipated that my fieldwork would bring me emotions and inspiring encounters. My expectations were largely exceeded. I have fond memories of my fieldwork, and the voices of my interlocutors keep echoing in my mind.

I am grateful to Irene Maffi, my PhD supervisor, for her guidance from the early stages of my research to its completion. I am also particularly grateful to Fiona Dykes. Her work has been a major source of inspiration, and her support and enthusiasm over the years have been precious. I warmly thank the other members of my committee, Orit Avishai and Véronique Mottier, for their thorough and constructive review of my manuscript. Their writings and teaching have also stimulated my thinking early on and contributed to the elaboration of my research. All shortcomings are mine.

My colleagues at the Institute of Social Sciences of the University of Lausanne inspired me, stimulated my research, and sometimes reviewed draft chapters. I particularly thank Alexandra Afsary, Edmée Ballif, Daniela Cerqui, Solène Gouilhers, and Claire Vionnet. Aside from my research and teaching activities at the University of Lausanne, I contributed to the anthropological component of the interdisciplinary Swiss National Science Foundation research project: "Lactation in History: A Crosscultural Research on Suckling Practices, Representations of Breastfeeding and Politics in Maternity in a European Context". I thank the "Lactation in History" researchers from the University of Geneva and the University of Fribourg for the many conversations, meetings, and scientific events which gave me a lot of food for thought. Deepest thanks also to James Akre, for his friendship and support since the day we met as guests on Swiss national radio and who carefully edited my book proposal to Routledge.

I am honoured that Routledge selected my work to become part of the "Social Science Perspectives on Childbirth and Reproduction" series. I warmly thank Robbie Davis-Floyd, the Social Science Lead Editor for the series, and Routledge Editor Katherine Ong for their kind guidance and support through this process, as well as the editorial and production teams.

Finally, the support of my loved ones has been invaluable to complete this work. As solitary as the writing process is, being surrounded by caring people makes it a lot more bearable. Thank you, all of you. My deepest gratitude goes to Fred, my partner and most faithful reader. His constant support, genuine interest in my work, and tireless listening have lifted me throughout the long process of completing a book.

Introduction

It has clearly guided our role as parents. Especially for me. I do not know how I could have been a mother if I had not breastfed. Breastfeeding helped me build the connection with her, the communication with her. (interview with Léa, mother of Simone, two and a half years)

In Switzerland, pregnant women have the choice to give birth in the hospital, at home, or in a birth centre. Similarly, either an obstetrician or independent midwife can follow up on their pregnancies. Whatever the chosen option, fees are covered by health insurance, which is paid for and mandatory for everyone. In practice, however, a gynaecologist follows up on a vast majority of pregnant women, and midwife-led deliveries are scarce, namely 3.3 per cent of births in 2018, of which 3 per cent births were planned out of the hospital (Grylka & Pehlke-Milde 2019). These births are part of so-called holistic care by an independent midwife who monitors the entire birth process: pregnancy follow-up, childbirth, and postpartum care.

As in other industrialised countries, out-of-hospital births remain very marginal in Switzerland. In the current context of a biomedical risk-oriented comprehension of birth, delivery is conceived as a highly risky, unpredictable event that can only be considered "normal" in retrospect (Akrich & Pasveer 1996; Carricaburu 2007; Maffi 2012; Négrié & Cascales 2016; Scamell & Alaszewski 2012). As a result, out-of-hospital birth is mainly addressed in terms of risks. However, epidemiological studies support out-of-hospital delivery. Olsen and Clausen (2012) published a meta-analysis aiming to compare the issues of "planned hospital birth *versus* planned home birth". They conclude that "there is no strong evidence to favour either planned hospital delivery or planned home birth for selected, low-risks pregnant women" (Olsen & Clausen 2012: 8). In fact, home births lead to "fewer interventions, fewer complications and fewer neonatal problems" (ibid. 2012: 20). Faucon and Brillac's (2013) meta-analysis reached the same results: fewer medical interventions at home and no increase in perinatal issues. In light of these conducive results, the National Institute for Health and Care Excellence (NICE 2014) in the United Kingdom took a stand in favour of out-of-hospital births. The NICE recommends out-of-hospital

DOI: 10.4324/9781003124108-101

delivery for low-risk pregnant women in order to avoid potentially harmful medical and technical interventions during labour. In Switzerland, a comparative study between a maternity ward and a birth centre led by paediatrician Borel in Aigle, in the canton of Vaud, reached the same conclusions: low-risk pregnant women giving birth in the birth centre undergo significantly fewer interventions, particularly episiotomies and caesarean sections (Borel et al. 2010). Babies born in the birth centre are also significantly less often transferred to neonatology.

In spite of these favourable results, in industrialised countries, home birth women often find it difficult to be understood and respected by those around them because giving birth in the hospital remains a standard, difficult to question (Chautems 2011; MacDonald 2007; Sjöblom et al. 2012; Viisainen 2000).[1] Likewise, independent midwives who practise out-of-hospital deliveries face the misunderstanding of their peers. Hospital staff are occasionally reluctant to collaborate with them. They are sometimes unwelcome, as well as their clients,[2] in the case of a transfer to the hospital during labour, for example (Davis-Floyd & Johnson 2006 MacDonald 2007; Matsuoka & Hinokuma 2009).

I took a particular interest in this marginalised minority of the Swiss perinatal landscape—that is, those who choose to give birth out of the hospital and under the supervision of an independent midwife. I specifically focused on the postpartum period, which in the birth process has been left little investigated generally, and especially for this care model (Dykes 2006; Perrenoud 2016). Between May 2014 and February 2017, I conducted an ethnography with the participation of 11 independent midwives, whom I followed during postnatal home visits in the canton of Vaud, Switzerland. Switzerland is one of the rare countries where the healthcare system offers a free-at-home postpartum follow-up for all women giving birth in the country, until 56 days after birth. Should this be a premature birth, multiple birth, or a caesarean section birth, women can benefit from up to 16 postnatal home consultations during that period, as well as up to ten postnatal home consultations in any other case. In my fieldwork, these postpartum visits took place exclusively in the context of "holistic care",[3] where the same midwife also ensures continuous care of pregnancy and childbirth. I analysed a local and specific modality of this care approach, based on the criteria of the care providers: holistic care is midwife-led care, with specific temporalities—especially the continuity of care during the entire birth process—and a specific place of childbirth and postpartum care—at home.[4] As I will develop later, the holistic care model also includes a particular view on infant care, including breastfeeding.

I approached the postpartum consultations with a primary interest in breastfeeding. Conceived as the "natural" continuity of childbirth without intervention, it is central in the midwife's follow-up and the parents' concerns. Shadowing independent midwives during their postpartum visits, I had the opportunity to document their care practices and observe discussions and negotiations with parents in case of a specific issue, as well as ordinary, routine behaviours. In addition to the participant observation carried out during postnatal visits, I conducted in-depth interviews with parents, which took place at regular intervals from birth to weaning, allowing me to trace their breastfeeding journey and grasp the evolution of their practices and feelings over the longer term.

Dykes's (2006) ethnographic work, in a postnatal maternity ward in the United Kingdom, challenges "the suitability of the hospital [...] as the place in which women begin to establish breastfeeding" (179). As an alternative to this dominant model, breastfeeding initiation at home with independent midwives still remains little investigated. Furthermore, Dykes (2006) highlighted a "striking absence of ethnographic work conducted on postnatal wards and considerably less that focuses upon aspects of breastfeeding within the postnatal ward setting" (48). This absence is even more striking in the context of postnatal follow-ups at home. For example, what happens when there are no set protocols to determine when to weigh the infant? Given that parents are alone with their newborn within a few hours after birth, how does it affect their accountability and empowerment? How do parents manage their autonomy, including regarding breastfeeding, in the first days of their baby's life? During a postpartum stay at the maternity ward, health professionals are constantly reachable. On the contrary, after an out-of-hospital birth, midwives are only present one or two hours a day, and between two consultations, even if midwives stay available by phone, parents are on their own in taking care of their newborn.

Independent midwifery enables the practice of holistic care, embodying a certain "ideal-type" of the profession, and the entire range of their prerogatives to be fully exercised (Charrier 2004; Paumier 2003; Vuille 2000). One-to-one care (one midwife/one woman) is also recommended as an optimal practice for "intrapartum care for healthy women and babies" by the NICE (2014). In the context of holistic care, this one-to-one model extends to prenatal and postnatal care. The terms of holistic care also tend to reconfigure relationships between health professionals and parents, breaking with the technocratic hierarchy that implicates the subordination of the individual to the institution and the practitioners representing it (Davis-Floyd & St. John 1998). Moreover, midwives and parents start from a shared value base, making communication smoother (Perrenoud 2016). Even if my main focus is on mothers' and parents' perspective, my research aims to explore the specificities of independent midwifery working conditions in a home postnatal setting.

Some researchers working in different European and North American countries have shown that independent midwifery is built in opposition to the dominant technocratic model and claims a non-invasive care approach, protecting the physiology of birth (Akrich & Pasveer 1996; Davis-Floyd et al. 2009; Katz Rothman 1982; MacDonald 2007). Nevertheless, in Switzerland, independent midwives' practice lies within and not on the margins of the biomedical system. Their initial training is embedded in the biomedical field, and whatever their divergences from the technocratic model, they speak the same language as hospital midwives or obstetricians. Furthermore, they work autonomously but are also held accountable, seeking the help of other health professionals whenever abnormalities appear during the postpartum period. For example, in the case of a breastfed newborn's failure to thrive, if there is no improvement after implementing the first corrective steps, they have to report to a lactation consultant or paediatrician.[5]

Becoming parents in Switzerland: navigating gender inequality and heteronormativity

The socioeconomic organisation in Switzerland is structured by gender inequalities and heteronormativity. Swiss women gained the right to vote in 1971, and military or civilian service is still mandatory for men in 2021. It was not until 1981 that gender equality was included in the Swiss Constitution, and it was only in 1996 that a Swiss law against gender discrimination was enacted. If same-sex couples are still excluded from marriage, a registered partnership has been open to them since 2007. However, it does not allow same-sex couples to adopt a child together (adoption is only open to heterosexual couples or single parents) or to access medically assisted reproduction. As a result, legally, filiation is not automatically recognised between a child and her or his parent's unregistered partner, but since 2018, registered partners are able to adopt their partner's child. The heteronormative character of parenting culture in Switzerland was manifest in my fieldwork because midwives' discourse often refers to gendered parental roles as complementary. I only met heterosexual couples, and no midwife mentioned former lesbian clients. More generally, if the transition to parenthood and experience of the perinatal period from the standpoint of fathers are the subject of health researchers' and health professionals' interest,[6] to my knowledge, no similar study has been conducted regarding same-sex couples in Switzerland so far.[7]

With a minimum paid maternity leave of 14 weeks, Switzerland lies in the lower third of European countries' rankings (Müller et al. 2017). In addition, while most European countries provide a paternity leave to which a paid (or sometimes unpaid) parental leave can be added in numerous European countries, the Swiss federal law has only included a paternity leave since 2021. Before the introduction of this two weeks leave, employers provided a minimum of one or two days off, but the duration of the paid leave varied and depended on their goodwill.

This long-inexistent paternity leave is symptomatic of the gender regime in Switzerland, named "neo-maternalism" by Giraud and Lucas (2009) and traditionally relying on women's assignment to the household and children care. The lack of day-care structures and their high cost encourage two-parent families to avoid these structures by deciding that one parent stops working and stays at home during the first years of the child's life. Since women's salaries are still 18.1 per cent lower than men's (Strub & Bannwart 2017), women are strongly incited to reduce or stop their professional activity. For a high proportion of women, the birth of a first child implies partial or total withdrawal of a paid activity.[8] Part-time work is the major modality of employment for women, concerning 59 per cent of working women in 2018, while only 17.6 per cent of working men are employed part-time (Federal Statistical Office 2019a). Consistently, infant care in Switzerland, especially during a child's first year of life, remains primarily under women's responsibility (Le Goff & Levy 2016).

The Swiss federal structure results in disparities between cantons regarding family support policies as well as gender inequalities. The canton of Vaud, where I conducted my fieldwork, provides specific services, which may have no strict equivalent in other cantons, such as postpartum home visits of an "early childhood nurse" after a midwife has completed her postpartum follow-up.[9]

More broadly, in comparison with other European countries, family policies in Switzerland remain sparse, restricting parenthood to a personal matter and enhancing individual responsibility (see, for example, Bühlmann, Elcheroth & Tettamanti 2010). This lack of family policy greatly hinders couples to adopt equalitarian parenting practices: the ideology of individual choice and autonomist values is structurally restricted by the absence of welfare policies supporting couples' equalitarian values (Le Goff & Levy 2016).

The breastfeeding project: an embodied parenting approach

Throughout the twentieth century, in most countries, breastfeeding has been recognised by public health agencies as well as nutrition and child health experts as the most appropriate infant-feeding mode (Millard 1990). Its promotion is an important public health concern.[10] Its terms and duration are also the subjects of specific guidance: the World Health Organization (WHO) recommends exclusive breastfeeding for the first six months of life (WHO 2001) and the continuation of breastfeeding, supplemented by other dietary and liquid intakes, until two years of age or beyond (WHO 2003). In the current perinatal context, dominated by a strong breastfeeding promotion message, an overwhelming majority of children are breastfed in Switzerland.[11] The total median duration of breastfeeding reaches 31 weeks, which exceeds the duration of maternity leave for most mothers (Dratva et al. 2014).

As a social anthropologist, I approached my subject with little interest in the health implications of breastfeeding for babies or mothers. Overall, the decision of whether or not to breastfeed was not a relevant issue in my fieldwork: as home birth users, all parents were committed to breastfeeding, conceptualised as the "natural" continuity of childbirth without intervention. That being said, I had the opportunity to observe some women struggling between the ideal of the birth model they chose, and their own feelings regarding breastfeeding, as a body practice they did not enjoy.

Choosing an out-of-hospital birth with an independent midwife is associated with specific parenting and care practices to the newborn, as well as a long-term education philosophy, outlining a "holistic care script".[12] This script partially summarises the ideological and practical principles of attachment parenting. Initiated by paediatrician William Sears and nurse Martha Sears, this parenting approach emerged in the 1980s in the United States and advocates for a child-centred, "proximal" parenting (Sears & Sears 2001). Attachment parenting relies on the work of British psychiatrist Bowlby (1969), conducted in the 1950s, on the effects of early maternal deprivation, which emphasises the determinant role of the continuous presence of the mother as the central figure of attachment for the child. In this perspective, Sears and Sears defend particular parenting practices, aiming for closeness between infants and their parents, such as "bed-sharing" (sharing the parental bed with one's children) or "babywearing" (instead of using a pushchair). Attachment parenting gives central importance to breastfeeding, ideally performed on demand and until child-led weaning— that is to say, typically for several years (Faircloth 2013).[13]

All the parents I met carried out babywearing and bed-sharing—practices often suggested and always supported by their midwife. These parenting habits would foster the development of a "secure" attachment for newborns, favouring their development, as well as their long-term wellbeing. Nevertheless, initially almost none of the parents had the ambition to breastfeed "to full term", meaning until their child did not need or want it anymore, thereby distancing themselves from the attachment parenting ideology.

I identified "natural motherhood", described by Bobel (2002) at the confluence of attachment parenting and "voluntary simplicity", as another important influence sketching the holistic care script. Parents' affiliation to this approach was reflected in shared critical perspectives on the neoliberal economic model expressed, for example, through environmental concerns and a desire to reduce their consumption, which they would translate into parenting choices, such as the use of washable cloth diapers. More generally, parents often chose to decrease their working time, with the purpose of increasing the time dedicated to their family.

In addition to a unanimous commitment to breastfeeding and a refusal to supply artificial milk to their child, most parents I met had a "breastfeeding project" established before birth.[14] Such projects were usually aligned with the WHO recommendations regarding how and how long to breastfeed—namely "on demand", following the child's own rhythm, and exclusively for roughly six months.[15] However, parents do not subscribe to the WHO recommendations regarding the total duration of breastfeeding (for two years and beyond) or at least not at first. Half of them eventually continued to breastfeed for about one year or beyond, largely exceeding the median breastfeeding duration in Switzerland. These long-term breastfeeding allowed me to observe the evolution of parents' breastfeeding practices as their child grows up and sometimes the negotiation taking place between mother and child around weaning.[16]

Memmi (2014) situated breastfeeding as part of a range of practices around birth and death implemented in Euro-American medical institutions during the 1990s, and which she described as a "revenge of the flesh".[17] These practices, which are rigidified in protocols, behaviour, and morally obliged gestures, contribute to manufacturing a "body-based" identity, for the concerned individuals. Through a work process of embodiment, the practice of breastfeeding thus contributes to the production of the new mother (ibid. 2014). In Memmi's (2014) perspective, my work aims to trace "the specific contribution of embodiment" to the identification work deployed by mothers, and to a lesser extent by fathers, as well as to show how midwives' follow-up takes part in this process (12).

Moreover, the parents I met fit in the "child by project" era (Boltanski 2004). This era emerged out of the liberalisation of contraception and the decriminalisation of abortion, and it corresponds, according to Boltanski (2004), to an investment in and attention to the child unmatched in the past. In this regard, the breastfeeding project is one of the most characteristic features of this commitment. Rather than acting on children to adapt them to their daily lives, for example, by imposing scheduled feedings, parents prefer to act on themselves by adjusting to the supposed needs of their child. They undertake a self-disciplinarisation in order to avoid having to "civilise" their baby (Dykes 2005, 2006). In line with Leboyer's (1974) philosophy, this perspective on infancy aims to limit any disturbance interfering with the "natural" rhythm or development of the child.

Home birth parents endeavour to consider their child as a full-fledged individual since birth. As a result, they do their best to develop communication tools to better understand her or his needs and desires and adjust to them. On-demand breastfeeding is perceived as central among the range of measures implemented to fill this purpose (to name a few of the most popular tools besides on-demand breastfeeding: "elimination communication",[18] massages, "baby-led weaning",[19] and sign language). To adopt an emic perspective on the babies I met during my fieldwork and based on Gottlieb's (2000) proposition to practise an "anthropology of infants", I aim to help fill the scholarly gap in socio-anthropological studies regarding babies in general, and especially as social actors on their own right. However, rather than a formal investigation of babies' behaviours per se, I intend to explore parents' and midwives' interpretations of infants' behaviours and the modes of communication around breastfeeding.

Women's commitment to breastfeeding is a necessary condition for "success" in terms of compliance with the WHO recommendations. However, other factors do not solely depend on them. Even in a social context that values breastfeeding, mothers have to deal with complicated and often conflicting sets of social rules, and they are subject to standards restricting the place, the time, the manner, and the duration of breastfeeding, as well as who may or may not see them breastfeed. As noticed by Dykes (2005), "breastfeeding practices within a given culture represent the ways in which women negotiate and incorporate dominant ideologies and institutional and cultural norms with the realities of their embodied experiences, personal circumstances and social support systems" (2283). Other bodies and actors are involved in this process. Familial, social, and economic contexts in which women are embedded strongly structure their breastfeeding experiences and practices, making their breastfeeding project more or less realistic and achievable. Thus, the conditions around maternity leave, their spouse's option to obtain work flexibility or leave, the presence of other children, and the proximity of family relatives and friends are factors determining the conditions of performing breastfeeding. In addition, the immediate postpartum situation heavily determines the course of breastfeeding initiation and continuation. Obermeyer and Castle (1996) emphasise the importance of a "helper" for breastfeeding mothers, providing information and supporting with household management. The social and structural circumstances surrounding birth can thus create or suppress opportunities.

In Switzerland, national and local independent organisations, as well as health professionals and hospitals, are actively promoting breastfeeding, influencing mothers' practices. In addition, at the regional level, the canton of Vaud has set up a programme to promote early childhood health.[20] In private obstetricians' offices and maternity wards, promotional material is usually available in the form of leaflets. Postnatal hospital staff and hospital guidelines strongly encourage breastfeeding to align with the WHO recommendations. At home, independent midwives practising holistic care do not need to convince parents of the breastfeeding benefits, but in a subtler way, they focus their efforts on breastfeeding methods, particularly regarding the notion of on-demand breastfeeding. For example, they remind parents that it is physiologically normal for a newborn to feed more than ten times a day, dismissing their potential wish to space the feedings.

Negotiated breastfeeding

Fassin and Memmi (2004) suggest to "reconsider the role of the state, perceived for a long time as a central place for rules formulation and action implementation with respect to the body, health, hygiene and prevention, serving as a standard for measuring the effectiveness of biopolitics" (23-24). They invite to investigate "the intermediate space of social and political regulation between the state and social practices" (ibid. 2004:24). The "breast is best" message has become a standard of good mothering practices now difficult to question (Wall 2001). Morally compelled to breastfeed, mothers internalise the standard, implementing a "self-government of oneself" (Memmi 2004: 151). In my research, I endeavour to report on the modalities of this self-government and the midwives' contributions to it. What kinds of parenthood practices emerge from a holistic care follow-up? To what extent are they shaped by midwives' discourses? How is parenthood built through breastfeeding practices? How do parents construct meanings about their parenting practices?

With a primary focus on breastfeeding, in this book, I examine more broadly the postpartum period as part of a holistic care and an out-of-hospital birth project. Built in response to the dominant biomedical model of care, the holistic care provided by independent midwives claims a physiology-centred gaze on birth. However, this care approach is anchored in the biomedical model, and midwives also rely on quantifying monitoring devices, namely weighing scales, in accordance with ordinary paediatric practices. Together with specific tools and body techniques, midwives actually deploy significant intervention measures to support the physiology of breastfeeding and lactation. In this way, they take part in the reproduction of a mechanistic conception of the female body, inherited from the Enlightenment (Martin 1987; Dykes 2005, 2006; Kukla 2005).

Since the 1990s, parenthood has been primarily addressed in terms of risk prevention and the corresponding "good" parenting practices thought to reduce risks. This risk-centred approach to child-rearing has justified an "intensification" of parenthood, discussed by numerous authors (Badinter 2010; Blum 1999; Büskens 2010; Douglas & Michaels 2005; Faircloth 2013; Hays 1996; Lee 2008; Lupton 2013a; Wolf 2007, 2011). Despite a growing involvement of fathers in parenthood and childcare during the twentieth century and a claimed equality in parental responsibilities, mothers remain primary caretakers, especially during the first year of the child's life (Le Goff & Levy 2016). As a result, this parenthood "intensification" proves to be primarily an intensification of motherhood, and early childhood professionals remain attached to the mother's primacy (Gojard 2010). However, based on my fieldwork observations, out-of-hospital birth parents tend to reflect upon their practices with the intention of avoiding an unequal tasks distribution. Furthermore, from my observations and discussions with them, independent midwives show a willingness to address parents in an inclusive way. In practice, however, this is not always the case.

Breastfeeding, as a morally obliged practice in the current biomedical context, constitutes a privileged observatory to examine parents' and, more directly, mothers' commitment to this intensified modality of parenthood. By focusing on a marginalised birth model, my research questions the dominant biomedical one, pointing out divergences and similarities in the discourses and practices of its proponents, practitioners, and users. My work explores transversal themes outlining how reproduction and parenting are carried out in Switzerland and are framed by the local cultural, political, and economic contexts, including the gender system and the resulting power relationships.

First, risk appears to be a central issue that structures both holistic and technocratic models. Parents and midwives often claim that giving birth out of the hospital defies a risk-centric definition of birth. However, my ethnography shows that home-birthing practices, including postpartum routines, still revolve around risk prevention and management. Although the logic of risk as a lever for action is not structurally challenged, the underlying arguments differ given that an "inversed" relation to risk is built into holistic care.[21] Risk culture and the biomedical approach to birth pervade all models of birth care.

Second, parenting reconfiguration, or parenting "intensification", a phenomenon permeating all strata of contemporary Euro-American parents and that translates into a "child-centred" approach (including long-term on-demand breastfeeding), achieves a particularly acute form within the holistic care model. This parenting niche approach acts as both a magnifying glass and a source of information about mainstream parenting trends and requirements. Inherited from child psychologists like Dolto (1985), a child-centred parenting style is driven by a strong commitment to listening and communicating with one's child and can be expressed through specific parenting practices such as on-demand breastfeeding or elimination communication. Interestingly, a child-centred parenting approach does not rule out disciplining children, thereby creating a degree of tension between an ideal for adjusting to the child's own rhythm and a desire to fit them into the parents' and midwives' schedules and personal agendas.

Third, if the child's behaviour is constrained by adult expectations, this disciplinary practice is even more obvious when considering bodies as loci of biopower (Foucault 1976). Primarily targeting women's bodies, this exercise of discipline also applies to babies' bodies.[22] In promotion discourses, breastfeeding is conceptualised as a "natural" practice, for which mothers and babies are innately skilled. However, this naturalist discourse stands in marked contrast to the body work deployed by mothers to perform breastfeeding, including techniques and specific tools designed to sustain it, and the discipline exerted on infants (through surveillance of their latch, for example) to ensure optimal milk transfer.

Therefore, breastfeeding initiation reveals a tension between "natural" and acquired skills, echoing broader debates about the naturalisation of mothers' skills through the notion of maternal "instinct", in a perinatal context governed by the idea that mothers have to rely on experts to perform adequate child-rearing. This tension also refers to divergent perspectives on children: on the one hand, in dominant medical discourses, babies are perceived as totally vulnerable beings in need of protection from their parents, but also from health professionals who are teaching parents how to do "right". On the other hand, infants are presented as "mammals" by natural childbirth supporters (Odent 2011 [1990]) whose perspective considers them as competent, but at the expense of their animalisation.

The dominant conception of breastfeeding as "natural" also conceals the body work achieved by mothers to engage in it, while justifying gender inequalities regarding parental responsibilities. If breastfeeding is "natural" for women, so, too, are other parenting tasks, since a woman's body is "naturally" designed to accomplish them. This mechanism both reflects and reinforces the Swiss sociocultural context and socioeconomic organisation, which are firmly structured by gender inequalities and heteronormativity.

Through all these aspects, breastfeeding appears as a "negotiated" practice between midwives and parents, between parents and babies, and inside the family. Furthermore, negotiations are also at play between parents and the holistic care script to which they subscribed (including their breastfeeding project), as they have to adjust their practices to comply with their everyday life requirements. The different protagonists are involved in a collective construction of meanings around breastfeeding, regarding risk and risk management, the child's "natural" rhythm and communication, or the construction of the lactating body and breastfeeding as "natural". As the meanings produced are not always shared by all protagonists, conflicts may appear, as I document in the empirical chapters of this book by addressing this question: how do parents, together with their midwife, construct meanings about their breastfeeding and parenting practices?

Finally, this book aims to contribute to a growing corpus of literature documenting women's experiences of body processes and practices. In line with Young's (2005) perspective on the exploration of women's specific modalities of being in the world in a female body, or with Froideveaux-Metterie's (2018) proposition of an "embodied feminism", I consider that human experiences are always embodied, situated, and immersed in a particular historical, cultural, political, and economic context. Froideveaux-Metterie (2018) describes her "embodied feminism" as a political project to redefine feminism as "simultaneously singular and plural, carrier of a specific experience but irreducible to any essentialisation, enduring social conditioning, but able to escape gender roles" (155). By analysing women's experiences and practices regarding their reproductive and maternal body, I aspire to capture and highlight their specific feelings as a lever of social awareness and political change.

Gender issues in holistic care

Based on the physical closeness between children and their parents, the parenting style I explored in my research, inspired by the "attachment" or "natural" parenting approaches, has been identified by some authors as strengthening gender inequalities between parents (Badinter 2010; Bobel 2002; Büskens 2010; Faircloth 2013). In the bonding theory, developed by Ainsworth and Bowlby, which constitutes the theoretical basis of the attachment parenting approach, the mother is indeed presented as the central figure of attachment (Bretherton 1992).

Anchored in the female body, breastfeeding was often described by my interlocutors, parents, and midwives as an innate, instinctive practice, creating a structural separation between parental tasks.[23] Consequently, it seemed to me even more important to adopt in this book an anti-essentialist stance and develop a critical gender perspective, informed by the theoretical work of Butler deconstructing the notion of gender:

> Gender is the apparatus by which the production and normalization of masculine and feminine take place along with the interstitial forms of hormonal, chromosomal, psychic, and performative that gender assumes. (Butler 2004: 42)

As argued by Laqueur (1990), the sexual body does not exist per se; it is rather an invention of biology, an object that legitimises biology as a scientific discipline. The sexual body is therefore "created by scientists as the object of scientific investigation" (Oudshoorn 1994: 4). In line with West and Zimmerman's (1987) thought, I perceive gender as "an emergent feature of social situations" (126). Gender emerges from social situations and is an ongoing process, achieved through bodily practices, behaviours, and discourses. In this perspective, gender is ubiquitous: in every social interaction, individuals' performance can be evaluated through the lens of gender, legitimating or discrediting their activities and social roles (Vuille et al. 2009). Breastfeeding therefore appears as a crucial gender performance, attesting to women's ability to fulfil their maternal role.

Relying on a critical gender perspective, I examine in this book how traditional gender regimes shape and are shaped by breastfeeding practices, both in midwives' discourses and in parents' accounts of their experiences and their everyday life organisation. In particular, I discuss the construction and implementation of gendered parental roles and responsibilities resulting from the female-body-anchored practice of breastfeeding, as well as how fathers endeavour to bypass this biological disparity by committing to each aspect of hands-on breastfeeding support and childcare.

Overview of the book

Chapter 1 contextualises out-of-hospital birth practices and the modalities of the holistic care model in Switzerland with its inherent opposition to a technocratic perspective on birth. This chapter also outlines the methodological approach taken, including access to the fieldwork and my research ethics, and the description of my research participants.

In Chapter 2, I briefly relate the circumstances of breastfeeding discredit, due to birth technologisation and the rise of formula, as well as its rehabilitation, with a focus on Switzerland. I then discuss the dominance of a risk-centric approach to parenting. For the last three decades, parenting practices have progressively become marked by a primary focus on risks to which children are exposed in the short and long term, and more specifically how "good" childcare practices can influence the prevention of these risks. The "intensification of motherhood" is one answer to these concerns. Crystallising maternal dedication and projection on the future, breastfeeding offers a privileged lens to observe this evolution. I also present in this chapter the authorities and evolving debates about breastfeeding practices, as well as how breastfeeding mothers deal with them.

Chapters 3, 4, and 5 are empirical chapters based on my ethnographic material, exploring parents' and midwives' breastfeeding practices and their discourses from the immediate postpartum until weaning. The three chapters are thematically organised in a non-linear way.

Chapter 3 is dedicated to the perception and management of risks revolving around breastfeeding: weight stagnation, weight loss, or weight gain perceived as inadequate by midwives based on medical guidelines.

In Chapter 4, I focus on the lactating body and the body work required from women to construct and maintain it in the long term, as well as fathers' involvement in the process.

Chapter 5 investigates how breastfeeding is considered by parents and midwives to be a communication tool, as well as the child's representations underlying this discourse.

Even if each chapter focuses on a specific aspect of the breastfeeding experience and performance, two transversal themes are omnipresent in the three chapters: first, the centrality of the body, that of women, that of babies and, to a lesser extent, that of fathers. The body is thought to be a major means for expressing parenthood, a vehicle of "skinship", an intimate bond created by physical contacts (Tahhan 2008, 2010). Parents' and especially mothers' dedication to the parenting model they elected is achieved through the provision of their bodies and through the body work they deploy. A second axis of analysis concerns the power relationships and the negotiations that take place between parents and midwives. The information that midwives transmit to parents also conveys certain values and expectations regarding childcare, potentially restricting parents' free choice and self-determination. At the same time, the continuity of care allows midwives to develop an in-depth, contextualised knowledge of the families and to create a trusting relationship with them: midwives undertake to involve parents in each decision, reducing the asymmetry between health professionals and clients.

To conclude this book, I discuss the differences and similarities of this marginal model of care with the dominant biomedical one. By doing so, I explore the transversal themes of risk, its anticipation and management, alongside birth temporalities, and bodies and technologies. I conclude by sharing considerations on gender regimes in holistic care, and I raise questions of a broader scope on this modality of care.

Notes

1 In this book, I use the expression "home birth parents" or "home birth mother/father" for convenience; this also includes "birth centre parents".

2 In my fieldwork, independent midwives always refer to their "clients" and never to their "patients".

3 The terminology "holistic care" is my English translation of the French emic expression *suivi global*.

4 I do not differentiate between home birth and delivery in a birth centre. First, in the case of a birth-centre delivery, return to home usually takes place a few hours after delivery. Second, given that both options provide the same possibilities regarding medical equipment, it appears to me that parents orient their choice mostly for practical reasons (apartment perceived as poorly soundproofed, concerns about cleanliness, difficulty conducting a pool birth in their home, etc.) that are not significant with regard to my research interests.

5 The International Lactation Consultant Association (ILCA) offers training intended for all health professionals. In practice, the graduates of the International Board of Certified Lactation Consultants (IBCLC) most often have an initial nurse or midwifery training. There are no physicians specialised in breastfeeding: the prerogatives of gynaecologists stop at delivery, while paediatricians focus on the health of children, including nutrition, but are often incompetent regarding breastfeeding itself. In general, physicians are poorly informed about breastfeeding management and the physiology of lactation (Dettwyler 1995b; Wolf 2006; Sandre-Pereira 2005; Palmer 2009 [1988]; Faircloth 2013).

6 See, for example, the 2019 documentary movie *La naissance d'un père* (A father's birth) realised by a research team of the School of Health Sciences of Vaud (HESAV) in collaboration with the fathers' association Männer.ch.

7 As I only met heterosexual couples, in the rest of this work, I will evoke "fathers" or spouses by using the masculine form.

8 Almost one in seven women stops working after giving birth to her first child, while the others reduce on average their occupation rate by 20 per cent after becoming mothers (Bläuer Herrmann & Murier 2016).

9 These professionals (*Infirmières Petite Enfance* in French) take over from the independent midwives after their postpartum follow-up. In Vaud, they offer state-covered home visits by appointment, as well as free weekly consultations open to everyone without appointment. These consultations are mostly used by parents as an opportunity to weigh their baby. For an in-depth analysis, see Sachs (2005) in the United Kingdom, or Vervatidis (2016) in Switzerland.

10 Here I will succinctly describe the main health benefits associated with breastfeeding: exclusive breastfeeding for up to six months tends to reduce the risk of gastrointestinal and respiratory diseases, otolaryngological and urinary infections, necrotising enterocolitis, and diabetes or atopic diseases in family history, and dental malocclusions (Galton Bachrach, Schwartz & Bachrach 2003; Duffy et al. 1997; Jackson 2004; Lawrence 1995; Oddy 2001; Owen et al. 2006; Quigley, Kelly & Sacker 2007; Sadauskaite-Kuehne et al. 2004; Scariati, Grummer-Strawn & Fein 1997; Victora et al. 2016). Breastfed children are also more rarely overweight (Grummer-Strawn & Mei 2004; Harder et al. 2005; Victora et al. 2016; WHO 2007). In the long term, people who have been breastfed have lower blood pressure and cholesterol levels (WHO 2007). The recent Lancet series on breastfeeding especially stresses the lifelong effect of breastfeeding on these issues (Victora et al. 2016). For mothers, breastfeeding, especially long-term breastfeeding, appears to reduce the risk of breast and ovarian cancer, as well as osteoporosis and diabetes (Blum 1999; Galtry 1997; Stuart-Macadam 1995; Victora et al. 2016; Wolf 2006). Health professionals and child psychologists also emphasise the importance of breastfeeding in establishing the mother–child relationship (Blum 1999; Lawrence 1995; Sheehan & Schmied 2011; Victora et al. 2016).

11 The latest statistical study showed that initiation of breastfeeding in Switzerland is more than well established: 95 per cent of newborns were breastfed at birth in 2014 (Dratva et al. 2014).

12 I borrowed the notion of "script" from Gagnon (2008), used in the context of the analysis of a sexual relationship. For a detailed discussion of the "holistic care script", see Chapter 1.

13 Breastfeeding on demand implies that infants can have unlimited access to their mothers' breasts and are able to regulate their food intake by themselves.

14 I borrowed this expression from Avishai (2007, 2011), based on her research on middle-class, white American mothers who are strongly committed to breastfeeding and setting specific objectives regarding their breastfeeding practices.

15 It can be noticed that in the last version of the Baby-Friendly Hospital Initiative (BFHI), in 2018, the terminology "responsive feeding" replaced the expression "on-demand breastfeeding" (WHO 2018). However, in my fieldwork, which ran from 2014 to 2017, midwives and parents were still using the expression "on-demand breastfeeding" (*allaitement à la demande* in French), which is why I chose to stick to this emic expression in this book. To my knowledge, this terminology has not evolved since I ended my fieldwork.

16 Based on my fieldwork and an emic typology of breastfeeding, I decided to define "long-term breastfeeding" as breastfeeding after one year of the child's life.

17 All French quotations have been translated by me.

18 Elimination communication is a method with which caregivers try to identify babies' clues to address their elimination needs, enabling them to urinate or defecate in a chosen place (e.g., a toilet, potty, or another container) when they are purposely not wearing a diaper.

19 This notion refers to a method of introducing solid foods in a baby's diet. Parents or caretakers offer infants a range of fruits or cooked vegetable pieces, cut to be easily grasped, so that they can eat autonomously. In opposition, in the dominant "parents-led weaning" method, children are more passive and fed with a spoon by their caretakers. According to the "baby-led weaning" approach, infants are encouraged to decide what to eat, in which order, and at what rhythm. To me, the French expression literally transcribed "child-led diversification" seems more accurate, since varying a baby's diet does not imply weaning her or him but only the end of exclusive breastfeeding.

20 The "Cantonal program for health promotion and infants primary prevention (0–6 years) – parents" (*Programme cantonal de promotion de la santé et de prévention primaire enfants (0–6 ans) – parents* in French), was established in 2006 by the public health and the youth protection departments. It is designed for health institutions and practitioners with the aim of standardising and coordinating health services intended for families (Diserens et al. 2006).

21 See Chapter 3.

22 See Chapter 4.

23 With stimulation and hormonal treatment, male lactation can be induced. This possibility remains very marginally realised, and it was never discussed among the couples I met during my fieldwork.

1 Holistic care in Switzerland and my ethnographic study

My fieldwork took place in the deeply intimate setting of the early hours or days after a home birth. Most parents chose holistic care, especially for the unique continuity of care, ensuring preservation of their intimacy, as their midwife remained the only professional protagonist of their follow-up. The postpartum period is made up of the vulnerability of bodies and minds, literally and figuratively left naked by the intense experience they just lived through. I took up the challenge of fitting into this sensitive time and being accepted by parents as an external witness with whom they would share their feelings and experiences. The ethnographic method, relying on participant observation and long-term immersion or "impregnation" (Olivier de Sardan 1995), was particularly well suited to these circumstances and allowed me to earn the trust of my interlocutors and build a reliable relationship with them.

In this chapter, I detail how I access fieldwork and how it unfolded. I then discuss my researcher stance and relationships with my interlocutors, including my ethical position. I also clarify the different methodological devices I used, as well as their articulations, to produce my ethnographic material.

In the second part, I describe the population of home birth parents who participated in my research. I develop the holistic care script underlining their childbirth and parenting choices, endorsed to varying degrees by parents.

In the last part of the chapter, I recount the emergence of modern midwifery practice in Switzerland, as well as contextualise natural childbirth and out-of-hospital birth practices. I present the common features and connections between the independent midwives I followed during their postpartum consultations. I give some insights on the modalities of independent midwifery in Switzerland in regard to work temporalities, and I discuss the notions of authoritative and experiential knowledge in the context of holistic care.

Fieldwork and method

Fieldwork entry

In 2010 and 2011, I conducted a comparative study aiming to investigate the influence of birthplace and pregnancy follow-up on pregnant women's

DOI: 10.4324/9781003124108-1

experiences and birth-preparation practices (Chautems 2011). This preliminary research, based on 20 interviews with pregnant women, motivated me to continue exploring out-of-hospital birth management and perinatal care. I had already observed during this initial research that the out-of-hospital birth model fosters a specific reflection about how to welcome and take care of a child. During the preparation of this research, I reconnected with Sandra,[1] a home birth mother I had met during the course of my previous fieldwork when she was pregnant with her first child.

Sandra was then in her mid-thirties and had given birth at home to her second child, Mathis. Sandra had a nursing degree but defined herself as an artist. She stopped working as a nurse after her first child's birth. She and her husband moved away from the town where they lived to a mountain locality where lower rents allowed Sandra to be a stay-at-home mother. They abstained from owning a car, so her husband commuted by public transportation to work in the complementary health sector in town. We met in their new home to talk about her breastfeeding experience. Mathis was five months old. Sandra explained her choice to stay at home:

> To be with my child, I would do anything. I would stop working, I would not even go to the hairdresser; well, I'm already not, but ... If I could cut back on this, if I could cut back on outings, I would save wherever I can, so I would be sure that I can fulfil my role and have fun in this role. Because that role is so intimate with the child, and it lasts for about two or three years; afterwards, it's over. You can't get back to it; the child has moved on. And, I don't know, it's nothing: two years, three years. It's nothing; I mean, in a lifetime, it's nothing.[2] (interview with Sandra, transcription)

After a smooth experience with her first child, Sandra was struggling with some breastfeeding complications with Mathis, exclusively breastfed, who had reflux and thrush issues. As a result, Mathis often vomited after feeding and his weight was stagnating. Sandra had to hold him vertically during feeding, making it impossible to feed him when lying in bed. She regretted not being able to feed him on demand as she did with her first baby. Concerning the thrush, she first unsuccessfully attempted to treat it with sodium bicarbonate on her nipples and in Mathis's mouth. Then, she asked for advice from her midwife, who concocted a specific ointment for her. She went to the paediatrician, a homoeopath, and a kinesiologist, as well as took some probiotics and homoeopathic remedies. She also completely reconsidered her diet, hoping to improve Mathis's digestion: she eliminated dairy, onion, garlic, cruciferous vegetables, pulses, and sugar. Five months after birth, the situation began to improve. Still, she continued to carry with her a jar of vinegar to smear on her breasts before proposing them to Mathis when going out. Her commitment to making breastfeeding work and combined methods of biomedicine and holistic medicine sparked my interest.

Furthermore, the body work she deployed contrasted with arguments used in her discourse that focused on the idea of breastfeeding as "so natural".

> For me, it was so natural to breastfeed. Maybe it's due to my travel experiences where I have seen lots of women[3] take their boobs out, and then [suckling noise] they feed their child like that, naturally. That's where I learned. (interview with Sandra, transcription)

This tension between naturalist arguments and active body management had already appeared in the discourse of Sandra, as well as other mothers, who had planned an out-of-hospital birth on the previous fieldwork I conducted. Other authors highlighted it as well (Gouilhers-Hertig 2014, 2017; Viisainen 2000, 2001). The choice to give birth out of the hospital reflects, on the one hand, a desire to respect the body's physiological processes like childbirth or lactation. On the other hand, these processes are actively supported by a range of practices implemented by women themselves—often advised by their midwife—which significantly change their daily lives. Involving different birth-preparation classes and workshops (yoga, haptonomy, and sophrology), these practices include holistic medicine treatments (homoeopathy, acupuncture, and naturopathy), perineal massage, use of the "Epi-no" (device for stretching pelvic muscles), specific diet (rich in vitamin K), and consumption of herbal tea (raspberry bush).

I discussed my research project to follow independent midwives during postnatal home visits in order to observe speeches and practices around breastfeeding in the early postpartum period with Sandra. She gave me the telephone number of her midwife, Adeline.

A short time afterwards, I contacted Adeline, who warmly accepted to meet me. She invited me to her house to discuss and have lunch together. I hesitated and told her that I would accept with pleasure; however, as a vegan, I was worried that it would be complicated for her to cook. She answered that it was fine because she was also vegan.

This really smooth entry was a harbinger of my fieldwork afterwards. My personal sympathy for the model of care proposed by independent midwives—being followed by an independent midwife and giving birth out of the hospital—certainly contributed to this easy integration. Without saying it loud and clear, midwives and parents knew implicitly, based on my reactions and over the course of our meetings and discussions, that I was fully supporting their birth choices. Sometimes, a midwife or a parent directly asked me what I would choose for myself if I were the one pregnant. I would answer honestly that I would opt for holistic care and an out-of-hospital birth with an independent midwife. As mentioned earlier, giving birth out of the hospital is a marginal choice in Switzerland. Parents often have to deal with disapproving judgements, as highlighted in other countries (MacDonald 2007; Sjöblom et al. 2012; Viisainen 2000). I believe that my transparent support has been critical to establishing trusting relationships with my interlocutors. Naepels called this intimate relationship some-times created between the researcher and her or his informers "friendship" (1998). Unlike in other research contexts, it was not difficult for me to feel close to and "like" my "locals" (Avanza 2008), with whom I often shared some characteristics and sympathies, at least in regard to birth manage-ment. These affinities have certainly facilitated my insertion and my ability to understand their viewpoint.

Without a doubt, my female gender greatly facilitated my insertion: my interest and legitimacy in dealing with such an intimate subject have never been questioned. Similarly, it never seemed to be a problem for women to expose their naked breasts in front of me. As a woman without children, I was nevertheless an outsider. This position was interesting. On the one hand, it prevented any comparison with my own experience and put me in the role of an apprentice: I had a lot to learn from midwives, but also from parents, as I had no parenting experience myself. On the other hand, I was frequently brought back, mostly by parents, to being a potential future mother. Parents assumed that my fieldwork, involving constant exposition to newborns and (often-exhausted) new parents, would necessarily influ-ence my reproductive projects. For example, one of the mothers pointed out several times that, fortunately, I was still meeting mothers long after the immediate postpartum, perceived as a chaotic and difficult period, so that I would not be discouraged to have a baby myself.

Let's go back to my first meeting with Adeline. She lived in a small town in the countryside. She offered to join me at the bus station. It was in mid-December, and I remember being very surprised to see her wearing sandals and no socks. I would realise later on that she would be barefoot or wearing sandals all year long. With a long skirt, henna-dyed hair, and barefoot, she matched a common "hippie" stereotyped representation of home birth users and practitioners. In my fieldwork, however, she was an exception, as the majority of the midwives and parents I met did not fit at all with this ste-reotype and obviously did not identify with "hippie" esthetical or cultural codes.

Once we arrived at her home, she offered me tea, and we started talking about breastfeeding. She was strongly interested in the subject and vehe-mently defended the specificity of out-of-hospital breastfeeding initiation:

> In comparison, at the hospital, what is annoying are the protocols: a baby that weighs that much is allowed to only go at the breast, but if s/he weighs less, s/he must be "completed" [with formula].[4] If s/he weighs more, s/he must also be completed ... So it's interfering with breastfeed-ing. And then there are all the old trainings, which imply that a baby should not go at the breast every hour.[5] If it is her or his request, s/he will be "completed", so s/he will be given sugar water at the beginning and formula after. So all of this thwarts breastfeeding a little. At home, for example ... I, in my practice, don't weigh the child every day. I know

there is a weight loss, so I'm not going to do anything about it, I just know it.[6] Nothing will be done against it, it's physiological. (interview with Adeline, transcription)

Adeline identified hospital protocols as a primary cause of interference with the physiological course of breastfeeding. Therefore, she presented a postpartum stay at the maternity ward and home birth postnatal follow-up as two radically different settings, each ruled by their own features and organisation to initiate breastfeeding. In her perspective, time is not an organising principle of breastfeeding. For example, she explained that she didn't pay attention to the lapse of time between birth and the first feed, unlike what she had experienced in the hospital, where the first feed took place within 30 minutes after birth, primarily to accelerate the placenta delivery. She described a mechanical way to put the baby at the breast immediately after birth:

> They want the baby to be at the breast, and it's true that the way it is done, I just can't do it! In any case, I don't do it like that! In my practice, I can't seize the breast, touch it like that. If I really have to help the mother, if she asks me, and if I really see that it's complicated, I'll tell her "do you want me to help you?" and if I have to touch her, I'll ask her, but it is true that there are very, very abrupt gestures [implied at the hospital]. (interview with Adeline, transcription)

Adeline's report reflected her own specific experience and perception of hospital care. Her interpretation and critical judgement also justified her decision to distance herself from the hospital model of birth management. Therefore, in contrast, she described her approach as non-invasive and respectful of the "natural" rhythm of delivery and the mother's intimacy.

Adeline gave me the contact details of women she followed in the frame of her holistic care practice and whom she thought had a particularly interesting breastfeeding experience. I met several of these women to conduct exploratory interviews, helping me to build my research. Adeline also offered to write an email to her independent midwife colleagues to present my research project and encourage them to collaborate with me. Indeed, on the very evening we met, she sent the email. Even if no midwife answered directly, when I contacted them later, they remembered the message and already had an idea of who I was and what I was about to ask them. Adeline's eagerness to help me and ease my fieldwork access can also be connected to a desire to legitimise and make visible her professional practices and the specificity of the care independent midwives provide to families.

In May 2014, I was ready to start my fieldwork and contacted Adeline again. While she would have gladly accepted my presence at her side during her postnatal visits, she had taken an "assistant" in the meantime and did not feel comfortable with the idea of the three of us arriving at the parent's home, outnumbering them.[7] Since her holistic care follow-ups were not accessible to me anymore, she offered for me to shadow her "assistant", during postnatal visits following hospital births. Indeed, alongside their holistic care practice, independent midwives are also assigned to postnatal visits at families discharged from the hospital. A duty system has been put in place in collaboration with hospitals in the area, where hospital staff call independent midwives to notify all discharged cases and organise the postpartum home follow-up. These follow-ups are often perceived by the midwives I met as more strenuous than the holistic care follow-ups. Through them, they are confronted with the hospital model and the fragmentation of care from which they have chosen to distance themselves: hospital birth mothers have spoken to a number of different practitioners and have received contradictory information as well. This early stage of my research allowed me to become familiar with independent midwives' professional practice, the physiology of lactation, and breastfeeding, as well as gain a basic understanding of newborns' development and abilities.[8] During the first months of my fieldwork, I also contacted other midwives and started working with them, attending both types of follow-ups (in holistic care and after hospital delivery). However, I did not immediately have the opportunity to follow a family through the entire breastfeeding experience, from initiation to weaning, like I would do later with the 27 core participant families to my research. I stopped attending "hospital discharged cases"[9] follow-ups to focus on holistic care postnatal visits in September 2014 once I was able to closely observe a holistic follow-up for the first time.

With two midwives, the collaboration stopped abruptly after one or two visits. In hindsight, they probably simply did not see the interest of my approach, especially in regard to their midwifery practice. I did not have the opportunity to meet them again and talk about it. With the nine other midwives, I felt very welcome. When we first met, I explained to them my research investigation and approach. Then, they talked to their expecting clients about my fieldwork and asked them if they were interested in participating and willing to have me present during the postnatal visits. At the couple's agreement, I would meet them for the first time after delivery, at the moment of the first postnatal visit I could attend.

Postnatal visits in holistic care

In September 2014, the first woman who had agreed to participate in my research gave birth to her baby. From September 2014 to May 2016, I attended 118 postpartum visits. For each family that I followed, I attended between one and eight consultations. This variability was due to each midwife's work habits (midwives do not make the same number of consultations), to the specificities of each family situation and, to a lesser extent, to my availability at the time of the postpartum follow-up. Depending on the situation and on the parents' needs, midwives generally did not come every day, but the postnatal home visits usually extended over the first ten days of the newborn's life. In the case of specific concerns or on parents' demand, the follow-up might continue during the child's first two months. Once the postpartum follow-up was completed, parents were still entitled to three additional free visits dedicated to breastfeeding support. These visits could be carried out by the midwife or a lactation consultant. According to my observations and discussions with parents and midwives, it was rare that parents requested these visits. I had the opportunity to attend such visits only twice, with two different families. In addition to the observations made during postnatal visits, I also attended postnatal classes (five sessions in total) given by one of the midwives. Because she organised these group classes, this midwife had a clear tendency to make fewer postpartum visits. The postnatal classes allowed me to have a more comprehensive vision of her approach.

The midwives' visits all lasted between one and two hours, which almost always gave the midwife the opportunity to observe a feeding session. Since all of these home birth parents intended to breastfeed their baby, and since obstacles can emerge at the time of its initiation, leaving parents disconcerted, breastfeeding was at the centre of the postpartum follow-up. Overall, the visits were usually organised in two parts: a conversation between the midwife and the parents, and a clinical examination of the baby and mother. The holistic care modalities, as well as the shared set of values between midwife and parents, based on non-interventionism and respect for the parents' autonomy, gave a friendly dimension to the midwife's visits, as also observed by Perrenoud (2016). Moreover, midwives strived to involve parents in every decision process, explaining in detail each test and procedure so they could make "enlightened" decisions (Gouilhers-Hertig 2017; Perrenoud 2016).[10]

Depending on whether the baby was awake or asleep when the midwife arrived, the visit would start with either the discussion or actions involving the baby: undressing and weighing, clinical examination, and, more rarely, giving the baby her or his first bath. During the moments of discussion, I was generally sitting with the midwife and parents, in the living room, on a sofa or armchair, arranged in a circle around a coffee table. The father often offered coffee to the midwife and me as the discussion started with the mother.[11] This configuration allowed me to observe all participants, to feel included in the situation, and, occasionally, to take part in the conversation. On rare occasions, this discussion time took place in the parents' bedroom, where we would sit on the floor around the bed, or at the edge of the bed, depending on the mother's preference.

In the same warm way that they received their midwife, all parents greeted me with a kiss and were on first-name terms with me (in French *tu* instead of *vous*). Their friendly attitude and ease of speaking with me demonstrated that my presence was welcome, also confirmed by some particular attentions. For example, a father remarked that I was the only one who had not held the baby in my arms and offered for me to hold her. Overall, they seemed eager to prove the efficiency of their birth model and parenting style. My presence was for them an opportunity to legitimise and give visibility to their birth choices and infant care practices, still marginalised in Switzerland. As their relatives were not always supportive, our meetings offered them a safe space to share their stories, feelings, and experiences. Some of them told me that they appreciated these regular "reports" allowed by our meetings as a way to put recent events back into perspective.

As independent midwives perform their postnatal care alone, their practices remain quite confidential and only witnessed by involved families. One of the midwives I met during my fieldwork insisted on this dimension, saying that it would be valuable if I could combine in a single volume all the tricks of independent midwives I witnessed—for example, cutting up disposable postpartum underwear to transform it into a nursing bra or using a diaper filled with hot water to warm a baby's foot before a blood sample. In this perspective, in my fieldwork, I was not only perceived as an apprentice but also a documentarist.

For some, I also played the role of a facilitator because I had the opportunity to make myself useful by centralising and sharing information I collected during the postpartum consultations. For example, I gave parents the name of an infant sleep specialist or informed them about a home delivery cleaner service for cloth diapers, resources I had heard about from midwives or other parents. Another emblematic anecdote occurred with Lauriane, one of the mothers I met when she gave birth to her second child. She asked me for help after giving birth to her third child. Initially, she sent a message to announce the birth and informed me that she had a severe postpartum haemorrhage and had to be transferred to the hospital after delivery. Having been exposed to radiation to stop the bleeding, she was unable to breastfeed her baby for the next 24 hours and was looking for a milk donation. I contacted another mother who was living close to the hospital and whom I knew had previously donated her milk. The newborn eventually received some milk from another mother, but Lauriane appreciated my effort and involvement.

My researcher stance

My researcher stance is part of the reflexive epistemology initiated by the interpretive approach (see for example Bensa 2006; Clifford 1983; Olivier de Sardan 1995, 2008; Schwartz 1993):

> Interpretive anthropology demystifies much of what had previously passed unexamined in the construction of ethnographic narratives, types, observations, and descriptions. It contributes to an increasing visibility of the creative (and in a broad sense, poetic) processes by which

"cultural" objects are invented and treated as meaningful. (Clifford 1983: 130)

By revealing the different stages of my reflection and the way I approached and proceeded in my fieldwork, tracing the story of my research is part of this reflexive process. In my writing, I applied myself to quote my interlocutors, often and at length, in order to highlight the collaborative character of my research and the multiplicity of voices intervening in the ethnographic knowledge production.

My fieldwork took place in the French-speaking part of Switzerland. My interlocutors spoke in French, and I translated their words into English. The translation of some French emic expressions was challenging, such as the *montée de lait*, an essential notion in the midwives' postpartum follow-up, which designates the moment when the colostrum turns into milk a few days after birth. In this specific case, I used the expression "when the milk comes in" and chose to avoid a substantive form.

I am aware that, in the translation process, I inevitably lost some subtleties and local particularities. However, I applied myself to reproduce my interlocutors' words, as faithfully as possible, to preserve their oral character, and I precisely recontextualised them by describing the context and the social situation from which they were extracted. Safeguarding against overinterpretation and generalisation, this contextualisation effort is crucial in the writing process (Beaud & Weber 1997). According to Bensa (2008), "opting, from a resolutely empirical perspective, for the primacy of the detail, the local and the circumstantial, is refusing to deindex the facts of their comments" (324). My attention was centred on what my interlocutors "do one by one as unique subjects and reasons for their actions within a specific social space" (ibid. 2008: 324). This focus on people and their individual, contextualised actions avoids the swallowing of the individual in the collective.

The analyses produced by research cannot be dissociated from the conditions in which they are produced (Bensa 2006). Through my choices, sensibilities, affinities, and readings at each step of the research process, I built my fieldwork and produced data specific to this context. These data are the result of "the transformation into objectified traces of 'pieces of reality' as they have been selected and perceived by the researcher" (Olivier de Sardan 1995: 74). From this perspective, I consider my analyses not as "results" but rather interpretations. As other interpretive social scientists, I think that observation without participation is an illusion of externality and objectivity: the mere presence of the researcher is already a form of "participation" in the observed social situation (Olivier de Sardan 1995, 2008; Schwartz 1993; Weber 1989). Therefore, researchers are part of their fieldwork, and their interlocutors assign them a role. This role allows researchers to understand what they represent in the eyes of their interlocutors and then to know "to whom one is talking" when talking to them. In this way, any fieldwork therefore contains a part of self-analysis.

Fieldwork ethics and relationships

To develop the ethical framework of my research, I relied on the Swiss Anthropological Association's (2010) stance on ethics in anthropological research, which suggests a set of "good practices" (149). The authors conceive their statement as "an instrument for reflection and discussion on ethnographic practice and commitment and not a list of normative and binding recommendations" (Swiss Anthropological Association 2010: 150). Ethics issues emerge at each stage of the anthropological work and all cannot be anticipated upstream. They must hence be treated in a contextualised way when they present themselves to the researcher. For these reasons, the Swiss Anthropological Association questions the relevance of the "informed consent" device regarding the anthropological approach. Indeed, requiring researchers to inform their interlocutors as clearly as possible about the objectives, implications, and dissemination means of the analysis is a necessary condition for ethnographic practice. Nevertheless, the initial questioning may evolve and the fieldwork events may open up on unforeseen observations and themes. Researchers must hence negotiate their presence and position on the field and ensure participants' agreement throughout the research process.

I conducted my fieldwork with independent midwives. They were not tied to any medical institution or formal organisation; they directly gave me their consent. In addition, I submitted my research project to the cantonal ethics committee on research involving humans (CER-VD), who granted my project with a certificate of no objection.

As suggested by Fassin (2008), I agree with a notion of "ethics as practice", as opposed to a regular notion of ethics "in terms of principles" (120-121). Ethics is thus built up as the research progresses and "through negotiation with those who participate in it" (ibid. 2008: 120). I did not submit to the "bureaucratic gesture" to have an informed consent form signed before each interview (ibid. 2008: 126). Instead, I presented my research, answered the questions, and discussed the conditions of their participation—and their possible withdrawal—at each stage of the fieldwork.

Requesting families' consent took place through several stages. I had prepared a written document presenting my project, containing my contact information, and proposed it to midwives. Some of them used it, and others preferred to explain my research in their own words.

Midwives first asked families before birth if they agreed to me attending their postpartum home visits. I was ideally present for the midwife's first postpartum visit, only 12 or 24 hours after birth. Sometimes I met the parents a few days after birth, in the case of a hospital transfer or for other reasons (if the midwife forgot to inform me of the birth or if I was not available at the time of her first visit).

Some mothers who had received the document proactively contacted me to inform me of their agreement to participate in my research, as well as their due date. After delivery, they reached out to me and communicated the time of the midwife's scheduled visit. This strategy allowed me to meet two mothers before their delivery. They were pregnant with their second and third child and already had a breastfeeding experience that they offered to share with me before starting a new breastfeeding journey.

At my first meeting with the parents, I introduced myself and presented my research. On that occasion, I made sure they agreed to participate, clarifying my research methods and answering questions. Once they had given their consent, I remained careful in offering them additional opportunities to withdraw. After the first visit, I asked if they agreed to me returning with their midwife for another consultation. At the end of the postpartum follow-up, I again asked for their agreement to be contacted a few weeks or months later for an interview. After each meeting, I ensured they were willing to see me again, until the last meeting, corresponding with their child's weaning.

At the beginning of my fieldwork, I did not know to what extent the parents would agree to participate in my research. Even though I hoped to follow families through their entire breastfeeding journey from initiation to weaning, I wanted to avoid scaring them away and first only mentioned one consultation and one interview. As I met with parents, I realised that my presence fitted easily into the midwives' consultations, as I had hoped would be the case. As a result, and to enrich my ethnographic material, I continued to follow them more closely and in the longer term. I was amazed to discover that most of the families became committed to participating in my research, largely exceeding my modest initial expectations.

In two situations, parents decided to stop their participation after one or two visits. They were not feeling comfortable with my presence and wished to preserve the intimacy they had created with the midwife. I was not surprised, as I too felt uncomfortable with these families: my attempts to engage in conversations sounded wrong, I did not know where to stand or sit, and my body felt cumbersome. It was the only real situations of discomfort in my fieldwork.

Overall, my fieldwork unfolded smoothly. I did not experience "the discomfort of the fieldwork" as described by de La Soudière (1988). I agree with him on the idea that "the field is (almost) never really disturbed, and this illusion arises from the discomfort of the fieldwork" (La Soudière 1988: 6). For my part, I did not feel that my presence changed the course of the visits or the content of the discussions. My fieldwork allowed me to socialise with the families and the midwives for quite a long period of time. Midwives and parents seemed proud in allowing a researcher to document their "niche" practices and perhaps contribute to their increased visibility. I was lucky enough to meet with some of them over a period of two years. This enabled the production of contextualised data rooted in "real life", "at the closest to the subjects' usual life situations" (Olivier de Sardan 1995: 73).

As mentioned above, one part of the visit was action oriented, often involving a clinical examination and weighing of the baby. These actions usually took place in the often-cramped bathroom, where it was difficult to fit more than one person. Even in these moments, my presence did not feel unsuitable. In general, I allowed myself to ask the midwife or parents questions for accuracy or clarification. Sometimes, the discussion deviated from the postnatal follow-up, and I openly took part in it. The parents spoke to me spontaneously, and in return, I also revealed myself, allowing them to know me better and reducing the artificiality of having a foreigner attending their consultations.

Sometimes, a clinical examination of the perineum was needed. In these cases, either I would leave the room or the midwife and the mother would go to another room. These moments were occasionally an opportunity to discuss with the father. The breast's nudity never seemed to be embarrassing for mothers. On several occasions, the midwife explicitly asked for the mother's agreement before examining her breast in my presence—for example, when there was a crack on the nipple.

I often had the occasion to perform small favours for participants: helping the midwife carry her equipment, holding the baby or keeping an eye on her or him when the midwife and mother were in another room for a clinical examination of the perineum, fetching an object located in another room of the house, taking a picture, and so on. These actions also provided me with a role in the field and facilitated my integration in the course of the visits.

On an organisational level, depending on the midwives, scheduling a visit could be quite challenging. Between the "hospital discharged cases" postpartum follow-ups, which midwives are not able to plan, and the unpredictable deliveries of their holistic care follow-ups, they are often very busy. Even if they were willing to do it, it was inconvenient to fit me into their schedule. Sometimes, I would only know the time and location of the appointment a few hours beforehand. I did not have a car or even a driver's licence, and some parents lived in villages difficult to reach by public transport. Depending on the location of the parents' home, the midwife's place of residence, and her itinerary of the day, either I joined her directly at the parents' home or we would fix a meeting place and travel together in her car. Overall, I spent a lot of time waiting for midwives. On the other hand, the many hours spent with midwives in their car constituted quality conversation time, during which we discussed their care approach and work organisation. More specifically, the midwife could give me information about the family we were visiting and their situation or summarise what had happened since we had last seen them. We would also debrief on the visit just completed, and it would give me the opportunity to ask for some clarifications. These moments of informal discussions constituted such a rich material that I did not feel the need to conduct formal interviews with all of them.

I assured all participants' anonymity. The names of the midwives, parents, and children have been changed to protect their identities. I avoided mentioning certain characteristics, such as the exact age of my interlocutors or our meeting dates, to prevent them from being identifiable. However, these measures were not sufficient to ensure the anonymity of all participants, especially the midwives, as my fieldwork took place on a relatively small territory with a local context of strong inter-acquaintance. For this reason, several midwives appear with two different pseudonyms so that they cannot be identified.

The midwives with whom I collaborated do not strictly form a collective, and because of their busy and very random schedules, it did not seem possible to give them a collective restitution. Neither was this request ever made to me. I had opportunities to discuss with some midwives about my field observations and to receive their feedback. One of the midwives, Sophie Guerra, became a friend and a highly valued interlocutor with whom I had multiple discussions at each stage of my work.[12] We undertook together several collaborative and interdisciplinary presentations and writing projects.[13] After the last meeting with the parents, I also asked them if they were interested in learning about the communications and publications on my work.[14]

Observing intimacy, sharing feelings

This was my very first postnatal visit. I had met Capucine, the midwife, 15 minutes earlier, and we arrived together at the front door of the house. The mother, Barbara, had arranged Capucine's visit at her parents' home because of noisy renovation works at her home, which had already started during her pregnancy. When we arrived, the parents and baby were not there yet, so the grandparents offered us coffee and we sat at the kitchen table to wait for them.

When the parents, who were obviously much stressed, arrived with the newborn, we stood up to greet them, and Barbara burst into tears. She was exhausted by the noise of the renovations and very insecure about the care of her daughter, especially in regard to breastfeeding. Capucine took her in her arms and gave her comforting words. She offered to sit down and talk quietly about her worries. I felt deeply moved by Barbara's distress. Even if she had given her prior consent to Capucine, I wondered if she had preferred that I were absent. On the contrary, Barbara and her spouse's very warm attitude towards me very quickly reassured me that my presence was welcome.

This type of scene was repeated many times during my fieldwork. I was surprised by the way I was affected by my interlocutors' emotions, often moved and empathetically involved in their struggles and doubts. Parents were tired, and breastfeeding issues or doubts often brought very strong emotions to mothers. I also listened to heart-breaking stories during interviews. Each time, I felt much moved, and I occasionally shed tears with them. My emotions, which I could not hide, caused me to feel exposed and distanced me from my role as a researcher. In these moments, I let myself "be affected" (Favret-Saada 2009).

> The researcher on her or his fieldwork is (hopefully) not only a researcher, and s/he also carries with her or him a personal world that

comes into contact with the personal worlds of those with whom s/ he works and lives, for a time. This aspect of being on the fieldwork is (fortunately) impossible to professionalise in the strict sense, that is to say, normalisable by professional standards, although it undoubtedly influences the professional production. Of everyone, depending on one's character, tastes, affects, intuitions, sensitivity, capacity of contact. (Olivier de Sardan 2000: 434-435)

According to Gallenga (2008), empathy felt by the researcher towards her or his interlocutors is sometimes perceived in ethnographic methodology guides as "a method, even a way to access the other person's world view" (115). My fieldwork pushed me to find my place in very intimate moments, during which my interlocutors often laid themselves bare, literally and emotionally. In this context, my own exposed emotions helped reduce the asymmetry of the research situation and the hint of voyeurism that can be associated with it: I was not only an observer, I was also "taken", to use the terms of Favret-Saada, by the situation, overwhelmed by the emotions it generated. This mutual sharing of emotions, which temporarily distanced me from my "project of knowledge", was also a condition for gaining access to it (Favret-Saada 2009: 159).

Over successive postnatal visits and discussions with midwives, my perspective and sensitivity have evolved through a process of "impregnation" highlighted by Olivier de Sardan (2000: 434). For example, incorporating the prophylactic discourse midwives delivered to mothers, I became quite attentive to protecting my own perineum, changing my way of moving, crouching, or carrying heavy loads. My fieldwork remained in my mind long after it was over. More broadly, after listening to so many out-of-hospital birth stories, the modalities of this type of birth management and experience seem to have become the norm for me: although experiences differ greatly from one woman to another, I believe that similarities remain in these stories because of practical and spatial modalities (no epidural, no hospital bed, etc.). I remember, for example, feeling surprised when a friend told me about her birth experience in a maternity ward. She noticed my incredulity and asked me what bothered me, to which I replied: "how did you manage to push while lying down?" I was used to hearing reports of the expulsion stage taking place in a birthing pool, with the mother often squatting, and I was having trouble imagining how pushing the newborn out in this lying posture was possible.

Ethnographic material

As highlighted by Geertz (1973), field notes form a "thick description" of the observed situations. They constitute a written record of fieldwork observations, a description of the acts, gestures, and discourses. During the fieldwork, I managed to write actions and observations as well as literal quotes on the spot. After each fieldwork session, I also read my notes again and completed them.

The different types of ethnographic materials, observations, and interviews complement one another.[15] On the one hand, combining observations and interviews makes it possible to confront discourses and practices, and make visible coherence or contradictions. On the other hand, interviews provide access to the way in which interlocutors give meaning to their behaviour and actions, which is not possible with observations alone.

The quantity and quality of my ethnographic material vary from one family to another. In some cases, I was able to attend a significant number of postnatal visits. In others, I could only attend one midwife's visit, but I continued to meet with mothers or parents for an extended period of time and had very fruitful discussions with them. With some families, I had the opportunity to have both: rich observation-based material during the postpartum consultations and substantial interview-based material. As a result, some families may appear as central characters more than others in my analyses.

Before conducting my exploratory interviews, I had made an interview guide, which mainly served as a reminder of the themes I wanted to address. Pretty quickly, I stopped using this guide. I adopted an open interview framework that resembled a conversation more than an interview (Kaufmann 2004; Olivier de Sardan 1995, 2008).

I recorded and accurately transcribed the exploratory interviews. However, once the second stage of my fieldwork began, I decided not to record my interviews anymore but to take notes in my fieldwork journal instead. First, for practical reasons, it was more convenient to have all my data immediately available and not unusable data waiting to be transcribed. Second, parents and midwives were used to seeing me writing in a notebook during our meetings and seemed very comfortable with this observation device.

Except for two interviews performed before birth, as mentioned above, all of the interviews were conducted after the observations and hence after the midwife's follow-up had ended. I already knew the parents quite well and was glad to meet them again to catch up. After some small talk about various topics, I asked them to tell me how things went for them with their baby, especially how their breastfeeding experience had been going since our last meeting. I prepared each interview by reading all the notes I had taken on the specific family beforehand. On the basis of this rereading, I invited them to talk to me about the points left unresolved or to recall an observed situation and enlighten me on their feelings regarding it. In most situations, the last interview corresponded approximately to the time at which weaning occurred.

I first approached families through mothers, who were my primary interlocutors. I often spent much more time talking with them than with their spouses. Fathers participated in my research at various levels and in different ways. Some of them were able and willing to be present at each interview, whereas others could not or were not interested in getting involved in these meetings. Among the 19 holistic postnatal follow-ups I observed in which the father was present, eight fathers also participated in one or more interviews. When the father did not seem interested in taking part in the interviews, I did not insist. I met my interlocutors according to their interests and availabilities, staying tuned to their feelings and desires. At the time of the interviews, most fathers had returned to work, and it seemed difficult and too demanding to arrange a meeting during their restricted free time. All eight fathers who were present at the interviews continued after they had returned to work as well. However, most of them worked part-time, and their schedule was flexible so that the interviews did not overlap with their evenings and weekends. Sometimes, the meeting occurred near their workplace, on their lunch break, and they would be eating during the interview. I did not arrange any interview with a father without the mother present.

I conducted two to six interviews with each mother or couple, mostly depending on the breastfeeding duration. My interviews were flexibly scheduled at regular intervals. The first interview usually took place a few weeks after the end of the midwife postpartum follow-up and the second a few months later, often after mothers had returned to work and the baby had experienced a day-care system. The following interviews were roughly scheduled every six months. The interviews usually lasted between two and three hours. They mostly took place at the parents' home or in a café, very rarely at my home, according to the parents' preference. During these meetings, we usually shared coffee or tea, sometimes a meal. At their home, mothers or parents continued to attend their usual activities: breastfeeding, diaper changing, meal preparing, feeding their older children with solid foods, and playing. I got involved in these activities, trying to make myself useful when I could. I held babies, played with them, and went for a walk with mothers. In that sense, these meetings were not only interviews but also sources of field observation notes. Since I decided to stop interviews after weaning, the last meeting was often bittersweet, as I enjoyed meeting them on a regular basis.

Concluding my fieldwork was not an easy decision, and I felt quite nostalgic about my regular discussions with parents, as well as with midwives. Interestingly, if accessing the fieldwork has been problematised extensively (see for example Darmon 2005), exiting the fieldwork is less often discussed. Yet, in the case of my research, I struggled more with concluding my fieldwork than with accessing it.

Who are these people who give birth at home? Challenging categorisation

Home birth parents have been described by other social science researchers as middle class, well educated, and economically privileged (Gouilhers-Hertig

2017; Hildingsson et al. 2006; Jacques 2007; Perrenoud 2016; Pruvost 2016; Quagliariello 2017b; Viisainen 2001). I observed that access to holistic care requires parents to search for information "prematurely and actively", excluding the most socio-economically disadvantaged families, which is consistent with the analysis of Perrenoud (2016: 150). If not actively pursued, information about holistic care and an out-of-hospital birth will probably not be provided by professionals. Obstetricians, if not solicited on the topic—and often even if they are asked about it—will not spontaneously supply detailed information on this modality of care. Nevertheless, information tends to become more accessible. For example, in French-speaking Switzerland and during my fieldwork, out-of-hospital birth was the topic of articles in national supermarket chain magazines as well as broadcasts on national radio and television. It still requires an ability to understand and read French.

My research population was significantly more heterogeneous than described by the abovementioned authors. Based on my discussions with midwives, this heterogeneity was representative of their clientele. The core participants in my research were 27 mothers, 19 fathers, and their children. In eight situations, the father was not included in my fieldwork observations, and I never met the father in four of these situations. One was living abroad: the mother, Jeanne, had planned to give birth in Switzerland and to join him a couple of months after birth. Three fathers had already resumed work at the time of the midwife postnatal visits. In the four other situations, I barely met the father who was taking care of older children during the visits, in a separate room than the mother, the midwife, the baby, and me.

The parents were between 20 and 40 years old. The families were all composed of a heterosexual parental couple and one to three children (including the newborn). I did not meet or even hear about lesbian couples during my fieldwork. Based on discussions with some midwives, it seems to reflect a general absence of experiences with the follow-up of same-sex couples. In Switzerland, parenting information of all forms, including birth preparation classes and leaflets provided by health professionals and institutions, are heavily loaded with heteronormative content, including an abundance of happy pictures of heterosexual parents. As a result, same-sex couples may understandably feel excluded. Unlike the dominant biomedical model, the holistic care model in Switzerland does not provide such written information and graphic content, which might accidentally help lesbian couples to feel more welcome. Nevertheless, the midwives' discourse remains strongly heterocentric—for example, by always referring to "the father" to theoretically designate the mother's partner instead of selecting a more inclusive term. Since I left my fieldwork, I have addressed this topic with another midwife, who told me that she was following the pregnancy of a lesbian couple for the first time. She informed them that while she would happily be their midwife, she was worried about occasionally making some heterocentric comments due to her lack of experience and that they would have to signal it to her. She commented that she appreciated the conversation dynamic between the three of them, refreshingly contrasting with the usual gendered heterosexual parental dynamic.

In general, if the holistic care model is heteronormative, in my view, it is merely a reflection of the Swiss cultural context, in which the perinatal care fits. I believe that the care continuity and individualisation in the holistic model make it more inclusive than the dominant technocratic one. In comparison, the follow-up of each family at the hospital is standardised, and there is a constant changeover of health providers. As a result, there is less room to nuance the dominant heterocentric culture and reference framework. Overall, and to my knowledge, there is no socio-anthropological work on the issue of the access and experiences of holistic care by lesbian couples, and it remains to be investigated.

The parents I met were of various nationalities (Swiss, French, Bosnian, Spanish, Italian, Peruvian, and Filipino). Twenty mothers or fathers were foreigners on a total of 54 parents, namely more than a third of them. This is consistent with the general Swiss population: with a proportion of 29.6 per cent of foreigners, Switzerland was in 2017 the country with the highest rate of foreign population in Europe, behind some microstates, such as Luxembourg, Monaco, and Liechtenstein (United Nations 2017). Since the second half of the twentieth century, the contribution of immigration to the population growth has been stronger in Switzerland than in formal immigration countries such as the United States, Canada, or Australia (Bolzman 2002). In Switzerland, the issue of race is not as pervasive as, for instance, in the United States. All the foreign parents I met were well integrated into the local population. In each family, at least one parent perfectly mastered French, enabling easy access to information regarding the model of care they chose and more broadly to local health systems. In addition, all of my allophone interlocutors were able to work in French. I did not discuss with midwives the nationalities of their usual clientele, so I cannot comment about the proportion of allophone or racialised people they work with. I generally believe that the ability to understand French remains an essential prerequisite to access the model of care they offer.

Among the parents, 15 families out of 27 were living in a city; the others were living in small towns or in the countryside. The parents were from various socio-economic backgrounds as well. If some parents were indeed well educated, having both high economic and cultural capital, a significant part (more than one third) of my interlocutors did not match this profile. Their education levels and fields varied, from health care to entertainment, teaching, or farming. Two families were in a precarious situation and received financial aid from social services. Based on my discussions with midwives, such families do not constitute an exception. For example, one midwife attended several homebirths with a family "at psychosocial risk" from a biomedical perspective. After a difficult hospital experience for the birth of their first child—they felt discredited by hospital staff—they had decided to avoid the hospital and opted for holistic care with an independent midwife for the births of their other children. The continuity of care and the intimacy of a homebirth fostered a feeling of trust and safety because they were able to bond with their midwife in a way unachievable with a standard, fragmented care. Consistent with a previous research I carried out (Chautems 2011), I noticed a prominence of occupations related to health care among the mothers I met (three midwives, three psychologists, two nurses, two early childhood educators, and one nursing auxiliary). The vast majority of mothers worked part-time, two mothers were unemployed by choice, one was in the process of stopping her independent activity, and one was temporarily unemployed at the time of my fieldwork. Among the 27 families, fathers also often worked part-time (11 of them), eight fathers were self-employed (for example, sports coach, landscape gardener, filmmaker, or farmer), thus allowing some flexibility in the organisation of work schedules.

Like the "natural" parents observed by Bobel (2002), my interlocutors mostly adhered to the "voluntary simplicity" lifestyle, advocating for a relative austerity and aiming to reduce their consumption, including on account of environmental concerns (Elgin 1993). Schor establishes a distinction between "simple livers" and "downshifters". Simple livers "establish a maximum level of outcomes beyond which it is unacceptable to live" for moral or environmental reasons (Schor 1998, cited by Bobel 2002: 52). In comparison, downshifters settle for a "trade-off between time and money, deciding that their time is more valuable than their income and that they will therefore live with less" (Bobel 2002: 52). In relation to this distinction, my interpretation is that most parents I met were rather taking part in the downshifter movement, even though they often expressed environmental sensitivity, especially through their consumption choices (organic and local food and washable diapers). They choose to work less and accept to rethink their consumption practices in order to spend more time taking care of their family. For example, one of the families was living in a caravan, in the garden of a squat (where they had access to a bathroom and kitchen), to save on rent. This downshifting strategy allowed nine families to avoid placing their child in a childcare centre.

All parents I met shared a holistic approach towards their health and body, as well as sceptical thoughts regarding biomedicine. Their out-of-hospital birth choice was part of this reasoning. As a result, parents primarily relied on their diet (often organic, local, vegetarian, or vegan) and on complementary medicine (homoeopathy, aromatherapy, osteopathy, or acupuncture being the most regularly cited) to treat themselves when going through minor health issues or discomfort, including during pregnancy and the postpartum period.

As part of the holistic care philosophy, all the families embraced proximal parenting at varying degrees and agreed with common childcare practices, including "babywearing" and "bed-sharing", practised by all the parents. However, the term "attachment parenting"—or "parentage proximal" in

French—was never used. Instead, parents sometimes used the term "maternage" (mothering), referring to parenting practices actually carried out by both mothers and fathers.

Thirteen families had planned home birth and 13 had chosen a birth centre. One couple, Carole and Michaël, opted for pregnancy and postnatal care with an independent midwife but preferred to give birth at a maternity ward with hospital midwives. I decided to include them in my study, even if their process was quite different. Their situation (a sleepy baby who had trouble gaining weight) was interesting, and contact with the parents was immediately very smooth. The project to give birth at home or in a birth centre was completed for 19 couples. The other eight deliveries took place at the maternity ward, either in a planned way following the detection of a condition that tilts pregnancy on the side of pathology (for example, gestational diabetes) or unexpectedly after a transfer during labour. Four mothers who gave birth in a hospital setting had a caesarean section.

The holistic care script

Relying on my observations and discussions with parents and midwives, I propose that the holistic care model presumes a particular script, regarding postpartum and infant care practices. This script partially aggregates the principles of the attachment parenting approach (Sears & Sears 2001), based on Bowlby's attachment theory, but also includes influences from the "natural motherhood" movement as described by Bobel (2002). However, it appeared to me that, contrary to Bobel's observations, fathers in my fieldwork were central stakeholders of this parenting project, engaging in all aspects of childcare, including breastfeeding.

Also based on local specificities of the Swiss perinatal landscape, the content of the script is transmitted to parents vertically by independent midwives forming a "community of practice" (Jordan 2014), and horizontally through common readings or online communities of home birth parents. Breastfeeding acts as a pillar of the holistic care script during the postpartum period, while other parenting practices being considered by midwives and parents as related to or facilitating breastfeeding.

Schematically described, the holistic care script supposes that parents choose to give birth outside the hospital with an independent midwife and sometimes a doula.[16] Once the baby is born, parents breastfeed her or him on demand, according to their breastfeeding project (i.e. roughly six months of exclusive breastfeeding) based on the WHO recommendations, then on-demand non-exclusive breastfeeding for about one year, or beyond for some families. Following a child-centred approach, some parents diversify their child's diet using the baby-led weaning method. The baby sleeps in the parents' bed at least during the first weeks after birth in order to support breastfeeding initiation and to facilitate night-time breastfeeding. Favouring bodily contacts with her or him, parents carry their baby on their bodies instead of putting her or him in a pushchair. In the same perspective, many parents massage their baby. Some of the parents extend the principle of on-demand breastfeeding to the elimination needs of their child, practising "elimination communication", whereas others would learn sign language to favour an early non-verbal communication with their infant. Infant care and parenting consumption choices are also part of the holistic care script, parents favouring ecological or organic products and more generally "downshifting" their consumption habits to reduce their waste, but also for some of them to decrease their working hours. For example, choosing washable diapers instead of disposable ones addresses all these concerns. Finally, in line with a will to avoid interfering with the physiology of the birth process, parents question all interventions on their baby; they would typically refuse to have her or him vaccinated, supplemented with vitamin K, and bathed directly after birth.

This description of the holistic care script corresponds to an ideal type of the model: in practice, parents adjust and negotiate this script with each other, their baby, and their midwives, depending on the specificities of their life circumstances and requirements. As a result, the script application crystallises tensions between the holistic care parenting model and its everyday implementation, highlighting the model's contradictions and inconsistencies within a modern neoliberal organisation.

Contextualising midwifery care

Midwifery in Switzerland: a historical perspective

Until the nineteenth century, in Switzerland, as in most other European countries, deliveries usually took place under the supervision of a "matron"— a traditional midwife—at the parturient's home (Charrier & Clavandier 2013; Fuschetto 2017; Gélis 1988; Moscucci 1990; Shorter 1984). The knowledge of these matrons was often based on their empirical experience only: they had not undergone any formal medical training (Rieder 2007a). This home care model, also prevalent in the North American perinatal landscape, is qualified as "social childbirth" by Wertz and Wertz (1989 [1977]) and allowed new mothers to "lie-in", whereas "other women took over responsibility of the household" (4). Hospital delivery was then perceived, in Europe and the United States, as a solution reserved for the most disadvantaged women—poor, unhealthy, or single (Fuschetto 2017; Praz 2005; Rieder 2007b; Wertz & Wertz 1989). In addition to the social stigma, hospitals represented health threats, such as puerperal fever and other contagious diseases.

In most European countries, the rise of medicine during the nineteenth century led to a reconfiguration of the event of birth. Previously considered a "normal" event and intrinsically linked to the private sphere, it became part of the public space and subject to medical care (Gélis 1988). In France, hoping to lower the perinatal mortality rate, surgeons, supported by the state, established an "art of childbirth" to supervise the activity of midwives. As described by Gélis, a "fight" of legitimacy began between the professional groups of midwives or "matrons" on one side and of surgeons on the other, resolving in favour of the latter (1988). In Switzerland, as was the case in France, the surgeons' medical knowledge gained definite legitimacy and outshined that of midwives during the twentieth century, downgrading midwives' skills and building a negative image of the midwife as "ignorant, superstitious and entangled in tradition" (Rieder 2007a: 19).

In addition, midwives were battling not only against physicians to protect their expertise area but also against visiting nurses, who had specialised training in childcare and were emerging during the interwar period in most European countries (Droux 2005; Marland & Rafferty 1997; Thébaud 1986). During the interwar years, the Europe-wide falling birth rate also severely threatened the midwifery profession. Finally, the economic crisis of the interwar period, which hit all European countries, led women to opt for cheaper, unqualified birth attendants and thus reject trained midwives (ibid. 1997).

Since the beginning of the twentieth century, improvements in hygiene protocols marked the end of puerperal fever in the maternity wards of most industrialised countries. The hospital's image improved and the proportion of institutional deliveries increased across all social standings. Hospital-based obstetricians developed new medical skills and techniques. From there, birth hospitalisation progressively began to spread, imposing itself as a guarantee of safety and rest for new mothers. Nevertheless, until approximately the middle of the twentieth century, most women in Switzerland, and in other European countries, still gave birth at home under the supervision of a midwife (Favre 2009, Gélis 1988, Morel 2016).

The medicalisation of birth marked a decisive turning point in midwives' activity: they henceforth have had to undergo medical training and have been subordinated to physicians. Subsequently, the midwifery profession was marginalised to varying degrees in Europe (De Vries 1996; Thébaud 1986), these disparities reflecting the national differences regarding midwives' tasks and responsibilities (Marland & Rafferty 1997).

In this context, the figure of the "male midwife" emerged in Europe. Profiled as experts, male midwives held anatomical knowledge and innovative medical skills (Moscucci 1990). At their instigation, institutions intended for labour and delivery with medical care, the maternity wards, emerged and multiplied, welcoming into their midst a new training programme designed for midwives (Rieder 2007b). Midwives in Switzerland were then largely integrated into these new structures, whereas liberal practices became scarce (ibid. 2007).

However, this integrative model strongly contrasts with the American context, where midwives tend to position themselves as a counter-power to the dominant technocratic model. Overall, the crisis of the midwifery profession in Switzerland was incomparable to the situation in the United States, where the profession was under the threat of extinction for the same reasons (Katz Rothman 1991 [1982], Wertz & Wertz 1989 [1977]). Today, a large majority of hospital deliveries still take place under the supervision of a midwife in Switzerland.

In most European countries, the division of labour between midwives and obstetricians is primarily based on a division between physiology and pathology (Akrich & Pasveer 1996; Gélis 1988). The medicalisation of childbirth induced an institutionalisation of the division of prerogatives between doctors and midwives. Eutocia, namely physiological pregnancies and deliveries, is the midwives' responsibility, whereas doctors take care of dystocia—that is, the pathological childbirth. The latter are responsible for not only curing the pathology but also preventing its occurrence. It is admitted that "although it remains unpredictable, risk can, in most cases, be detected and evaluated by close surveillance" (Carricaburu, 2007: 128). Midwives position themselves as specialists in physiological pregnancy and eutocic delivery. However, as Cavalli and Gouilhers-Hertig (2014) have shown, in Switzerland, the operability of this distribution must be nuanced, and rivalries and tensions between the two professions persist.

Praz (2005) conducted a study of perinatal health in the canton of Vaud between 1860 and 1930. She found that awareness of the key role of midwives in reducing maternal and infant mortality emerged early on within health institutions and practitioners of Vaud. Consistently, the first European midwifery school opened in 1778, in Orbe, Vaud, under the direction of surgeon Jean-André Venel. The school was transferred to Lausanne in 1792 and was established at the cantonal hospital in 1886. The training duration extended from four months in 1883 to two years in 1919. Located in the very premises of the cantonal hospital, students constituted a free workforce, available night and day.

In 1894, midwives united and created the *Fédération Suisse des Sages-femmes* (Swiss Federation of Midwives). The publication of an official journal, *Die Schweize Hebamme*, started in 1903 and is still active (Bosson 2002). These corporatist initiatives aimed at reducing the precariousness of the midwives' remuneration and obtaining a better recognition of their specific skills and knowledge. The midwifery profession experienced a "crisis", particularly marked in the Geneva canton, in connection with the institutionalisation process of childbirth, which greatly restricted home care by a midwife (Droux 2007a). Nevertheless, given their immediate integration into maternity wards, midwives never stop practising (Rieder 2007b).

The demographic momentum of the post-Second World War period increased the need for midwives (Droux 2007a). However, it was only in 1961 that a real reform occurred in the training of Geneva midwives, including remuneration, leave, and pre-established educational programmes (ibid 2007a). The reform in training attracted new recruits to the profession.

Midwives are trained to monitor the entire birth process, from the beginning of pregnancy to postpartum. In Switzerland, however, it is currently only possible for them to provide continuous care if they practice as independent midwives. In addition, a minority of women choose to entrust the monitoring of their pregnancy to an independent midwife instead of an obstetrician. At the hospital, the work of midwives is limited to the monitoring of births under the supervision of obstetricians. Thus, they may feel torn between their training-inherited conception of birth care and the one imposed on them by the institution to which they belong (Ólafsdóttir & Kirkham 2009). Moreover, in the maternity ward, physicians maintain a strict monopoly regarding the creation and update of protocols. As Gouilhers (2010) explains, "in Switzerland, it is true that the role of midwives is reduced. They have neither their own skills nor a monopoly over doctors" (241). However, as shown by Scamell (2011), hospital midwives are not necessarily in opposition to institutional protocols and birth management: they are also actively contributing to the transmission and reproduction of a technocratic and risk-centred approach to birth.

"Natural" and out-of-hospital birth: convergences and divergences

In the 1970s, some birth practitioners in Europe and the United States advocated for a "humanisation" and a de-medicalisation of birth, emphasising the idea of pregnancy and childbirth "as physiological and natural events" (Paumier & Richardson 2003: 247). However, the understanding of the term "natural childbirth", first coined in 1933 by British obstetrician Grantly Dick-Read, greatly varies depending on the actors involved (users and practitioners), the place of delivery, the country, and the historical time, in a spectrum ranging from a hospital-monitored vaginal delivery to an out-of-hospital birth without any medical or technical intervention at all (Macdonald 2006, 2007; Mansfield 2008; Moscucci 2002; Quagliariello 2017b). As argued by Quagliariello, "natural childbirth" thus appears as an individual "creative craft", a compromise with a blurred definition, allowing women to incorporate or reject medical or technical components in their birth experience (within constraints from the place of birth, the birth attendants, and the commodities available). In addition, Mansfield (2008) demonstrates that, in addition to technical criteria, the "naturalness" of "natural" childbirth is accomplished through a range of social practices: active birth preparation, gestures and movements during childbirth, and adequate social support. For example, since the beginning of the "natural" birth movement, fathers' involvement in birth preparation and during delivery is constitutive of these social practices.

In North America and most European countries,[17] the social movement for de-hospitalisation challenges the hegemony of biomedicine and urges women to regain power over their own bodies.[18] In this perspective, the activity of independent midwives is often understood as part of this movement of re-appropriation of the birth experience by women. According to MacDonald (2007), independent midwives are also seen as fervent activists for the de-medicalisation and de-technologisation of birth.

This interpretation describes independent midwives and their practices at odds with the technocratic model, which is not the case. Independent midwives have a biomedical background: their care practice is integrated into the medical system. As reminded by Macdonald (2006), whether at home or in the hospital, midwives do use technical and medical interventions, either during the pregnancy follow-up or during delivery. In Switzerland, overall, there are few variations in the examinations that punctuate the pregnancy follow-up, whether the pregnancy is attended by a midwife or obstetrician. For example, midwives prescribe ultrasounds. Even if they cannot perform the scan themselves, they refer their clients to an obstetrician or an imagery centre. Likewise, for out-of-hospital births, their standard equipment always includes oxygen and a resuscitation kit, as well as synthetic oxytocin injection in the case of uterus bleeding.

Furthermore, elements of the "natural" birth philosophy, such as the father's involvement during childbirth, skin-to-skin contact, breastfeeding immediately after birth, and the recommendation to breastfeed on demand rather than according to a pre-established schedule, have been incorporated into hospital practices in many European countries and in the United States (Maffi 2013). An interpenetration of the two models can thus be noted.

The notion of "natural childbirth" refers to a certain approach to birth as a natural and physiological process that every woman "knows" innately how to perform (Paumier 2006). For the defenders of this "demedicalised" conception of birth, the hospital, even if "humanised", is not an adequate place to perform a natural birth (Paumier & Richardson 2003). As a result, during the 1970s, some out-of-hospital birth centres opened in North America, and women could access a homelike birth experience there, attended by midwives and significant others. The Farm Midwifery Center, created in 1971 in Tennessee by the midwife Ina May Gaskin, was a pioneer and emblematic example of such an extra-institutional birthplace in the United States (Gaskin 1975).

In parallel to the establishment of these birth centres, initiatives to create spaces suitable for a "natural childbirth" within some maternity wards emerged in Europe and North America. For example, in the fall of 1975, the Maternity Center Association of New York City opened a birth centre "offering obstetrical and nurse-midwife care during labour and delivery in a homelike setting, which, however, had 'safety equipment' at hand" (Wertz & Wertz 1989 [1977]: 284). This centre appeared as a compromise: intended to feel like home, it offered an alternative to women who would not trust home birth as safe.

In Europe, Odent is considered one of the leading figures of the movement for the de-medicalisation of birth. In the late 1970s, he set up de-medicalised birthing rooms in the maternity ward of Pithiviers, France, in order to accommodate women who wished to have a delivery without medical intervention. In his interpretation of "natural" childbirth, Odent placed central importance on the environment in which the birth takes place. To establish his precepts, he was inspired in particular by Frédérick Leboyer, also a French obstetrician and author of the bestseller *Birth without Violence*, published in 1974. In this book, Leboyer advocated for a delivery free of medical intervention so that the lived experience of birth could be as serene as possible not only for parturients but especially for newborns. Odent's initiative has both inspired and been echoed in other maternity wards in Europe and North America, where changes have been made accordingly. For example, in Italy, at the instigation of the obstetrician Brenda Grandi, a "natural childbirth room" was set up in 1984, in the maternity ward of Poggibonsi (Quagliariello 2017b). According to Brenda Grandi, this room was inspired by natural childbirth predecessors, including Ina May Gaskin and Michel Odent (ibid. 2017b). These examples are non-exhaustive, but they mark the milestones of natural childbirth development and reflect the diversity of meanings around this birth model.

Even if birth centres encountered administrative and legal difficulties in obtaining insurance cover, including professional insurance for employed midwives, by 1988, 150 birth centres were opened across the United States. A lot of them were run by obstetricians, using more technical interventions than the midwife-led ones. Such "compromise solutions" seem specific to the North American context, with birth centres in Europe being led by independent midwives.

In Switzerland, the first birth centre opened in 1983 in Lenzburg in the canton of Aargau (Vouilloz Burnier 2010 in Gouilhers-Hertig 2017). Currently, ten birth centres are in operation in French-speaking Switzerland, including four in the canton of Vaud, where I conducted my research. These centres are all midwife-led and independent from hospitals. Unlike in the French or American contexts, in Switzerland, independent midwives performing extra-hospital deliveries can be covered by their professional insurance.

Independent midwives providing holistic care

Among the 11 midwives who participated in my research, ten were trained in Switzerland and one was trained in France.[19] They all worked in a maternity ward during their training internships, but also after they graduated. Indeed, Swiss midwives must first complete two years of hospital practice or "assistantship" with an independent midwife already established before obtaining their "concordat number" and becoming authorised to reimburse their services through health insurances.

The Swiss midwifery school programme is hospital oriented in different ways. Independent midwives remain a minority in the teaching staff. Even if out-of-hospital deliveries are mentioned in classes as a valid and safe option, in line with the NICE (2014) and Cochrane guidelines (Olsen & Clausen

2012), the representation of out-of-hospital practice is marginal in the content of the training (Perrenoud 2016). Internships in independent practice were only included in the study programme in 2012 and still remain infrequent. According to European regulations, midwife students must attend at least 40 deliveries before graduation, an objective they can fulfil much faster with hospital internships.

Consequently, independent midwives learn to accomplish clinical examinations and obstetrical and postpartum care acts in a hospital setting, remaining more or less imbued with these hospital references depending on their professional trajectory. Once engaged in an out-of-hospital practice, they must reinvent their practice in a home setting. For example, their training does not confront them with specificities of a postpartum follow-up that is longer than the few days of hospital stay. In addition to their initial medical training, independent midwives have often undertaken certifying training in holistic care approaches (homoeopathy, aromatherapy, and massages), which they use in their work depending on each situation and the parents' wishes.

Bowlby's work, and psychoanalytic approaches in general, occupy a primary position in the Swiss medical curriculum, deeply framing health professionals' discourses, including midwives' (Ballif 2020). As demonstrated by Ballif (2020), in favour of a holistic approach to the perinatal period, midwives also rely on psychological theories as a criticism of the dominant biomedical approach. On the other hand, Sears and Sears's "attachment parenting" model is not mentioned in Swiss midwifery schools. Ensuing recommendations and practices of independent midwives regarding infant care and parenting, which I witnessed in my fieldwork, are not formally taught during training. Moreover, no midwife clearly quoted Sears and Sears or used the term "attachment parenting" to qualify her approach. The practices affiliated with attachment parenting that I observed, such as "baby-wearing" or "bed-sharing", were integrated by midwives separately from their training and based on their own personal interest, as well as transmitted orally and by observing other independent midwives.

Indeed, the midwives who participated in my research frequently worked with each other. During a home birth, for example, a second midwife usually joined her colleague at the expulsion stage of labour. Several midwives were previously other midwives' "assistants"; in these cases, they worked in close collaboration for an extended period of time, before starting their independent practice. In addition to these collaborations, some midwives regularly held meetings, organised in one of the birth centres in the area, in order to discuss their practice, develop common guidelines, and thus alleviate the professional isolation caused by the status of independent worker. They did not attend all these meetings, and their participation was random, depending on each of their agendas and interests. Although they did not provide documents collectively written for their clients, the midwives attending these meetings created together an "eco-bag", conceived of as a response to the "birth kit" provided by maternity wards, as a giveaway for parents. The hospital birth kit varies but might include free information, samples of formula milk and baby food,[20] and a baby bottle. Independent midwives decided on the eco-bag contents together. The bag included informative leaflets on local parenting support resources, as well as locally crafted objects and organic products they favoured for newborn and mother's postpartum care, including breastfeeding support.[21]

Even though independent midwives were autonomous in each situation they supervised and their personal approach differed, they advocated for the same newborn care practices, gave similar advice to parents, and favoured the same remedies and products. In this sense and through the different types of exchanges and collaborations mentioned above, they formed a "community of practice" and knowledge about childbirth (Jordan 2014).

In Switzerland, different categories of independent midwives coexist. Only a small minority of independent midwives offer holistic care. Most independent midwives dedicate their time to home postpartum consultations following a hospital birth. They do not necessarily subscribe to a holistic birth approach, and, as a result, they can attend home postpartum follow-ups while remaining very close to institutional schedules and protocols, for example. Independent midwives who practise holistic care commit themselves to a marginalised work modality. Some of them have had this desire since the beginning of their studies. For others, this choice was born out of frustration for hospital practice. As noticed by Perrenoud (2016), time management is one of the most important differences between hospital and independent practices; hence, the opportunity to take the necessary time with each mother and family is a primary motivation to become an independent midwife.

Counting time in holistic care

According to McCourt and Dykes (2009), the predominance of the technocratic model is part of the broader context of social and cultural changes brought about by industrialisation, which particularly affects how the concept of time is considered. Before the modern period, time was apprehended as cyclic, in relation to seasons and agricultural work. The advent of capitalism and industrialisation profoundly altered this organisation. Work, which was previously subjected to the imperatives of seasons, has become organised in a fragmented way. The different tasks to be performed have become separated from one another and "may not respond to the worker's perception of what needs to be done" (McCourt & Dykes 2009: 19). Similarly, workers often find it difficult to see the broader process to which their work contributes. These changes also affect health-related professions, where previously personalised and comprehensive follow-ups have shifted towards fragmented and often-repetitive, protocol-based activities serving many patients simultaneously (ibid. 2009). Martin (1987) also emphasises the causal relationship between industrialisation and the hospitalisation of birth. She establishes links between the Marxist analysis of the effects of capitalism on the organisation of work and the fragmented experience of birth caused by its hospitalisation. In this parallel, the fragmented nature of hospital care would cause alienating effects on parturients, whose dispossession of their delivery is compared to workers' dispossession of their work as a result of labour division. Detached from the overall process over which they have no control, the task performed is meaningless.

In the context of hospital birth care, time acts as an organising principle that requires deliveries to match institutional standards. The various interventions that parturients experience in most industrialised countries aim to format deliveries so that they fall within these standards. As early as the 1970s, the systematic use of time-related interventions, such as synthetic oxytocin injection to accelerate labour, was the focus of criticism of birth medicalisation and hospitalisation (McCourt & Dykes 2009, Négrié & Cascales 2016).

Despite such criticism, the principle of active management of labour (AML), first used in 1980 (O'Driscoll, Meagher & Boylan 1980), continues to be applied. Originally designed in Ireland as a way to shorten the duration of labour for nulliparous women, AML was rapidly used in most industrialised countries (Maffi 2016). AML was introduced in Switzerland in the 1990s, with the objective of stopping the increase of births by caesarean section. However, the caesarean section rate has not been reduced, quite the contrary. This surgery represented a third of all births in Switzerland (Federal Statistical Office 2019b), a rate much superior to the 10 to 15 per cent recommended by the WHO (2015).

AML prescribes a precise measurement of the labour progress, which must comply with established and internationally recognised time standards, as well as the systematic use of medical and technical interventions in the case of non-compliance with these standards and without consideration for the parturients' feelings (McCourt and Dykes 2009). This monitoring is particularly illustrative of the manner in which women's individual bodily experience is ignored and delegitimised in favour of the respect of standards enacted by biomedicine. AML lies on the presumption of a "universal" female body and physiology that ignores specific sociocultural and economic contexts in which women are integrated, and that denies the influence of these social factors on the birth process (Maffi 2016). Today, AML is mainly used as a work organisation facilitator for hospital staff, converting the physiological time of labour to an institutional time (ibid. 2016).

Dykes conducted an ethnographic study in two postnatal wards in northern England between 2000 and 2004. Her observations highlighted the challenging work conditions of hospital midwives, "heavily constrained by linear time, in that their work was unpredictable and rushed, coping with women who were usually complete strangers" (Dykes 2006: 168). Hospital organisation and protocols, both implicit and explicit, greatly restrain midwives' autonomy. They consequently develop coping strategy, to navigate through their workday, using routines to adjust to their work rhythm and communicating to parturients in a straightforward way. As deplored by Dykes (2005), "the focus appeared to be upon the need of the institution first, women and babies second" (168). Davis-Floyd and St. John (1998) also denounce the alienating effect of the technocratic model on hospital staff. Surrounded by a medical paradigm underpinned by the principle of separation, health professionals feel at the same time disconnected from their patients and from themselves. On the one hand, as the technocratic model "does not recognise any role for the emotions in illness and disease, it logically follows that there is no reason to deal with the patient's emotions at all" (ibid. 1998: 25). On the other hand, health professionals are encouraged since medical school to cut themselves from their emotions and treat their own bodies as machines in order to deal with intense levels of stress and workload.

At home, since they are not required to respond to AML, the independent midwives I met generally attach little importance to determining exactly when labour begins. They accept to manage the uncertainty and to have no guarantee on the duration of the process they supervise. Simonds' (2002) analysis of obstetrics textbooks and reference books in perinatality suggests that independent midwives, who have a holistic approach to care, have an "expansive" conception of time, which differs from dominant linear time in hospitals (569). This "expansive" conception of time contrasts sharply with the hospital's technocratic and restrictive management of time.

Authoritative knowledge, experiential knowledge

In childbirth care, biomedicine and resulting protocols represent "authoritative knowledge", a system of thought developed from recognised knowledge, integrated as legitimate by members of a given society (Jordan 1997). Considered the most reliable and effective form of knowledge, it has established itself as the only valid system, becoming the norm and the only acceptable reference, especially with regard to the management of birth. According to Jordan (1997), "the constitution of authoritative knowledge is an ongoing social process that both builds and reflects power relationships within a community of practice" (56).

As representative of medical authority, independent midwives embody and reproduce authoritative knowledge but also question its normative protocols in the frame of out-of-hospital birth. Relying on their experiential knowledge, based on an in-depth observation of the childbirth process and the parturients' behaviour in general, as well as a thorough knowledge of their particular patient, they challenge the dominant understanding of what is authoritative knowledge in birth.

In this context, the notion of "continuity of care" is particularly important: only one person is taking care of pregnancy, childbirth, and postpartum follow-up. The application of this principle contrasts with the practices favoured by the dominant technocratic model in which these different stages are fragmented and left to the care of different people. In Switzerland, in most cases, the pregnant woman's obstetrician provides pregnancy monitoring. Midwives, obstetricians, and anaesthetists of the chosen institution monitor the delivery. Moreover, since midwives have a work shift schedule for organisational reasons, it is not necessarily the same staff present from the beginning until the end of the delivery, which, in the perspective of the midwifery model of care, can negatively affect the parturient (Davis-Floyd et al. 2009; Katz Rothman 1982). Finally, once the new mother and her newborn have returned home, a different midwife takes care of the postpartum follow-up.

Furthermore, in line with the standardisation of care, medical care systems in Euro-American societies are dominated by evidence-based medicine. Coupled with the high expectations of users' certainty and safety, the practice of evidence-based medicine leads to the creation of hospital protocols, based on the principle that scientific "evidence" is applicable to every individual without limitations (Downe & McCourt 2008). In addition to causing a significant increase in interventions during delivery, this standardisation of medical treatments also threatens the autonomy of practitioners (Burton-Jeangros, Hammer, Manaï & Issenhuth-Scharly 2010). This process causes the negation of practitioners' experiential knowledge (Perrenoud 2016).

In the context of evidence-based medicine, midwives' follow-up must be evaluated "in terms of efficiency and effectiveness" (Perrenoud 2016: 25), and the interventions implemented during the follow-up are subject to evaluation by means of a randomised controlled trial. Because they are not affiliated with an institution, independent midwives have somehow escaped "a standardisation of the intervention constituted by the follow-up" (ibid. 2016: 25). Their follow-up has not been subjected to such control yet, so they retain more space for manoeuvring. This additional "freedom" is, however, limited by legal constraints, determining, for example, the conditions to transfer a labouring woman to the hospital or to transfer a case to a paediatrician in the event of a newborn failing to thrive.

For an ethnography of holistic postpartum care

Childbirth care, including the history of its medicalisation and power relations between birth professionals, has been the subject of abundant work in social science. Among the classics, the work of Davis-Floyd (1992) and Jordan (1978, 1997) can be cited, as well as that of Katz Rothman (1991 [1982]) and Oakley (1984). However, the postpartum period is surprisingly little explored in this body of work. Hence, there is a certain gap in the social science literature in the analysis of the links between pregnancy and the birth model of care, as well as postpartum care, including breastfeeding initiation. More specifically, the abovementioned authors have contributed to the emergence of a significant body of literature on pregnancy and childbirth as part of holistic care with a midwife, but they have not explored in detail the postpartum period in the frame of this particular model of care. As for historical works, there is a body of literature on childbirth care, but it does not address the postpartum period (Gélis 1988; Thébaud 1986; Wertz & Wertz 1989 [1977]). Other history works focus on advice and recommendations for childcare, including breastfeeding, but do not consider childbirth care (Apple 1987; 2014; Hardyment 2007).

Studies on out-of-hospital birth mostly focus on pregnancy follow-up and childbirth, often related to the question of risk management (Gouilhers-Hertig 2017; Viisainen 2000, 2001). Katz Rothman (1991[1982], 2007b) is one of the few authors who has elaborated on home postnatal care but without especially focusing on breastfeeding.

As highlighted by Martin (1987), modern obstetrics rely on a mechanistic conception of the female body as a "machine" prone to failure and requiring close medical monitoring, inherited from the Enlightenment. The "woman-as-machine" metaphor, conceiving the mother as a machine, and thus the child as a product, implies that the mother and the child are apprehended as two distinct entities whose interests are not necessarily compatible (Davis-Floyd 1992; Martin 1987).

In this perspective, the biomedical model establishes a physical and conceptual separation between the mother and newborn whose postpartum needs are considered incompatible: the mother needs to recover, pregnancy and birth being perceived as gruelling events, whereas the newborn is seen as a disturbance preventing his mother from resting. As a result, the routine separation of mothers and babies has long been the norm during hospital stays. While the "room-in" nowadays dominates hospital practices in Switzerland, it is still common to propose that the mothers take their baby to the nursery so they can rest. At home, the mother and child are never separated: the midwife is responsible for the health of both "as an interdependent unit" whose needs are complementary (Katz Rothman 2007b: 73).

In holistic care, childbirth does not mark a break: mother and child are understood as one physiological unit, as was the case during pregnancy (Katz Rothman 1991 [1982]). After a conclusive clinical examination of the newborn, the midwife transfers the responsibility of monitoring the baby to the parents, telling them to which clues they should pay attention. Parents are considered legitimate to observe their baby and to pass on the information to their midwife. In the hospital, however, this legitimacy is questioned, especially as an objection to parental wishes for same-day discharges.

Notes

1 All names are pseudonyms.
2 All literal quotes from the fieldwork were initially said in French and later translated by me. At the end of the quotes, I specify "transcription" when the

interview was recorded and then accurately transcribed. When I indicate "notes" after the quote, the discussion was not recorded but transcribed on the moment with handwritten notes in a notebook.

3 Sandra and her spouse made a three-year journey almost exclusively on foot from Switzerland to Nepal.

4 I chose to adopt inclusive writing in this book, including in my French-to-English translations, whether the quotes are from the fieldwork or from the literature. I translate the generic *il* presumed to indicate both the feminine and masculine in French by "s/he", *lui* by "her or him", and *son* by "her or his", in order to make the feminine members of the collectives visible.

5 Adeline is referring to the various backgrounds of the hospital staff and the knowledge of breastfeeding. In addition, hospital midwives are exempted from continuing education, unlike liberal midwives who follow updating module classes on specific topics such as breastfeeding.

6 In Switzerland, hospital protocols require breastfed newborns who lose more than 10 per cent of birth weight to be "completed" with formula. At home, in the absence of institutional protocols, independent midwives have to set their own limits of what is an "acceptable risk".

7 Swiss midwives must first complete two years of hospital practice or "assist-antship" with an independent midwife already established before obtaining their "concordat number" and becoming authorised to reimburse their services through health insurances.

8 I explored this ethnographic material in a separate publication (Chautems 2019).

9 Translated from the emic French expression *les sorties de l'hôpital*.

10 See Chapter 3 for a discussion on the limitations of the notion of "choice" and Chapter 5 for an analysis of situated negotiations between midwives and parents.

11 Even if the midwife's intention was to speak to both parents and fully include the father in consultations, the focus of attention was clearly on the mother and baby, as a dyad supposed to function in synergy, especially through breastfeeding.

12 She will appear with a pseudonym throughout the rest of the book.

13 See Chautems and Guerra (2021a, 2021b).

14 I shared information when I participated in local events or contributed to media contents to communicate on my research.

15 Independent midwives did not provide any written document intended for the parents. Unlike researches conducted in an institution, I was therefore unable to add this type of material to my analysis.

16 A doula is a non-medical birth para-professional who provides emotional and informative support to mothers and parents during the perinatal period, includ-ing being present at delivery. In Switzerland, doulas are accepted in all maternity wards in addition to the birthing mother's partner. However, they still consti-tute an emergent category of birth protagonist, in comparison, for example, to North America, where their role is better established. For detailed ethnographic accounts on the doula's care and relationships with parents, see, for example, Casteñeda and Johnson Searcy (2015).

17 The Netherlands is an exception in the European perinatal landscape, since home births are seamlessly integrated to the care system: in the case of a low-risk, phys-iological pregnancy, only a midwife's follow-up is reimbursed by health insur-ances (De Vries et al. 2009).

18 In contrast, French materialist feminists like Badinter (2010) consider the natural birth movement as a decline in gender equality and a reassignment of women to the domestic sphere. In this perspective, technical interventions like epidurals are perceived as a means for women to emancipate from their biological destiny.

19 The midwives trained in France came to Switzerland specifically to practice holistic care and out-of-hospital deliveries, since it has become nearly impossible

to do it in France (for more on this topic, see Sestito 2017). The annual rates offered to French midwives by insurance companies have become exorbitant (25,000 euros per year in 2016) as a result of the Perruche case law judgement of September 17, 2000. However, since 2002, all health professionals practising independently must have public liability insurance to be able to compensate the possible victims of medical accidents. Any midwife exercising as a liberal must therefore contract an insurance of this type. Since January 1, 2004, failure to meet this obligation may lead to disciplinary sanctions, up to a 45,000-euro fine and prohibition on practising (Négrié & Cascales 2016).

20 According to the Code for the Marketing of Breast Milk Substitutes (WHO 1981), the distribution of formula samples is prohibited. This prohibition is however often circumvented by distributing "second age milk" or diversification foods.

21 A discussion on tools and remedies favoured by independent midwives has been developed with Sophie Guerra in an upcoming publication (Chautems & Guerra 2021a).

2 Reinventing parenthood through breastfeeding

Risk-centric society and embodied parenting

As a bodily practice closely monitored by the medical gaze and ingrained in the parenting project, breastfeeding appears to be a locus of convergence between socio-anthropological literature on reproduction and the body, on the one hand, and parenting studies, on the other hand. I hereby propose to build bridges between these two areas of research that usually seem to have little dialogue. Through this selected and non-exhaustive review, I focus on specific issues raised by the literature, of which I propose an in-depth and contextualised analysis in Chapters 3, 4, and 5. I thereby develop the notion of risk, its anticipation and management, alongside birth temporalities, mothers' bodies, and birth technologies. These three major issues influence one another, with time acting as a pillar in risk management during both childbirth and the postpartum period, while the use—or rejection—of medical technologies is mostly justified by risk prevention concerns.

I first recount in this chapter the circumstances of breastfeeding's decline and rehabilitation, with a focus on Switzerland, in order to contextualise the Swiss breastfeeding culture and the construction of current recommendations regarding infant-feeding practices. These processes are tied with the biomedicalisation of birth and "scientifisation" of motherhood as well as the biopower exerted on mothers' bodies and constructed as public and political bodies. The biomedical model of birth shaped the medical monitoring of breastfeeding, centred on the transfer of maternal milk from mother to newborn. This vision is part of a mechanistic conception of the female body inherited from the Enlightenment (Martin 1987; Dykes 2005, 2006; Kukla 2005).

Additionally, risk prevention has become central to parenting choices in an attempt to reduce children's health and emotional risk exposure in the short and long terms through "good" childcare practices. The "intensification of motherhood", highlighted by numerous authors (Badinter 2010; Blum 1999; Büskens 2010; Douglas & Michaels 2005; Faircloth 2013; Hays 1996; Lee 2008; Lupton 2013a; Wolf 2007, 2011), is one answer to these concerns. Crystallising maternal dedication and a projection in the future, breastfeeding offers a privileged lens for observing this evolution.

DOI: 10.4324/9781003124108-2

I discuss in this chapter the authorities and debates evolving about breast-feeding practices and the way breastfeeding mothers address them.

Rehabilitation of breastfeeding: mothers' bodies and the state

In this section, I reconstruct the historical context that has allowed for the rehabilitation of breastfeeding, mainly focusing on Switzerland, but also outlining a larger picture, based on the works of French historians (Badinter 1980; Knibiehler 2012; Lett & Morel 2016), as well as American historians (Apple 1987; Blum 1999; Hardyment 2007; Kukla 2005). Relatively few sources report specifically on the history of the decline and rehabilitation of breastfeeding in Switzerland. Some Swiss historians address this topic as a peripheral issue of their primary focus (Bosson 2002; Droux 2005, 2007a, 2007b; Praz 2005), while Swiss historian Scholl focuses on breastfeeding but also uses sources from neighbouring France (2017).

In France, as early as the seventeenth century, a medical discourse emerged about the benefits of breast milk: doctors encouraged mothers to breastfeed their own children instead of wet nursing (Kukla 2005). The moral reconceptualisation and reforming of the family entailed by the Enlightenment, under the impulse of philosophers such as Rousseau, strengthened this tendency. Children were to be taken back from wet nurses in order to bring the family back together: this was not just about feeding, but more widely, about mothers being closely involved in their children's education. This reappropriation of motherhood is realised through the mother's body:

> Rousseau changed the symbolic and imaginative value and function of the maternal body; sparked revisions in the standards and social arrangements governing mothering practices; brought together medical, aesthetic, and political discourses with respect to maternal bodies; and transformed these bodies from private, almost furtive matters into vivid centers of public management, surveillance, celebration, approbation, and regulation. (Kukla 2005: 53)

Since the eighteenth century, the liberal state has had a well-established preoccupation for procreation: "the notion that reproduction ought to be managed and directed by human rationality lends itself to an instrumental view of pregnancy and child-rearing that is characteristic of capitalist liberal societies" (Ruhl 2002: 647). Supervision of infant-feeding practices by medical authorities was part of the process of reproduction management by the state in order to produce healthier citizens, more likely to serve the nation's interests. In this perspective, breastfeeding became mothers' first duty not only towards their children but also towards society, as citizens. Medical discourses on maternal bodies—"heavily burdened with civic hopes and responsibilities"—were then profoundly shaped by moral and political concerns (Kukla 2005: 53). According to Kukla (2005), this representation has remained: even today, "maternal bodies are imagined, represented, and treated within a fundamentally Rousseauian framework" (53).

Because the future of society depends on it, the maternal body is thought of as a public and political body, a locus of biopower, and a new centre of power that appeared in the middle of the eighteenth century (Foucault 1976). Reproduction has become an issue of knowledge and power that medicine and public health aim to improve and regulate. Thereby, in addition to the power exerted on individuals through the discipline of their bodies (Foucault 1975), biopolitics is also exerted on populations. In this second phase, overall biological processes are targeted.

Eugenics, strongly influential in Switzerland between the end of the nineteenth century and the middle of the twentieth century, was one mode of expression of biopolitics. Based on the assumption that physical and mental features, those thought of as both "positive" and "negative", are genetically inherited, eugenics emerged as a science and a social movement with the purpose of improving a national population. While dissuading some groups of the population—perceived as genetically "inferior"—from procreating, the eugenics movement encouraged other groups—thought as genetically "superior"—to have children, based on the theories of the English scientist Galton, who coined the term and pioneered the movement in the late nineteenth century (Mottier 2000). As a result, the regulation of sexuality, as the locus of reproduction, became a central preoccupation of public health policies (Foucault 1976). Switzerland was at the leading edge of eugenics: Swiss eugenics theorists contributed importantly to the international debates, while enforcement measures and policies were implemented (Mottier 2000). These preoccupations were associated with concerns about the degeneration of the Swiss "breed" and "racial hygiene". In Switzerland, criminals and people judged "immoral", such as those active in prostitution, with a mental illness, or with a disease such as tuberculosis or haemophilia, Jews, "vagrant" people and gypsies, were the target of forced sterilisation practices (Mottier 2000). As Mottier (2000) highlights, by primarily focusing on women as the nation's "breeders", forced sterilisation was a distinctly gendered practice, acting as a means to regulate women's bodies and sexualities.

Surveillance of infant-feeding choices and maternal practices by medical authorities, acting as the "intermediate space of social and political regulation" between mothers and the state (Fassin & Memmi 2004: 24), can be interpreted as a less intrusive form of eugenics, motivated by the same ideal of "improving" the quality of the population.

Emergence of paediatrics and infant nutrition science

The practice of wet nursing remained widespread in Europe until the nineteenth century (Badinter 1980; Knibiehler 2012; Lett & Morel 2016). Prior to the nineteenth century, the medical profession had little interest in childhood, and high rates of infant mortality were considered inevitable (Bosson 2002). In the mid-nineteenth century, in Europe as well as in North America, paediatrics emerged as a specific branch of medicine. Concerns about the high infant mortality rate due to poor nutrition drove physicians' interest in the topic of infant feeding (Apple 1987; Bosson 2002). Bosson (2002) points out that prevention measures in Switzerland resulted in lower infant mortality compared to other European countries. Furthermore, important differences existed between "rural, catholic and conservative" cantons like Valais or Fribourg, and "industrialist, protestant and liberal" cantons like Vaud or Geneva, the latter experiencing a greater decline in mortality at the beginning of the twentieth century (ibid. 2002: 100).

In 1880, in the canton of Vaud, health institutions were concerned by infant-feeding practices using cow's milk of inappropriate composition or unhygienic preparation (Praz 2005). In the Vaud countryside, at the end of the nineteenth century, midwives played a key role in the transmission of health and hygiene practices to families, establishing themselves as "the auxiliaries of the doctor or the surgeon" (Praz 2005: 467). Midwives' prerogatives were not limited to childbirth and the immediate post-partum period but extended to childcare, which they taught mothers (Bosson 2002). In doing so, midwives became "the ideal advocate[s] for breastfeeding" (ibid. 2002: 115). At that time, a large number of science popularisation leaflets written by physicians to spread the nascent rules of childcare to the general public began to appear (Bosson 2002; Droux 2005; Praz 2005). Breastfeeding was unanimously recommended in these writings. In parallel to the spread of information, basic medical facilities for perinatal health and childcare facilities were established (Bosson 2002). These facilities provided not only care but also advice to strengthen the above-mentioned prophylactic mission.

In addition, in France, infant weighing by public health workers became a key practice of infant health monitoring in the 1880s, based on a medical consensus according to which infants' weight is an accurate indicator of their overall health (Brosco 2001). This weighing practice spread throughout Europe and North America during the 1890s under the impulsion of national infant welfare movements aimed at the reduction of infant mortality rates.

By the early twentieth century, infant feeding and more broadly infant care became a "science": proper infant care required the application of scientific health principles, simplified into rules laid down by experts and diffused to all mothers. At the midwifery school of Lausanne, Vaud, a learning module of "rational childcare" was added to the midwives' training in 1919 (Praz 2005). According to Kukla (2005), the health benefits of breast milk were already known in North America as well as in Europe, but "the scientific turn brought with it a new interest in quantifying and monitoring the breastfeeding process" (94).

Even though breastfeeding was perceived as the ideal infant-feeding method, the nineteenth century saw the emergence of concern about milk quality and sufficiency. Physicians believed many women did not have enough milk, in some cases even in the first days after delivery. Moreover, women's milk would be "satisfactory only if the mother's diet was well-balanced and adequate. Even then, dietary supplements were needed" (Apple 1987: 36). Furthermore, during the twentieth century, in Europe and North America, children's nutrition was the subject of multiple, often contradictory, statements and recommendations by health professionals (Apple 1987; Hardyment 2007). These changing recommendations resulted from complicated conjunction of scientific, medical, economic, and cultural factors and, therefore, cannot be understood as a reflection of a linear progression towards an ever better understanding of the children's needs (Apple 1987; Murphy 2000). In this context, Blum (1999) noted that "the mid-twentieth century break in which artificial feeding predominated, in fact, was only a brief hiatus, and, on scrutiny, it was more rather than less continuous with this history at the breast" (19).

Under the spell of formula

In the late nineteenth century, Pasteur's discoveries on heating cow's milk made bottle-feeding safer, and the wet nursing business declined (Blum 1999). At the same time, the dairy industry was growing, producing large quantities of surplus milk in industrialised countries (Palmer 2009 [1988]). Nevertheless, physicians did not unanimously consider pure, unmodified cow's milk appropriate for babies: it required scientific manipulations to improve its composition (Scholl 2017). These manipulations relate, on one hand, to dairy cows' breeding conditions, especially regarding the cows' food and the barns' hygiene, and, on the other hand, to specific recommendations regarding the bottle preparation. Through the industrialisation of these processes, cow's milk became a scientifically validated food, "an artificial version of this liquid, standardised by more and more accurate standards, as they constitute a system" (Scholl 2017: 118).

The formula milk industry began to develop efficiently. In particular, several world-renowned formula milk industries, like Nestlé and Guigoz, were founded in the French-speaking part of Switzerland. It seems that as a result, formula feeding was widespread through all social classes in Switzerland as early as the beginning of the twentieth century, despite a medical emphasis on the importance of breastfeeding (Bosson 2002). In the 1920s, formula companies contributed heavily to the decline of breastfeeding. Through widespread advertising and marketing, they rallied support from practitioners, who received much more information about formula than about breastfeeding and became more familiar and comfortable with it. Similarly, they targeted mothers, relying on informative material about the proper use of formula, or infant nutrition, and hygiene books (Bosson 2002; Palmer 2009 [1988]).

As a result, in industrialised countries, trust in formula feeding grew rapidly during the first half of the twentieth century, even though physicians continued to encourage mothers to breastfeed until the Second World War (Blum 1999). By the mid-twentieth century, their confidence in formula feeding had reached its peak: "practitioners have moved from a belief that bottle-feeding could healthfully augment or replace breast feeding to a conviction that artificial feeding generally had positive benefits for infant health" (Apple 1987: 72). They came to see formula not only as a corrective treatment for unsuitable lactation but also as a "healthful, positive form of infant nutrition" (ibid. 1987: 73). In addition, formula feeding had the significant advantage of showing the exact quantity of milk ingested, consistent with the medical preference for a weight-centric assessment of infants' feeding.

In industrialised countries, in conjunction with the shift from home to institutional births, mothers were presented with formula as a necessity during their postpartum hospital stays. Institutional standards separated newborns from their mothers, except for predefined feeding sessions. Breastfed babies were weighed before and after each feeding to determine the amount of formula needed to "supplement" breast milk, showing mothers that their milk was never enough for their babies to thrive. Healthcare facilities became an ideal showcase for formula businesses, as they engaged in a fruitful collaboration with physicians: marketing directly through hospitals was the most efficient way to convince mothers of the safety of formula milk, since it was obviously doctor-approved (Palmer 2009 [1988]).

However, just like the medicalisation and hospitalisation of childbirth did not unfold as a linear process imposed on women through physicians' authority (Wertz & Wertz 1989 [1977]), women also actively participated in the rise of formula:

> Breastfeeding cannot be seen as a "simple" activity that was conducted exclusively by all mothers until utterly disrupted by science and medicine. While techno-medicine and commercialisation have indeed contributed to a striking disruption of breastfeeding and a dramatic loss of intergenerational, community-based knowledge, this needs to be viewed in connection with the socio-cultural context of women's lives. (Dykes 2005: 26)

Formula feeding met the expectations of women, who perceived it as a possibility to be emancipated or to gain more control over their everyday lives. Furthermore, as Carter (1995) notes, based on a study of breastfeeding practices and experiences in a working-class neighbourhood in England between 1920 and 1980, many women breastfed while at the same time giving formula to their babies. For Carter (1995), the desire to establish neat categories of breast and bottle feeders is based on a confusion between "breastfeeding" and "exclusive breastfeeding", the latter referring to women who do not give any food other than breast milk to their babies. Moreover, as Obermeyer and Castle (1996) highlight, "The idea of the universal practice of exclusive breastfeeding by mothers is not supported by evidence on pre-industrial societies" (48). They deconstructed the idea of "natural", exclusive breastfeeding, disrupted by industrialisation, by showing through numerous European historical examples that exceptions to the norm of the exclusively breastfed baby are abundant and that early supplementation with solids or liquids is perceived as an essential part of babies' diets in contemporary societies (for example, in various African countries or Indonesia).

Furthermore, the notion of "decision-making", which is applied to infant-feeding practices and serves as the basis for the majority of studies and policies on the topic, is seemingly irrelevant from a positivist perspective. The "decision-making" process can only be understood in relation to women's life circumstances, like household arrangements, as well as to the larger cultural context that surrounds them, which Carter (1995) designates "working circumstances"—circumstances in which the breastfeeding "work" is done.

From formula regulation to breastfeeding promotion

Enthusiasm for formula was dramatically challenged by the Nestlé scandal that occurred in the 1970s.

> Church and university-based coalitions uncovered the corrupt practices of infant formula producers selling to the Third World. The coalitions pressed corporations to change their policies and led the highly publicized boycott against Nestle, the Swiss-based multinational that dominated the two-billion-dollar world market. (Blum 1999: 44)

Breastfeeding became highly politicised on a global scale. International attention was drawn to the rise of formula feeding in Third World countries through the publication of "The Baby Killer", a pamphlet published in 1974 in Great Britain (Müller 1974). The report demonstrated that the rise of infant mortality in low-income communities with insufficient sanitation and medical care was correlated with the decline of breastfeeding. For the first time, protests did not target mothers but a company. In conjunction with the Nestlé boycott, the Women's Health Movement and the environmentalist movement emerging in the 1970s "added a subversive anti-capitalist interpretation to the 'natural' mothering" (Blum 1999: 44).

This mobilisation supported the creation of a code to regulate formula advertising. It led to the creation of the International Baby Food Action Network (IBFAN), which aimed to promote breastfeeding worldwide and "eliminate irresponsible marketing of infant foods, bottles, and teats" (Van Esterik 1995: 152). In 1981, the World Health Assembly adopted the

International Code of Marketing of Breast Milk Substitutes. The code marks the beginning of a series of breastfeeding promotion initiatives implemented by the WHO and UNICEF. In 1991, the Innocenti Declaration edited by the WHO and UNICEF came out with the purpose of defining a unified international policy on breastfeeding. In 1992, the WHO and UNICEF set up the Baby Friendly Hospital Initiative (BFHI), which was implemented in Switzerland in 1993. The goal of this initiative was to create the conditions for optimal breastfeeding initiation in all maternity wards. In 2017, twenty-nine Swiss maternity wards held the BFHI label, of which only four were in the French-speaking part of Switzerland (UNICEF 2017).

Since the mid-1970s, studies have been conducted on the composition of breast milk, the physiology of lactation, and the links between breastfeeding and various medical conditions and diseases (Avishai 2011; Faircloth 2013). These studies showed the positive impact of breast milk on the prevention of a number of health problems, as mentioned in the introduction. These discoveries were synthesised in the popular slogan "breast is best", widely circulated in the context of government campaigns to promote breastfeeding and also used in the literature intended for future parents. Promoting breastfeeding has become a priority for public health campaigns (Gatrell 2011). Initially focused on improving the initiation rate of breastfeeding, the efforts now focus on increasing the duration of breastfeeding. This shift corresponds to the WHO's implementation of new guidelines recommending exclusive breastfeeding for the first six months after birth (2001) and the continuation of breastfeeding, combined with other dietary and fluid intake, for up to two years of age or older (2003).

Advocating for the "liquid gold" and the individual choice paradigm

Hall Smith, Hausman, and Labbok (2012) argue that because of the lack of a feminist stance on breastfeeding, breastfeeding promotion policies have been primarily defined by capitalist values and interests. These authors deplore that the recommendations of public health organisations, geared towards changing individual behaviour, ignore the diversity of mothers' life situations, which are often limited by structural and organisational factors that out of their control. The ideological paradigm of individual choice, favoured by breastfeeding promotion campaigns, fails to account for the constraints that influence and weigh on maternal practices and have the effect of making mothers feel responsible for breastfeeding failure. Their attention is focused on their own bodies, perceived as deficient, rather than on the social system that fails to support their goals and practices (Hausman 2012). Insufficient milk, for example, is typically perceived by mothers as a biological failure, whereas it usually results from inadequate lactation management. The physiological abilities of mothers are thus shaped by social and cultural influences. In this regard, Hausman (2004) refers to the "reproductive burden" on women, of which breastfeeding is an important component, as a fundamental element for a comprehensive reflection on gender equality:

> Proclaiming an equality with men that mandates the ability to act as men in the social sphere (that is, to be autonomous individuals without physiologically dependent on others) is to impoverish our expectation of what sexual equality should be. Certainly, such an understanding of equality forgets, ignores, or never knew the exigencies of breastfeeding as an embodied practice. (Hausman 2004: 281)

On the other hand, Hall Smith, Hausman, and Labbok (2012) report an uprising of feminist "antibreastfeeding" voices, which oppose a moral injunction to breastfeeding as a result of promotional campaigns. These breastfeeding detractors would adhere to a conceptualisation of formula as a vector of freedom and self-determination for mothers and perceive the injunction to breastfeed as a way of "entrapping" women in their maternal role (ibid. 2012: xii). Hall Smith, Hausman, and Labbok (2012) regret that instead of looking at breastfeeding difficulties as a consequence of an over-arching system which generates gender discrimination and keeps women out of the labour market and away from public spaces, it is breastfeeding itself that is designated as an impediment to women's freedom and sexual equality.

Blum (1999) uses the notion of "exclusive motherhood" to refer to the ideology that mothers need to prioritise their children's needs and provide "intensive" attention and care to meet their physiological and emotional needs, which include breastfeeding. This exclusive motherhood is identified by American feminists as a "life project" of white middle-class women, who seldom work outside their homes (Blum 1999; Wolf 2011). These women joined the ecological movements emerging in the 1970s, which advocated a "natural" approach to motherhood and strongly valued breastfeeding (Quandt 1995). In general, it appears that white middle-class mothers with tertiary education are more likely to breastfeed their children than mothers with lower levels of education (Galtry 1997; Sandre-Pereira 2005; Faircloth 2013).

In contrast, in North America and Europe, women from less favoured backgrounds do not share this positive "natural" view and prefer to feed their children with formula milk (Blum 1999; Carter 1995). These women usually do not retain favourable working conditions for reconciling their professional activities with breastfeeding (Galtry 1997). Overall, continuing to breastfeed in the longer term requires a supportive environment and some material resources, which tend to be a privilege reserved for mothers from the most favoured backgrounds (Carpenter 2006). Breastfeeding can there-fore also be considered a significant social marker of inequalities between mothers.

Breastfeeding promotional campaigns present breast milk as "liq-uid gold", important not only for the children's health but also for their emotional well-being. This strategy postulates that because mothers want the best for their child, they will opt for breastfeeding and follow the recommendations of public health organisations in terms of breastfeeding duration and modalities (Sheehan & Schmied 2011).

The "natural" attributes of breastfeeding are also valued, as are its "practical" aspects: breastfeeding dispenses with the sterilisation of bottles, and breast milk is always at the right temperature (Breastfeeding Promotion Switzerland 2017). Breastfeeding promoters also point out that breastfeeding enhances weight loss in the postpartum period (Avishai 2004; Blum 1999; Breastfeeding Promotion Switzerland 2017). Finally, the economic argument is put forward that breastfeeding helps reduce healthcare costs (Badinter 2010; Breastfeeding Promotion Switzerland 2017). From an individual point of view, however, breastfeeding is rarely free, as it generally involves a range of products, tools, and accessories to support lactation and facilitate the breastfeeding process.

However, this type of campaign does not consider the mothers' well-being or the material conditions that influence and structure their experience. Breastfeeding discourses focus on the behavioural choices of mothers, thereby obstructing other factors beyond the mothers' control that determine breastfeeding success (Murphy 2000). In breastfeeding promotion campaigns, it is, in fact, as if mothers have the sole responsibility for their child's nutrition, regardless of the family and social contexts around them (Gatrell 2011; Hall Smith, Hausman & Labbok 2012; Maher 1992). Furthermore, breastfeeding promotion discourses from public health agencies and child nutrition experts emphasise the benefits of breast milk for children's health; in other words, they focus on the product rather than on the relationship (Hall Smith, Hausman & Labbok 2012).

Additionally, a significant gap can be observed between the fantasy breastfeeding picture spread by promotion campaigns and the actual experience of mothers (Schmied & Lupton 2001). By focusing only on breastfeeding's positive aspects, promotion campaigns tend to give an idealised image of breastfeeding. To convince mothers that breastfeeding is easy, activists mobilise an often-naturalising discourse showing breastfeeding as a "natural" and "normal" activity that does not cause any particular difficulties, except for small, easily overcome obstacles (Gatrell 2011).

Breastfeeding support and organisations in Switzerland

Different organisations are working to promote breastfeeding in Switzerland. In 2000, UNICEF Swiss and the Federal Office for Public Health founded the Swiss foundation Breastfeeding Promotion Switzerland with the priority objective of putting the WHO's "Global Strategy for Infants and Young Child Feeding" into practice. The foundation's main strategies are "the objective information of the population, in particular parents, the fight for a better conciliation between breastfeeding and work and creating places that are suitable for breastfeeding in the public space, as well as monitoring the marketing of infant products" (Breastfeeding Promotion Switzerland 2015). It released informative leaflets and the smartphone application Mamamap, which lists public areas dedicated to breastfeeding.

The Geneva Infant Feeding Association (GIFA) was created in 1979 to protect and promote breastfeeding, serving as a liaison office for the IBFAN. This association also collaborates with local nutrition and breastfeeding promotion projects such as *Marchez et mangez malin!* (walk and eat smart) with the *Fondation promotion santé Suisse* (Swiss Health Promotion Foundation), which promotes healthy nutrition and regular physical activity. The organisation La Leche League was established in Switzerland in 1972 and collaborates with Breastfeeding Promotion Switzerland and GIFA.[1] Delegates of this organisation propose local support group meetings for mothers.

In 2014, Swiss law encouraged breastfeeding for working mothers by providing paid breaks of up to one and a half hours per working day during the child's first year of life. In addition, employers must make available a private room suitable for breastfeeding and a refrigerator for storing breast-milk. As a "right still unknown", in practice, the law's application is far from obvious (Ruz 2018). Female employees often encounter hostile reactions from their employers and colleagues, making the possibility of pumping their milk at the workplace or being absent to breastfeed their child difficult or impossible. In addition, and in Vaud only, a one-month paid breastfeeding leave can be obtained at the end of the four-month maternity leave. A medical certificate attesting that the woman is actually breastfeeding must be supplied to her employer.

Techno-medicalised motherhood and breastfeeding

At the beginning of the nineteenth century, the conception of the female body as fragile and potentially defective dominated Western scientific and medical discourses (Martin 1987; Dykes 2005; Kukla 2005). Since the late nineteenth century, the medicalisation of society intensified the desire for control of the female body as a whole and the reproductive processes in particular, as reflected in the systematic and widespread hospitalisation for childbirth (Blum 1999; Dykes 2005; Kukla 2005; Jacques 2007; Oakley 1984). Birth was redefined from a "normal" aspect of women's lives to a biomedical event that was likely to fail, was dangerous and unpredictable, and required medical supervision (Dykes 2006; Oakley 1984). Lactation and breastfeeding were not immune to this desire for control.

As an extension of the metaphor of the "woman-as-machine" Martin (1987) exposes in the context of pregnancy and childbirth—according to which the foetus is a "product" of the female body and the doctor a "repairer"—breast milk is perceived as a commodity produced by the maternal body but detached from it. In this new configuration, breastfeeding becomes the production process of which breast milk is the product. This objectification of the body is also present in the mothers' discourse as they, in turn, tend to conceive their breasts as "potentially faulty machines" (Dykes 2005: 2287). From this perspective, the use of perinatal experts, such as midwives, paediatricians, or lactation consultants, has become indispensable for overseeing breastfeeding. It can also be noted that these experts have a certain monopoly in the area of breastfeeding information, since mothers are part of a contemporary cultural context of bottle-feeding (Dykes 2006). Mothers have little personal experience with breastfeeding as they have often not been breastfed themselves and have rarely witnessed other mothers breastfeed. This lack of cultural experience is an opportunity for biomedicine to position itself as the unique source of knowledge on breastfeeding (ibid. 2006).

Measuring breastfeeding

Biomedical culture favours "seeing" over "feeling", particularly in the field of perinatality. Already during pregnancy and at the time of delivery, women are conditioned to feel dependent "upon visual verification and validation of embodied experiences" (Dykes 2006: 84). In the context of breastfeeding, this verification results in a careful measurement of infant growth. The need to rationalise their breastfeeding experience is thus very present in mothers' minds. For example, the quantification of the milk absorbed by their baby is a major preoccupation (Avishai 2007; Mahon-Daly & Andrews 2002 Marshall, Godfrey & Renfrew 2007). The regular weighing of infants, largely encouraged by professionals (Dykes 2005, 2006; Maher 1992), appears as the only way to palliate this uncertainty: babies' weight gain constitutes "objective" and "scientific" evidence of their good health and the "success" of breastfeeding.

From birth, newborns undergo medical observation and measurement and are compared to other babies in their developmental stage. "Height, weight, and head circumference are measured, plotted, and evaluated in relation to 'average' growth" (Wolf 2011: 87). Even if the child is perfectly healthy, this process implies the ever-present fear of "deviance". Children are subject to regular medical checks to ensure that they remain within the margins of normalcy. In this context, the infant's body and its (good) growth become tokens of maternal skills, while a lower weight gain is interpreted as a breastfeeding failure and a sign of maternal incompetence (Lupton 1996, cited by Dykes & Williams 1999). Since mothers are rarely equipped with appropriate scales, babies are most often weighed by professionals. While knowing the child's weight is generally perceived as reassuring, over-valuing this indicator to the detriment of other qualitative aspects such as the baby's behaviour can, however, undermine mothers' confidence. Rather than learning to trust their feelings, they rely on health professionals (Dykes & Williams 1999; Marshall, Godfrey & Renfrew 2007). In this regard,

Dykes (2006) notes a striking contradiction between the message issued by health professionals, who ask mothers to place their trust in breastfeeding and breast milk to meet the nutritional needs of their children fully, and the scientific precision offered by artificial milk, easily quantifiable. In this perspective, the latter would more adequately meet the requirements of the biomedical culture for visual verification.

Moreover, "insufficient milk syndrome", a medical syndrome identified since the early 1980s as culturally constructed, was still very often diagnosed in modern Euro-American societies until the beginning of the twenty-first century (Dykes & Williams 1999; Dykes 2002; Van Esterik 1988). It appeared as one of the most common reasons for mothers to stop breast-feeding (Blum 1999; Obermeyer & Castle 1996), which for some also had the advantage of being socially acceptable (Van Esterik 1988). Van Esterik (1988) highlights that this phenomenon was more present in cultures under the influence of a biomedical conception of breastfeeding—where breast milk is, first of all, a product valued for its nutritional composition—than in cultures favouring a holistic view of breastfeeding as a process. The institutional management of breastfeeding also contributed directly to the construction of this syndrome, notably through the encouragement of a strict breastfeeding schedule. Indeed, scheduled breastfeeding reduces the number of feedings and can inhibit the production of breast milk since the more the baby suckles, the more the breasts produce milk (Blum 1999; Wolf 2006).[2]

In addition, Van Esterik (1988) describes the syndrome as a "self-fulfilling prophecy", as mothers' anxiety can greatly contribute to reducing their milk production (101). From a physiological point of view, the milk ejection reflex is controlled by oxytocin, the diffusion of which can be influenced by emotional factors. The insufficient milk syndrome is a good example of how medical culture and health professionals' practices can interfere with the experiences of breastfeeding mothers. The "epidemic" of insufficient milk syndrome seems to be currently in decline, partly due to the influence of the WHO's new guidelines and breastfeeding awareness campaigns. However, as Wolf (2006) mentions, physicians' "misogynist theories of lactation failure portended a mistrust, which lingers even today, of lactation as a reliable body function" (406). Millard's (1990) analysis of American paediatric literature on infant feeding from 1897 to 1987 also shows that, more broadly, breastfeeding issues are actually often the result of inadequate recommendations issued by paediatricians. Accordingly, recommended restricted feeding regimes lead to insufficient milk supply but also increase infants' hunger and unsettlement, bringing doubts and feelings of incompetence to mothers' minds. In this perspective, as Millard (1990) notes, paediatric advice indirectly fosters bottle-feeding "despite biomedical and maternal goals to the contrary" (216).

This focus on quantitative criteria for judging infant health excludes any subjective competence mothers may have, as is already the case during pregnancy and childbirth. As such, breastfeeding can be considered a continuation of pregnancy and childbirth, a process subject to intensive control and supervised by the medical profession. Throughout their pregnancies, women are encouraged to dismiss their own feelings in favour of medical discourse. Once the moment to breastfeed has arrived, conditioned by this experience, they continue to seek medical approval (Maher 1992; Liamputtong 2011; Faircloth 2013). Mothers have indeed well internalised the idea that health professionals, who possess "authoritative knowledge" (Jordan 1997), always know better what is good for a woman's child. As a result, consulting a breastfeeding "expert" seems to have become unavoidable (Lee 2011). On the other hand, mothers' feelings of alienation from the objectification of their lactating body and its product, breast milk, are reinforced by the technical language adopted by professionals. Mothers are indeed remarkably absent from the biomedical literature on breastfeeding, as is any idea of a relationship between mother and child (Dykes 2006).

Moreover, the need to evaluate breastfeeding only on the basis of quantitative criteria excludes the subjective notion of pleasure (Maher 1992). An optimal breastfeeding is first and foremost effective and rationally managed, the affective dimension being secondary. It is also interesting to note that breastfeeding is primarily perceived by mothers, as by professionals, as a transfer of milk from mother to child and thus as a one-way relationship (Dykes 2006; Dykes & Flacking 2010). Considered as lacking reciprocity, breastfeeding is therefore experienced as particularly restrictive by mothers.

Standardised lactating bodies and time-related issues

The medical gaze on the body establishes what is "normal", "desirable", and what is not. Hospital protocols and practices thus lead to a power of "normalisation" for individuals. As Dykes (2006) notes, in reference to the work of Foucault (1977), the lactating body is a "'productive' yet 'subjected' body": mothers are "expected to be productive—producing breast milk, but their bodies are also subjected to surveillance of their performance and to dominant and authoritative forms of knowledge" (80). Birth hospitalisation implies a rationalisation of the process, subject to strict temporal norms. The initiation of breastfeeding in hospitals is part of this reasoning and responds to a logic of temporal controls without considering the distinctive features of each individual situation of mothers and babies (Dykes 2005, 2006; Maher 1992; Millard 1990). This conception of breastfeeding and the practices that result from it are particularly harmful to the initiation of breastfeeding and undermine the mothers' confidence in their ability to breastfeed (Dykes 2006). In terms of breastfeeding, however, the recommendations seem arbitrary and vary significantly from one paediatric manual to another depending on the institution or even between different members of a hospital staff within the same maternity ward (Maher 1992; Millard 1990; Palmer 2009 [1988]). One constant nevertheless remains: the perception of time as a structuring principle of breastfeeding (Millard 1990).

Scheduled feeding and "civilised" babies

The introduction of scheduled feeding also corresponds to a desire to produce "civilised" babies, who behave in a manner deemed appropriate, that is to say who are not "too" demanding, who do not cry excessively, who quickly sleep through the night, and who only ask for their mother's breast if they are truly hungry (Dykes 2005). The neoliberal subject is defined in terms of babies' autonomy, which is understood as a competence of self-determination expressed by the control of their behaviour and emotions. While all societies are making efforts to socialise their babies (Bonnet & Pourchez 2007; Conklin & Morgan 1996; Gottlieb 2004; Walentowitz 2013), the educational model favoured in a neoliberal context aims to produce children with early qualities of autonomy and self-regulation. For example, babies are taught from birth to sleep in a different room than their parents (Tomori 2015). Dykes (2006) used the term "civilising" to refer to the modality of socialisation that is at work to achieve the neoliberal model of individual. Her fieldwork observations showed that "mothers and midwives are still preoccupied to varying degrees with the baby being able to develop routines, be 'good', passive and docile. This involved the baby not being too demanding, sleeping for acceptable periods and not playing at the breast" (ibid. 2006: 102).

Time acts as a standard to appreciate the "civility" of infants. From birth, disciplinary measures are established so that the infants are able to regulate their feedings. The underlying objective is a concordance with the temporal structure of the parents' daily life, punctuated by three separate meals during the day, with the night being reserved for sleep. Already challenging in the first days after birth, the temporal "chaos" of the first weeks of a newborn's life quickly becomes unbearable from the point of view of both mothers and professionals. The baby is quickly expected to find a certain routine with established schedules and little variation (Balsamo et al. 1992; Dykes 2006; Lupton 2013a). In this perspective, scheduled breastfeeding can be seen as a social preparation for the temporal order that dominates our culture (Balsamo et al. 1992).

Dykes (2006) highlights the links between the desire to "civilise" babies and the industrialisation process, which involves the necessity to prepare individuals for factory working conditions. To achieve this purpose, enhancing authority and discipline is required from early childhood. In the 1920s, the growing popularity of behaviourism led to the application of its theories to child-rearing, and child behaviourists "reshaped norms of embodied attachment" as they dissuaded mothers from being too affectionate and permissive to the baby, especially in the case of "bad habits", like crying or being "too" demanding (Blum 1999: 31). Needless to say, this understanding of infants, in need of regularity and strict schedules, validates scheduled feeding. It was not until the 1950s that this approach would be radically challenged by Bowlby's (1969) work and his "bonding theory" (1969), preparing the grounds for the concept of breastfeeding "on demand".

On-demand feeding and the reconceptualisation of time

In Europe and North America in the 1970s, the biomedical approach to birth and its standardised vision of the female body started to be challenged by feminist and ecological movements advocating for women's reappropriation of their bodies, including a "natural" approach to birth (Blum 1999). The importance of breastfeeding in the construction of the mother–child bond was emphasised, and on-demand breastfeeding was beginning to gain favour (Rollet & Morel 2000; Dykes 2005; Quandt 1995; Woolridge 1995). Nevertheless, if the notion of on-demand breastfeeding appeared in the paediatric literature in the middle of the twentieth century (Millard 1990), it was not until the 1980s that it became largely recommended (Rollet & Morel 2000; Dykes 2006)—and even more so after the BFHI's introduction in 1992.

In the 2018 revised version of the BFHI, the expression "responsive feeding" replaced "on-demand breastfeeding" (World Health Organization 2018). This shift stresses the importance of the relational aspects of the breastfeeding process, inviting mothers to "recognize and respond to their infant's cues for feeding" (Aryeetey & Dykes 2018). This emphasis reflects a paradigm change among birth professionals regarding breastfeeding initiation and support (Dykes & Flacking 2010). Nevertheless, in my fieldwork, midwives and parents were still using "on-demand breastfeeding", an emic expression I thus chose to keep. Similarly, the "breast is best" message has been revised in official health policy guidelines in most Euro-American settings. However, it takes some time for health professionals and local institutions to adjust to a new rhetoric, and I observed that the "breast is best" message is still widely used in Switzerland, including by the Breastfeeding Promotion Switzerland Foundation (2020).

However, consistent with a persistent technical perspective of breastfeeding as a milk transfer, health professionals seem to remain attached to temporal benchmarks and quantitative data to evaluate the success of breastfeeding (Balsamo et al. 1992; Dykes 2006; Maher 1992; Dykes & Williams 1999; Dykes 2005; Palmer 2009 [1988]; Sachs 2013). They still encourage mothers to maintain a specific time-lapse between feedings, often adjusted to the baby's age. As Dykes (2006) shows, the notion of time remains central in on-demand breastfeeding, both in the biomedical literature and in the discourses of health professionals or mothers. Millard (1990) raises another issue that comes with on-demand breastfeeding: in infant-feeding advice, the term "demand" has generally not been defined. Therefore, depending on the professional, it can vary from "a vocal signal from the baby" to "outright crying" (217). Mothers are urged to breastfeed at their babies' demand, but only if they express "true hunger" and not solely for comfort. However, the definition of criteria indicating "true hunger" also remains unaddressed.

In industrialised societies deeply structured by time linearity, the notion of on-demand breastfeeding seems particularly problematic. Thus, even when mothers practise on-demand breastfeeding, the frequency and duration of feedings remain at the heart of their concerns. As Millard (1990) observes:

> Once the clock is seen as inherent in human behavior, adherence to the timetable becomes a standard for judging competence, adequacy and normality. Its presence in early infancy is a signal of its existence as a central touchstone in our cultural system for many themes, including the ascendancy of professionals, the maintenance of hierarchy, and the separation of lay people into categories of normal and abnormal, and adequate and inadequate. (1990: 219)

Time, through feeding patterns, acts as an organising principle, set to assess both the mother's and the infant's adequacy. According to Dykes (2006), this focus on the frequency and duration of feedings would also come from the widespread assumption that these temporal measures can indicate the amount of milk absorbed. This presumption is based on a common association between the notions of time and quantity, rooted in industrial production: at the factory, time is closely linked to the quantity produced (Adam 1992).

As an alternative framework of conceiving time, Kahn (1989) introduces the notion of "maialogical time", referring to the period of pregnancy, childbirth, and breastfeeding and understood as a time of mutuality and reciprocity between mothers and their children (27). According to Kahn (1989), linear time, which is part of an industrial logic, is opposed to cyclical, "maialogical" time, dictated by body rhythms and responding to an internal logic. Without any notion of linearity, infants would fit into the slow and cyclical rhythm of this "maialogical" time. In this perspective, the eagerness to establish a "routine" and return to a "normal" temporality—that is to say a linear one—as quickly as possible creates tension with respect to "maialogical" time. As Dykes (2006) points out, "If time is seen as linear and related to efficiency and productivity in the industrial sense, then women will see breastfeeding as time-consuming and potentially time-wasting" (113). In the dominant perception, the status of breastfeeding is confined to a transitional stage rather than having its own ontology. Bartlett (2010a) suggests that this restricted view of breastfeeding precludes an understanding of breastfeeding for itself. It also has the effect of removing its potential for a reconceptualisation of time that breaks categorically from the dominant conception of temporality.

From "scientific" to "intensive" motherhood

During the twentieth century, the medicalisation and hospitalisation of childbirth in industrialised countries and the scientification of infant care corresponded to the emergence of a "scientific motherhood", which supplanted the authority of mothers based on experience and favoured gestures and practices validated by experts (Apple 1987; Dykes 2006; Faircloth 2013; Kukla 2005).

> Scientific motherhood, like the "cult of domesticity", defined women in terms of their maternal role centred in the domestic sphere. At the same time, however, it increasingly emphasized the importance of scientific and medical expertise to the development of proper childrearing techniques. (Apple 1987: 97)

To perform adequate child-rearing, mothers needed to be scientifically trained, relying on childcare manuals and educational centres, where they could receive advice from physicians or nurses, or home economics and childcare courses in public schools (Apple 1987; Bosson 2002).

Such classes were actually established in Europe and the United States at the beginning of the twentieth century. In 1905, in Vaud at the request of the cantonal medicine society, childcare courses were added to primary school and integrated into girls' domestic economy classes (Praz 2005). The figure of the nurse-visitor, specially trained in childcare, appeared as early as the 1920s, and several nursing schools opened in Geneva to offer childcare-oriented classes (Droux 2005). Students were also sent to visit families at home, where they provided care for babies and mothers who had just given birth, spreading childhood hygiene practices. Once they had completed their training, young graduates were often placed in privileged families, as a radically medicalised version of the traditional nanny. Familiar with the latest medical knowledge, but not encroaching upon physicians' privilege, "the missing link between the great specialist and the mother in distress is finally found" (Droux 2005: 299). For young women, nursing school was also thought to be an educative step before marriage and motherhood. They accumulated knowledge to assist paediatricians effectively when they would themselves become mothers. Professional and personal ambitions intertwined, preparing women in an institutionalised way to achieve the goals of scientific motherhood.

From the beginning of the 1950s, maternal and child health centres appeared, offering childcare classes and targeting primarily a popular clientele, often from immigrant communities. Moreover, the success of these programmes—which have multiplied between 1950 and 1965—attest to the changing expectations of parents. From the passivity that had so far characterised healthcare relationships, parents wished to become "legitimate interlocutors of health professionals, and this throughout the whole reproductive cycle leading to childbirth" (Droux 2007b: 146). Better informed about technical and medical innovations, parents claimed access to available services, which could disturb the institutional routines. For example, in Switzerland, fathers were finally admitted in birthing rooms in the 1960s (ibid. 2007b).

Infant's nutrition constituted a privileged field for this new area of health education. Whatever their feeding choices, mothers were accountable to physicians, so that even though they were given greater responsibility for adequate infant feeding, they were not in positions to decide the ways to feed their own children. Contradictions emerged from the obsession of medical expertise on infant-feeding practices.

> On the one hand it accorded women status; they were responsible for the health and well-being of children and, by extension, for the nation's future. Modern mothers, responsible mothers, scientific mothers should use the advances of science and medicine to shape their infant-care routines. On the other hand, scientific motherhood denied women control over their own mothering practices; women were incapable of successfully fulfilling their maternal duties without expert advice. (Apple 1987: 132)

Although the content of the recommendations has significantly evolved—schematically from artificial milk administered on a pre-established schedule to on-demand breastfeeding—the underlying idea remains that a mother is not the most competent person for her own child's care and must rely on experts. As summarised by Perrenoud (2016), "The bonding process between child and parents, the transition from the conjugal couple to the parental couple, the learning of childcare, are the subject of educational or support measures as if they could not be experienced by the social actors within their intimate sphere" (21–22).

Besides, being a parent now requires some degree of expertise in perinatal and child health. It is expected that parents keep abreast of the latest recommendations issued by health professionals and public health authorities but know how to question these recommendations to position themselves as "informed consumers" who are able to exercise "informed choice" (Murphy 2003: 457). Parents are not only exhorted to learn in depth about children, their health and well-being, and proper care methods but must also be critical and reflexive about the information received. Thus, the injunction to read and learn about the recommendations in force is particularly significant and requires intensive dedication. It is the continuation of the pregnancy period and even, more broadly, of the perinatal period, during which parents, and especially mothers, are already urged to inform themselves to prevent any identified risk and adjust their behaviour and daily lives accordingly.

Intensive motherhood and breastfeeding

Various authors (Badinter 2010; Blum 1999; Büskens 2010; Douglas & Michaels 2005; Faircloth 2013; Hays 1996; Lee 2008; Lupton 2013a; Wolf 2007, 2011) highlight this "intensification" of parenthood, and more specifically of motherhood. They defined it as a trend, according to which the social role of the mother would largely exceed the prerogatives strictly related to raising children and would become a life project in itself. Daily routines, such as "touching, talking and feeding are no longer ends in themselves, but tools mothers are required to perfect to ensure optimal development" of their children (Faircloth 2013: 22). In this perspective, motherhood becomes a full-time occupation, often preventing an additional paid activity, at least in the first years of their children's lives. Intensive maternity thus constitutes a "life project" for economically privileged mothers (Blum 1999; Wolf, 2011). Consumption also plays a central role in this quest to optimise each aspect of the baby's life. To ensure proper development, "no dimension of baby's existence is without the potential to be optimized through consumption, and no purchase is devoid of long-term implications" (Wolf 2011: 88).

This "intensive" practice of motherhood, which advocates for a "child-centred" approach and not a "mother-centred" approach, would become the norm of "good motherhood" (Lee 2008: 469). At the same time, the ideology of intensive motherhood tends to consider motherhood as an activity too crucial to be left to the sole responsibility of mothers, which justifies the systematic recourse of experts (Hays 1996; Lee 2008).

Playing a prominent role in this ideology (Lee 2008; Wolf 2007), Faircloth (2013) identifies breastfeeding as an embodied criterion for evaluating intensive motherhood. How to feed one's child serves as an "embodied measure" of motherhood, which affects all other aspects of childcare, such as where the baby sleeps or who can take care of her or him. In this perspective, it is truly breastfeeding that "makes" the mother. It seems that breastfeeding materialises the set of skills and characteristics that constitute motherhood and literally "embodies" maternal love, a process defined by Faircloth (2013) as "identity work" (15).

Mothers would breastfeed because of not only the different benefits it brings to their children but also their desire to adhere to a certain "model" of maternity deemed superior and to which they identify. Wolf (2011) describes breastfeeding as a "fateful moment" in the construction of the mother's identity, one of the "turning points at which people must make highly consequential choices that speak to their identity, or who they are trying to be" (105). Giddens (1991) highlights the emergence, in late modern cultures, of a conception of the self as a "reflexive project" (32). In this "post-traditional order", identity is created and shaped by individuals' decisions and practices in their everyday lives: there is no inherited lifestyle to follow anymore. As written by Giddens (1991), "We are not what we are, but what we make of ourselves" (75). In this perspective, breastfeeding, among other parenting practices, fits into a specific lifestyle, defined by Giddens (1991) as "a more or less integrated set of practices which an individual embraces, not only because such practices fulfil utilitarian needs, but because they give material form to a particular narrative of self-identity" (81).

For some mothers, failing to breastfeed can be particularly difficult to overcome. From their perspective, breastfeeding is not only beneficial to the child's health but also a crucial element in the creation of the mother–child bond. Breastfeeding issues thus jeopardise their very capacity to be mothers and maternal identities (Lee 2008; Sheehan & Schmied 2011). This strong association between maternal identity and breastfeeding also explains women's motivations to continue breastfeeding despite the difficulties encountered and plays a role in the duration of breastfeeding (Sheehan & Schmied 2011).

In the case of infant feeding, as for any other health topic in the era of "informed choice", Lee points out, "'to choose' is not to pick between two valid options each with advantages. Rather, it is to opt to live life in a way judged preferable according to experts 'evidence', or to decide to continue living in a way that encourages illness and early death" (2011: 83). The cultural and political context into which mothers' decisions fit imposes breastfeeding as the only acceptable choice. Mothers who choose to formula feed tend to develop different argumentative strategies to justify their choice without jeopardising their legitimacy and maternal skills (Balsamo et al. 1992; Murphy 1999; Lee 2008).

Interestingly, besides numerous studies on the effects of breastfeeding on children's health, its effects on maternal health remain little explored (Blum 1999; Maher 1992). As Blum (1999) notes, a mother's altruism is supposed to be so strong that it seems inconceivable that this aspect may be taken into account in the decision process of how to feed their children; a mother is not supposed to breastfeed for her own sake. In modern Euro-American societies, the notion of the "good mother" generally implies accepting to put the needs and well-being of one's child ahead of one's own, which may explain why this type of breastfeeding promotion strategy is considered effective (Blum 1999; Murphy 1999; Schmied & Lupton 2001).

Wolf (2011) also notices that medical researches on breastfeeding are shaped in a way "that reflect and reinforce the principles of total motherhood, but the veneer of scientific objectivity conceals this moral bias and makes maternal sacrifice appear less ideological than pragmatic" (93). For example, other feeding practices specifically involving fathers are not investigated. The premise underlying breastfeeding research is that the mother is necessarily the primary caregiver. In this perspective, risks would be "most important to address when they can be managed by mothers, and, by extension, that mothers are culturally responsible for reducing risks to their children" (ibid. 2011: 94).

Breastfeeding and risk management

The prevalence of risk in the management of pregnancy and childbirth is part of a broader cultural context, focusing on risk as central to action thinking in our modern neoliberal societies. This predominance of risk, particularly expressed in the health field, seems paradoxical: "Modern societies feel increasingly vulnerable to biological, environmental and technological developments, despite decreasing mortality and morbidity rates" (Walsh, El-Nemer & Downe 2008: 118).

By breastfeeding their children, mothers respond to a logic of risk prevention, linked to the emergence of "surveillance medicine" and characterised by the extension of the medical field to processes previously considered "normal", such as pregnancy or child growth (Armstrong 1995). New measures were implemented, such as the use of screening devices and the development of health promotion campaigns. Already in utero, increased attention is given to the child and her or his physical and psychological development (ibid. 1995). Health education gradually focuses on "lifestyle", distinguishing between risks attributed to external causes over which individuals have no control and risks they create for themselves that are caused by their way of life (Lupton 1993). It would be everyone's responsibility to avoid this last type of risk.

This "privatization of risk management" typical of neoliberal societies also implies a transformation of the individual relationship to risk and health. It reconceptualises the notion of "behaviour", which becomes the result of responsible and well-considered individual choices, in the light of expert advice, to anticipate risks and secure the future (Rose 2006: 158). Ruhl (2002) denounces a "fetishization of the will" (651), through which socioeconomic disadvantages that limit individual agency are eclipsed by the neoliberal model of the autonomous citizen and are capable of self-determination. Once duly informed by authoritative experts in the concerned field, "the liberal subject is called on to exercise of self-subjection and self-regulation" to obtain the desired results (Murphy 2000: 306).

As Armstrong (1995) points out, the devices put in place by surveillance medicine—health promotion and screening campaigns and broad public health surveys—aim to "transform the future by changing the health attitudes and health behaviours of the present" (402). Projection into the more or less distant future is a decisive aspect of risk prevention, and a child offers a particularly favourable ground for this anticipation (Giddens 1990; Murphy 2000; Rose 1989). Giddens (1990) highlights the "colonization of the future" typical of modernity: individuals must plan their lives in a reflexive way, anticipating future risks. From this standpoint, parents' practices and behaviours determine future outcomes. In this way, breastfeeding is meant to provide a strong foundation for one's child, promising better health in the short and long term and optimal emotional development for a serene affective life in adulthood. As a result, "if good health in a risk culture is an indicator of a person's capacity to make wise choices, babies' physical and developmental well-being is a reflection of their mothers' discernment" (Wolf 2011: 86).

The responsibility for risk prevention is largely attributed to the individual, and the role of parents takes on a new dimension: it is now up to them to assume risk management by opting for appropriate educational and care practices, among which breastfeeding occupies a special place because of the multiple benefits it grants (Faircloth 2013). Furedi (2002) proposes the concept of "parental determinism" to designate this reconfiguration of parental responsibilities, understood as a form of determinism in which the daily activities and actions of parents are directly and causally associated with the possibility of failure or harm to their children and, more broadly, to society. Parents thus appear as "risk managers" who have the power to decide their child's fate depending on how they perform their parental tasks.

Moreover, the focus on risk in neoliberal societies contributes to the professionalisation of parenthood and the necessity to seek assistance from experts, as parents are perceived as incapable of effectively managing risks by themselves (Lee 2008). Assessing danger is a task for scientists and experts: "Risk society is marked by the pervasiveness of scientific authority and an endless production of data that either support or revise existing risk determinations" (Wolf 2007: 612). This expert guidance begins long before the baby's birth, right from the beginning of pregnancy—or even before conception—to ensure that the foetus is protected from potential risks caused by "bad" maternal behaviour.

Recent developments in epigenetics, supported by the Developmental Origins of Health and Disease hypothesis, further strengthen mothers' accountability (Kenney & Müller 2017; Richardson 2015). This new research area, focused on the periconceptional period until the child's second anniversary, "explores how the socio-economic environments individuals experience during gestation and early life significantly shape their susceptibility to a range of diseases in later life. Researchers in this field increasingly postulate epigenetic mechanisms as plausible causal explanations for their epidemiological and bio-anthropological observations" (Kenney & Müller 2017: 38). Mothers' bodies, thought of as "epigenetic vectors", and mothers' attitudes and practices in relation to their children's health hence become a privileged place of observation and investigation for researchers (Richardson 2015: 211). Attention is thus fully focused on the mother, a bias Kenney and Müller (2017) denounce as the "extended mother" phenomenon: the child's environment is reduced to her or his mother (10).

Conceptualising babies

It should be emphasised that children, while being at the centre of discourses promoting breastfeeding and claiming a "child-centred" approach, are also notably absent from them. In this type of speech, the child seems abstract, disembodied, or even standardised, particularly through the notion of the "civilised" baby. Rather than being perceived as a relational process involving two social actors—the mother and the child—breastfeeding is presented as the sole responsibility of the mother. Babies are not only absent from discourses on breastfeeding but also non-existent in socio-anthropological studies on breastfeeding and anthropological research in general. The epidemiological impact of breastfeeding on infant health has been the subject of many medical studies, while social scientists have instead focused on the mother's perspective.[3] From a socio-anthropological perspective, it seems that babies are never considered social actors in their own right, and their behaviours and modes of communication around breastfeeding have remained surprisingly unexplored. In general, interest in newborns as relevant subjects of study for social science developed only recently, along with the recognition of corporeal phenomena as culturally constructed (Gottlieb 2000). Until then, babies were rather perceived as pre-cultural beings: impervious to any cultural influence and excluded from any social interaction, they were removed "by nature" from anthropological concerns. Through her observations on Beng infants, Gottlieb shows that the cognitive, social, and motor development of newborns is culturally determined, which makes them culturally soaked, and invites the practice of an "anthropology of infants", rather than an "anthropology of infancy as seen by others" (2000: 127). Nevertheless, works on newborns and the care practices they receive in the immediate postpartum period remain scarce.[4]

The 1970s and the legalisation of abortion marked the advent of the "child by project" (Boltanski 2004; Charrier & Clavandier 2013). Until then, Charrier and Clavandier (2013) report the "poor place left to children for themselves. The history of birth does not include them as actors strictly speaking" (43). Children were perceived first and primarily as beings who should be efficiently managed. Child psychiatry, especially personified in Europe by Françoise Dolto (1985), played an important role in the recognition of infants as full-fledged individuals. From the end of the Second Word War, Dolto undertook the education of mothers to free children from traditional upbringings. The objective was more precisely to preserve them from "psychological risks" defined by psychoanalysts based on their clinical work (Garcia 2011). On this point, Garcia (2011) noticed a historical link between the important space held by child psychoanalysis and intensive motherhood. However, my observations showed that, even though it is "child-centred", the holistic model is not without discipline imposed on the child's body and behaviour. For example, as with the maternal body, the child's body is shaped to be suitable for breastfeeding. More broadly, the babies' behaviours—especially their rhythms regarding feedings or sleep patterns—are expected to fit within midwives' visits and parents' schedules.

Focused on the moment of birth, Leboyer (1974) defends the child's interests on another level. Focused on the baby's perspective of birth and immediate postpartum, Leboyer (1974) also claimed a vision of the baby as a "person", whose experience had to be taken into consideration. Understanding the baby as being vulnerable and in need of protection, Leboyer (1974) proposed a set of measures to avoid any form of aggression at the time of childbirth, for example, reducing lights and avoiding noise or abrupt movements. Infants are "people", but their vulnerabilities or ineptitudes are more often pointed out than their skills.

Breastfeeding promotion discourses reflect this conception and inform the perception of babies' bodies. The argument of the beneficial effect of breast-feeding on the infants' immune systems, for example, occupies a prominent place in these discourses. The notion of the immune system—conceptualised as particularly weak and deficient—has become central to the way babies' bodies are perceived (Brownlie & Sheach Leith 2011; Lupton 2013a). The outside world is perceived as a threat to newborns, whose body boundaries are seen as "porous" (Lupton 2013a: 44). To protect this defective immune system, aside from breastfeeding, different strategies are put in place to create a reassuring bubble of cleanliness around babies. For example, special attention is given to hygiene in the house: newborns are kept away from people or places perceived as potential contaminants, their clothes are regularly cleaned, and all objects intended to be put in their mouths are systematically sterilised.

Since the mid-1970s, in Europe (see, for example, in France, Herbinet & Busnel 2009 [1981]) and North America (Bradley & Mistretta 1975), a competitive perspective emerged with psycho-developmental theories, highlighting that foetuses already develop sensory skills in utero. This conception of newborns was also reflected in the discourses of the midwives I followed during my fieldwork, alongside a more usual representation of infants, primarily defined by their vulnerability.

According to Lupton (2013a), the interembodied relationship between a mother and her child is part of the surveillance measures set up around infants for monitoring and detecting any abnormalities. The mobilisation of an embodied knowledge induced by this interembodiment would make it possible to evaluate their physical well-being. Children are generally seen as vulnerable, requiring continuous parental control—most often operated by the mother—to ensure that they are healthy and develop normally. Based on this logic, the younger the children, then the more vulnerable and helpless they are. Nevertheless, the younger they are, the more often their mothers are their primary caregivers. The alarmist view of babies' bodies and immune systems combined with the emergence of intensive maternity results in expectations that mothers continuously monitor their babies and seek for signs of illness or "abnormal" development.

The concept of interembodiment is therefore central to understanding how mothers "think and feel about their infants' bodies" (Lupton 2013a: 39). Interembodiment implies that "apparently individuated and autonomous bodies are actually experienced at the phenomenological level as intertwined" (ibid. 2013a: 39). Individuals' bodies are not isolated units; on the contrary, they are inseparable from other bodies with which they interact. Because of the proximity and intimacy required, breastfeeding can be seen as an act of "extreme" interembodiment. This perspective identifies the infant as a social actor whose body is as active as her or his mother's is.

If interembodiment also applies to older children's and adults' bodies, it is particularly central in the apprehension of babies and their bodies. On the one hand, because infants do not yet master the verbal language, interembodiment is an important mode of expression. On the other hand, babies' bodies have high needs for care, which implies greater interembodiment between their parents or caregivers and them.

Praise for proximity

In contrast with the dominant ideology of separation that underpins the biomedical paradigm, as well as the cultural context of modern Euro-American societies, new parenting models such as "attachment parenting" have emerged. Attachment parenting originated in the 1980s in the Anglo-Saxon world, following Sears and Sears' (2001) successful publications among young parents. This current seems to have extended all over Euro-American countries and defends a child-centred, "proximal" parenting approach, with an emphasis on specific practices, such as bed-sharing or child wearing and particularly breastfeeding. As a polysemous notion, attachment parenting is subject to different interpretations and applications, depending on local cultural contexts. Through her comparative study of attachment mothers in the United Kingdom and Paris, Faircloth (2013) shows that, as the model is more marginalised in France than in the United Kingdom, French mothers who are engaged in attachment parenting manifest a stronger commitment and a more purist approach than British mothers do.

For proximal maternity supporters, proximity between mother and child is obviously central, if only for the establishment and continuation of breastfeeding, preferably performed on-demand and until child-led weaning. Kukla (2005) criticises this focus, as it would elevate mother–child closeness to a "mark of good mothering and the guarantor of well-ordered nature" (149). This simplification of motherhood to proximity, and then the simplification of this proximity to breastfeeding would minimise the complexity of motherhood by reducing it to "a static and inarticulate spatial bond" (ibid. 2005: 149).

For parents who practise attachment parenting during the first months and even years of life, children would specifically need their mother for biologically determined reasons: women would be "designed" for motherhood. Therefore, it seems only "natural" that the father maintains a paid job out of the domestic sphere, while the mother, "liberated" from the hazards of a livelihood, can stay with the child and be fully dedicated to her or him. More broadly, the father is expected to show support for childcare and especially breastfeeding, but in an indirect or passive way. He provides support by relieving the mother of material constraints, rather than fully participating in childcare. From this perspective, social and parental roles are a direct result of body design (Bobel 2002).

Proponents of attachment parenting rely on British psychiatrist Bowlby's work (1969), conducted in the 1950s, on the effects of early maternal deprivation. Bowlby's work was inspired by Lorenz's (1973) research based on animal studies and showed that children's first hours and weeks of life have a long-term impact on their development. Lorenz used the term *imprinting* to refer to the "sensitive period" during which it is crucial that mother and child "bond" (i.e., create emotional bonds). According to Lorenz, failure to bond during this time window would put the child's development at risk. On this basis, attachment theory, as developed by Bowlby and Ainsworth (Bretherton 1992), argues that the "constant presence of a loving and responsive attachment figure—typically the mother—was the foundation for lifelong mental health" (Faircloth 2013: 29).

Attachment theory found resounding success in the United States and Europe and continues to have a significant influence on perinatal health professionals and a prominent place in developmental psychology (Wall 2001). In these discourses, breastfeeding is identified as contributing to bonding between mother and child and is therefore part of the cultural norms of intensive motherhood (ibid. 2001). Widely integrated with popular representations of motherhood beyond its initial scientific definition, this notion of bonding echoed an ideological vision of the appropriate role of women, described by Garcia (2011) as "the ethics of maternal availability" (12). In the original bonding theory developed by Ainsworth and Bowlby, the mother is presented as the central figure of attachment (Bretherton 1992). This work has since been criticised, including by social scientists highlighting the adequacy of the attachment theory with ideological elements concerning the "appropriate" place of women in Euro-American societies (Crouch & Manderson 1995; Eyer 1993).

Nevertheless, even if the bonding theory and, more specifically, the "sensitive period theory" have lost popularity in scientific research from the 1980s, they persistently remain in the minds of health professionals and mainstream birth literature (Wall 2001). Bowlby's theory is still taught in Swiss midwifery schools, occupying a central place in the training. The notion of bonding is thus central in breastfeeding promotional discourses, presented as the continuity of the special link mothers had with their unborn baby.

> Breastfeeding, it is implied, is an extension of the natural, embodied, and intimate connection that presumably begins between mothers and babies during pregnancy. (Wall 2001: 599)

As a result, the bonding process should begin even before the child's birth. According to this "bonding-oriented" understanding of breastfeeding, the act of breastfeeding has benefits that spread far beyond the epidemiological considerations of breast milk's nutritional benefits. By promoting skin-to-skin contact and sensory stimulation, breastfeeding is presented by developmental psychology as a way to optimise the development of the child's brain, contributing to "build a better baby", destined to become a "better" individual when an adult (Wall 2001: 603). The physical closeness between mother and child is seen as "always positive" for both of them, and the "bond" that develops is an exclusive one that "only a (breastfeeding) mother and her baby can know" (ibid. 2001: 602). These preconceptions reflect and reinforce the myth of maternal "instinct", which is embedded in bonding theory. In this context, breastfeeding is undeniably a moral obligation for mothers, anchoring its authority "through its connection with cultural constructions of nature and motherhood" (Wall 2001: 605).

In case of failure in this bonding process, the long-term consequences would extend beyond the family sphere and are considered in terms of "social problems", criminal or deviant behaviour being commonly associated with emotional deprivation in the early years of life (Lee 2008). Kukla (2005) denounces this topic as a "rhetorical slide from the medical evidence supporting the benefits of breast milk as an infant food to the glorification of a romanticized vision of the actual act of breastfeeding, with little or no marking of where medical advice leaves off and ideological images of appropriate bonding begin" (170). Interestingly, the argument of a compromised psycho-emotional development is also used by natural childbirth advocates to warn about the harmful impact of the caesarean section on infants. Odent (2005), for example, linked caesarean section to "an alteration of the capacity to love" for concerned individuals, possibly leading to long-term damages, including social issues and unsuitability.

Breastfeeding toddlers

Studies in non-industrialised societies have shown that prolonged breast-feeding beyond the first year of the child's life is common practice—at the time of the authors' fieldworks anyway (Dettwyler 1995a, 1995b; Gottlieb 2004; Mabilia 2005; Maher 1992; Rao & Kanade 1992). However, it remains quite unusual in modern neoliberal societies. Regardless of medical recommendations, there seems to be an age culturally identified as adequate for weaning (Kukla 2005; Scott 2011). More than a defined chronological age, it is related to individual development and varies from one child to another (Scott, Binns & Arnold 1997). A social consensus appears to prevail, according to which breastfeeding an infant is normal but breastfeeding a toddler is not because he or she is a conscious individual and can ask to breastfeed. On this last point, Kukla (2005) suggests that the articulation of a child's desire to access the pleasure of breastfeeding is problematic because "it makes manifest the desire *of* one agent *for* satisfaction from the body of another" (205). In consequence, the breastfeeding session can no longer be seen as "a simple, mute unity of two bodies" (ibid. 2005: 205).

If the decision to breastfeed is an indicator of mothers' skills and morality, it seems that the continuation of breastfeeding beyond the socially appropriate age may, on the contrary, be perceived as "deviant" and expose mothers to social judgement once again (Gribble 2010; Murphy 1999; Sinnott 2010). As a result, in a cultural context where breasts are primarily sexualised and early weaning is standardised, mothers often wean their children earlier than they would have liked or continue to breastfeed while hiding themselves (Gribble 2010). Moreover, "prolonged" breastfeeding is often perceived by laypersons and health professionals, despite WHO guidelines, as having a negative impact on the psychological development of children, who would be voluntarily maintained in a state of dependency on their mothers, which is considered inappropriate (Sinnott 2010; Scott 2011). Prolonged breastfeeding is also problematic because of its potential incompatibility with the paid work of women and the sexual function attributed to breasts that must remain "available" for marital and (hetero) sexual relationships (Blum 1999).

In a neoliberal context, continuing to breastfeed beyond the first months of life is perceived as out of the ordinary. Mothers who breastfeed well beyond this time limit are often forced to justify themselves, and they develop different strategies for this purpose. According to Faircloth (2013), the invocation of "nature" occupies a central place in mothers' discourses: by relying on archaeology and primatology in an evolutionist perspective, or even on the contemporary practices of societies judged closer to an "original" human lifestyle, they find scientific validation of the prolongation of their breastfeeding. For example, mothers can rely on the work of Dettwyler (1995a), a physical anthropologist and a breastfeeding activist, who established a "natural" age of human weaning between two and a half and seven years based on comparative data about primates. She thus denounced a gap between our "evolutionary heritage" and the current paediatric recommendations and practices.

Ecological reasons are also mentioned to justify long-term breastfeeding because of its associated energy and waste reduction, as opposed to formula feeding based on cow's milk. Some mothers also resort to Bowlby and Ainsworth's attachment theory or neuroscience and the study of human brain development to validate their breastfeeding practices (Sinnott 2010). Another area of justification consists of arguments based on mothers' feelings and their subjective experiences: they continue to breastfeed because it seems "right" (Bobel 2002; Faircloth 2013).

Children are often absent from breastfeeding promotion discourses. Gribble (2010) proposes to explore breastfeeding from their point of view, thus giving a voice to the breastfed. Gribble (2010) shows that breastfed infants who are old enough to talk about breastfeeding "take pleasure, find comfort and relaxation and closeness with their mother in the process of obtaining milk, as well as enjoying the milk itself", considered by some children in the study "as good as chocolate" (75). These observations challenge the commonly held and often mediatised perception of mothers forcing their children to continue breastfeeding to fill an emotional void or refusing to accept the fact that their children are growing up and gradually breaking away from them.[5]

As Faircloth (2013) points out, in neoliberal societies dominated by individualistic values, breastfeeding—even more so "prolonged" breastfeeding—is problematic, in that it blurs the bodily boundaries between children and their mother. Yet, it is widely accepted that the body envelope acts as a separator between individuals: for there to be an individual, it is necessary to respect the boundaries of the body (Kukla 2005). Breastfeeding, which implies that a body fluid flows from one body to another, transgresses this order. Thus, it is a continuation of pregnancy and acts as a reminder of the "incorporation" of the child's body into that of her or his mother, which operated during pregnancy.

> In pregnancy, a woman's body/self becomes doubled—and breastfeeding, particularly for "extended" periods, serves as a reminder of this ability to reproduce and transgress these boundaries. (Faircloth 2013: 78)

Biomedicine, and more widely the functioning of neoliberal societies, strongly encourages mother–child separation from a conceptual as well as a pragmatic point of view. According to Davis-Floyd and Davis (1996), "the history of western obstetrics is the history of technologies of separation" (237). Already during pregnancy, ultrasound scans dissuade mothers from trusting their feelings: it is necessary to rely on an external intermediary to be aware of the presence of the foetus and to make sure that it is well. At birth, the umbilical cord is cut very quickly after delivery to "release" the newborn from her or his mother. At a societal level, maternity leave is designed for mothers to return to work a few months after their child's birth. Mahon-Daly and Andrews (2002) use the notion of "liminality" from van Gennep (1909) to qualify the experience of breastfeeding for women as a state of transition, inscribed in the continuity of the pregnancy and delivery. In this perspective, the end of breastfeeding corresponds to a return to "normality"—to ordinary, individual life. On the contrary, long-term breastfeeding appears as a subversive prolongation of the liminal state of postpartum for mothers: a period during which they have lost their former status of non-mother but have not yet entirely gained their new social identity of established mother. As long as they breastfeed, women are stuck in a transitional stage requiring space and time negotiations in everyday life, before acquiring the status of experienced mothers and having integrated their new identity and being now able to get back to "normal" life (ibid. 2002).

As discussed above, to meet the expectations of the "civilised" baby ideal, infants are also expected to integrate the notion of separation at a very early age, for example by sleeping alone in a separate room or learning to keep occupied by themselves. With this in mind, a concern can be raised from the mother's side as well as the professional's side to prevent the baby's emotional dependency on her or his mother's breast: the child must not use it as a pacifier[6] or request it for comfort (Dykes 2006). Even if breastfeeding is recognised as fostering the mother–child bond, it must first and foremost fulfil a nutritive function.

Natural mothers and criticism of capitalism

Bobel (2002) understands natural mothers as being at the intersection between "attachment parenting" and "voluntary simplicity", "while taking inspiration from cultural feminism" (48). Wolf (2011) describes natural motherhood as a "microcosm of total motherhood": "in a risk culture, when virtually everything from conception through childbirth can ostensibly be either controlled or optimised, nature becomes a beacon, a respite from the complexity of a highly specialized world" (82).

According to Bobel (2002), if "natural" mothers question neoliberalism in some regards by adopting an alternative lifestyle and educational approach, they do not challenge the structure and content of the gender system. The path they propose is, therefore, an adaptation to the ideology and patriarchal conception of male and female roles "including the gender division of labour and, more abstractly, the dualistic split between private and public spheres and the exaltation of biology as the shaper of human destiny" (ibid. 2002: 47).

The message that breastfeeding is free is often emphasised by its proponents (see for example Breastfeeding Promotion Switzerland 2017), in accordance with "voluntary simplicity". However, in practice, and for economically privileged mothers, breastfeeding generally implies acquiring more or less expensive specific consumer goods, such as nursing bras, breast pads, or breast pumps. Some mothers assign crucial importance to these objects in the course of their breastfeeding journeys and can no longer conceive breastfeeding without these material supports, a phenomenon Avishai (2007) refers to as the "fetish value" (147).

Wolf also nuanced the criticism of consumerism claimed by the movement.

> Natural baby catalogs and mail order businesses, for example, offer nursing wear, noncompetitive toys, and other merchandise designed to enhance natural living and to satisfy consumer urges. These products, in addition to advice that natural mothers will make their own baby food, wash cloth diapers, and constantly "wear" their babies in slings, ignore the time, income, and flexibility necessary for natural mothering, resources that are unavailable to single or working mothers or families dependent on two incomes. (Wolf 2011: 83)

The link between motherhood and consumerism is often perceived as disturbing, as highlighted by Taylor, Layne and Wozniak (2004). Indeed, motherhood has been ideologically perceived and naturalised as a matter of emotions that stand outside the capitalist consumption system. This association is even more troubling in the context of a natural mothering approach and remains largely unaddressed and unproblematised. In this perspective, Bobel (2002) emphasised the paradox between an "alternative mothering style" and a submission to biological determinism. Accepting to defer to the authority of "nature", but challenging that of the market economy, natural mothers "simultaneously resist and embrace the dictates of forces larger than themselves" (ibid. 2002: 140).

Kukla (2005) denounces the "normative weight attached to having a 'natural birth', which is neither based on the results of scientific research, nor on the desires of mothers for their comfort during pregnancy and childbirth, but on the quality attributed to the mother, who could be corrupted by interventions perceived as against 'nature'" (223). Kukla (2005) notes that "even the most 'natural' maternal practices occur in a cultural context in which pregnancy, labour, and mothering are regulated, disciplined and monitored at every stage" (223). In this way, "a few fetishized moments", mainly the delivery and infant-feeding times, are selected and elevated into "the markers of proper 'natural' mothering" (ibid. 2005: 223). Furthermore, the emphasis on nature tends to erase the fact that breast milk and breastfeeding practices are analysed and shaped by medical research: the so-called natural on-demand breastfeeding is also constructed and approved by experts (Wolf 2011: 97).

Büskens (2010) points out a paradox between a "natural" style of mothering (arguments based on evolutionary theories, references to childcare practices in non-industrialised cultures) and that mothers often discover and "learn" this style of mothering through books that are written by experts. Paradoxically, it would still be the experts who could explain to mothers how to be "natural", as is already the case in the context of natural childbirth (Büskens 2010, Wolf 2011). From this perspective, "proximal" or "natural" mothering makes no sense outside of industrialised societies, although its proponents often refer to mothering practices in non-industrialised societies to support their argument. This reasoning, according to which non-industrialised societies would be closer to an original "state of nature", is reminiscent of the myth of the "noble savage" that is well known in anthropology.

Similarly, the natural childbirth movement is based on a political and cultural criticism of the industrialised modern society lifestyle.

> The solution to these evils has been seen to lie in a return to "nature", variously defined as the country, the primitive, the spiritual and the instinctual. Nature has also been strongly associated with putatively feminine values such as love, cooperation and altruism, in opposition to the destructive qualities traditionally vested in the male. (Moscucci 2002:168)

According to this vision, inherited from the Enlightenment, civilisation has weakened women's bodies, so that they would no longer be able to give birth physiologically, explaining the rise in medical and technical interventions surrounding childbirth. This argument, first proposed by Dick-Read, combines "Darwinian themes, neuropsychological theories, and cultural stereotypes of childbirth among 'primitive' people" (Moscucci 2002: 171). In Dick-Read's view, the pain felt during childbirth rests upon cultural beliefs and behaviours towards childbirth rather than biological causes. Relying on anthropological literature from the late nineteenth century, Dick-Read assured that "primitive" women would give birth easily and without pain, in contrast with "civilised" women from modern industrialised societies.

More broadly, the nature versus culture dichotomy, and the resulting assignment of women to nature and men to culture, emerged in European thought in the eighteenth century (MacCormack 1980). Paradoxically, if "the status of 'nature' becomes much higher in this period than it had been in more traditional dialectics, where it was associated with the fall, savages and the failure of education" (Bloch & Bloch 1980: 27), the recognition of women as "closer to nature" did not equate to any promotion of their social or political role. They remained subordinated to men, such as "natural" creatures, enslaved by reproductive bodily processes and meant to be "mastered" (Bloch & Bloch 1980: 33). Writers from the enlightenment, Rousseau in particular, attributed an important role to women in the creation of a better society through investment in their maternal and domestic duties: "In the medical ideology to which the French eighteenth-century writers were heirs, women and nature were seen to be in a peculiarly close relationship, particularly with regard to childcare" (Bloch & Bloch 1980: 32). However, some women seemed to be "closer to nature" than others. For example, in Diderot's imaginary development, women from Tahiti freely expressed their sexual and procreative "instincts", allowing them to develop "natural" maternal feelings towards their children, unlike "civilised" women who did not accomplish their maternal roles (ibid. 1980).

Conclusion

As breastfeeding intersects reproduction and parenting, in this chapter I reconnected two corpuses of literature: medical socio-anthropology literature focusing on reproduction and the body and parenting studies. The themes I chose to highlight and develop—risk, temporalities, bodies, and birth technologies—are major issues crossing both literature. I identified risk as the main lever for action, justifying the technologisation and hospitalisation of birth, but also essential in the discourse of natural childbirth proponents. Similarly, risk prevention legitimates the rise of formula and the rehabilitation of breastfeeding.

The temporalities of birth management, governed by the AML principles, extend to the postpartum period and the initiation of breastfeeding. A mechanistic vision of the female body, translated into industrial metaphors, is manifest in the entire birth process management, relying heavily on health practitioners' interventions. Provided by independent midwives, the specific and local modality of care I observed, which I called "holistic care", stands against this technocratic approach of birth. However, as an expression of intensive motherhood, the holistic care model still relies on risk as the main motivator for women to embrace this high-maintenance path to motherhood.

Notes

1 La Leche League is a non-profit organization for the support and promotion of breastfeeding founded in the United States in 1956 by a group of Catholic mothers. The founding of La Leche League in 1956 constitutes an early response in protest to formula feeding under the supervision of physicians. La Leche League is based on the principle of peer support, consistent with various studies highlighting the importance of support by female relatives who have breastfeeding experience (Balsamo et al. 1992; Dykes & Williams 1999; Maher & Serini 1992; Marshall & Godfrey 2011). Other associations carry out breastfeeding promotion and support activities, but La Leche League remains the best known and has a large international network. Since 1981, the League has been collaborating with UNICEF and has been involved in the establishment of the Baby Friendly Hospital Initiative (Sandre-Pereira 2005). Specifically, La Leche League advocates for on-demand breastfeeding as opposed to scheduled breastfeeding for maximised physical contact between mother and child and for gradual weaning guided by the child's needs and individual evolution (Faircloth 2013; Blum 1999).

2 The term "produce", commonly used by medical textbooks and practitioners, refers to the industry and the production line, in the same vein as the metaphor of the "woman-as-machine" (Martin 1987). As done by Dykes (2005, 2006), I use this term with awareness of this background.

3 See for example (Avishai 2004, 2007, 2011; Blum 1999; Dykes and Williams 1999; Dykes 2005, 2006; Murphy 1999, 2000; Schmied and Lupton 2001). Nevertheless, Gribble's (2008, 2010) work, which explored breastfeeding from a child's point of view, thus giving a voice to those who are breastfed, is a rare exception.

4 On the topic of care practices of premature newborns by nurses in a neonatal unit, see Rochat (2014).

5 See for example on the website of the daily newspaper *20 minutes*: "She was breastfeeding her 7-year-old daughter, judged for sexual act", on December 26, 2016: http://www.20min.ch/ro/news/suisse/story/-Donner-le-sein-n-est-pas-un-a cte-sexuel--27608302 (accessed 14.11.2017)

6 A paradigm shift can be noted here with a transition from the pacifier that replaces the breasts to the breasts that replace the pacifier (Dykes 2006).

3 Feeding to thrive

In this chapter, I explore how parents and health professionals measure and appreciate breastfed newborns' growth. In the context of out-of-hospital birth, during the immediate postpartum period, midwives must evaluate newborns' health and development on their own. If hospital risk management is perceived as invasive and potentially harmful by out-of-hospital birth users and practitioners, how do independent midwives establish their own risk management models, and on what criteria do they base their assessment of breastfeeding's success? Moreover, how do they reconcile the hospital protocols they have been trained to apply, paediatrician's expectations regarding babies' growth curves, and parents' desire—as well as their own—to prioritise breastfeeding over supplementation with formula? Finally, how do they discuss and negotiate the implementation of interventions with parents in cases of failure to thrive?

Parents who give birth at home tend to create their own risk perception models, which they reveal through their specific breastfeeding practices, such as bed-sharing or "breastsleeping" (McKenna & Gettler 2016)[1] and milk sharing, as well as infant care choices such as non-vaccination or letting babies sleep on their stomachs, a position condemned in official health guidelines. Based on my observations, independent midwives support these practices, which are conceptualised as deviant from a biomedical perspective. These stances lead to an emotional perspective and risk management that complies with parents' sensibilities. Midwives perceive parents' feelings—as well as their own feelings and intuitions—as valuable information that serves as the basis for their decisions and actions. Supported by their midwives, but often criticised by other health professionals who do not share the same healthcare approach, home birth parents may feel torn between the defence of their practices and the dominant risk culture.

In this chapter, I analyse how midwives, along with home birth parents, create a "customised" risk management model during postpartum follow-ups. Before directly addressing the topic of infants' weight, it is necessary to discuss the perception and management of risks during childbirth to gain a contextualised understanding of risk management and negotiations during the postpartum period. I explain how parents construct their stances

DOI: 10.4324/9781003124108-3

towards the so-called issue of "failure to thrive" in the context of their out-of-hospital birth plans. From there, I first expand on how they explain and justify their out-of-hospital birth plans. In particular, I examine how they conceptualise the notion of risk in the light of their perception of hospitals as environments that jeopardise breastfeeding initiation. Second, I elaborate on how midwives evaluate breastfeeding achievement and their use of weighing scales in this process. I then discuss in-depth fieldwork situations of infants' weight loss or stagnation and how midwives and parents negotiate the management of these issues, including the involvement of paediatricians. Finally, I propose an emotion-based model of risk management that relies on midwives' experiential knowledge and parents' empirical observations and feelings.

As Perrenoud (2014, 2016) highlights, midwives' experiential knowledge results from social and environmental circumstances and depends on the practitioners' specific professional and personal trajectories. This kind of knowledge has been rejected by biomedical authorities, especially with the rise of evidence-based medicine, because of its subjectivity and variability (Perrenoud 2016). Indeed, "the quality of this knowledge depends on the personal and professional trajectories of the social actors, as well as the characteristics of the communities of practice that have sheltered them" (ibid. 2016: 141-142). Experiential knowledge appears to be highly valued and occupies a central place in holistic care and home birth. It drives midwives' care decisions and supports the development of a personalised interpretation of risk culture that they share with parents.

Between monitoring and negotiating: a comprehensive approach to risk

Tomori (2015) conducted a study on night-time breastfeeding and infant care practices among American middle-class families. Specifically, she focused on dilemmas arising from night-time breastfeeding. As she observed, during the night, parents "confront conflicting medical guidelines about breastfeeding and infant sleep as well as larger questions about middle-class personhood and the social relations among children and their parents entailed in these reproductive processes" (Tomori 2015: viii). On the one hand, parents prioritise breastfeeding, following recommendations from public health organisations and nutrition and infant care experts. To achieve their goals, they sleep with the baby in their bed. By reducing the distance between their baby and them, they favour their own rest and facilitate breastfeeding. On the other hand, parents find themselves at odds with medical guidelines about safe sleep for infants, and they fear endangering or hurting their children accidentally while asleep. Medical authorities have also identified bed-sharing as a "risk factor" for sudden infant death syndrome (SIDS) (ibid. 2015: 71).[2] Moreover, parents worry about their children's psychological development. In a cultural context that privileges early autonomy, solitary sleep is a basic principle that shapes infants' personhood and relationship with their parents to produce self-reliant, "civilised" children. Tomori (2015) developed the concept of "embodied culture dilemmas" that emerge from night-time breastfeeding "as a lens through which we can glean unique insight into the complex dynamics of American personhood, family relations, biomedicine, and the far-reaching effects of capitalism" (19).

Similarly, during the postpartum period, conflicts appear between maintaining breastfeeding and ensuring infants' weight gain. Formula feeding facilitates regular weight gain and a linear growth curve. Until 2006, the WHO adopted the US National Center of Health Statistics (NCHS) growth reference charts, which were based on data collected in Ohio in 1929 on formula-fed children, with early diversification with solid foods (Sachs, Dykes & Carter 2005). Studies conducted in the 1980s indicate "a consistent mismatch between the shape of growth trajectories of healthy breastfed infants, in various settings, and the shape of the centiles on this chart" (ibid. 2005: 66). In 2006, the WHO released a new growth chart based on breastfed babies from various countries (Brazil, Ghana, India, Norway, Oman, and the United States) to create a new standard for healthy breastfed babies (WHO 2006). Breastfed babies often have less regular weight gain compared to formula-fed babies. After birth, their weight gain is faster and steeper, but it slows down, or "breaks", below the chart centiles (Sachs, Dykes & Carter 2005). From this perspective, breastfeeding requires a risk management model that may not align with the dominant model developed for babies fed with formula milk.

Supporting mothers during breastfeeding initiation leads independent midwives to subscribe to a holistic birth model to create a "customised" risk management model,[3] especially concerning the sensitive topic of babies' weight gain. In Switzerland, hospital protocols require that breastfed newborns who lose more than 10 per cent of their birth weight be "completed" with formula. At home, independent midwives can distance themselves from institutional protocols and set their own limits regarding what constitutes an "acceptable risk". The choice to give birth outside the hospital results from a reflection led by parents and generally includes a breastfeeding project. Parents are therefore particularly committed to breastfeeding success and eager to achieve specific goals, such as exclusive breastfeeding during the first six months of life. When midwives identify a situation as risky, they negotiate with parents for an intervention, such as supplementation with formula.

In socio-anthropological works criticising the biomedical management of birth, midwives are identified as "guardians" of physiology and keepers of "normal" birth (Davis-Floyd 2009; Katz Rothman 1982; Macdonald 2007), a fortiori in the context of independent midwifery practice and out-of-hospital birth. Scamell (2011) shows that hospital-based midwives in the United Kingdom, however critical of the risk-centred understanding of birth, contribute to the transmission and reproduction of this model by their professional practices.

> On the surface the swan may look calm and serene, suggesting her confident belief that everything is fine, everything is normal; but only inches under the water (which is a transparent liquid making visibility easy), the swan's feet tell quite a different story. It is a story of risk amplification and risk avoidance driven by the so-called risk society (Beck 1992).
> (Scamell 2011: 990-991)

Independent midwives choose to distance themselves from hospital protocols and constraints. Nevertheless, they also have biomedical and institutional backgrounds, with which they remain more or less imbued, depending on the professional trajectory that led them to independent practice. Some of them pursued long institutional careers before starting their independent practices, whereas others worked in an out-of-hospital setting immediately after graduation, as "assistants" to established independent midwives. The duration of their hospital careers can influence their out-of-hospital practices, and their sensitivity varies regarding newborns' weight loss or weight stagnation management. I observed, for example, that midwives who worked for a long time in hospitals before transitioning to holistic care tend to stick more closely to hospital protocols regarding the daily weighing of newborns, in contrast with their colleagues who have never worked in maternity wards. However, this tendency cannot be generalised, as midwives' attitudes towards weight-related issues and, more broadly, risk management, also depend greatly on their character and personal experiences, both professional and non-professional. Perrenoud (2016: 290) observed that institutional experience comprises "a multitude of situations, relations, actions, feelings and emotions composing a phenomenological entity, which cannot be exhaustively thought and deconstructed". As a result, midwives are sometimes torn between their theoretical ideals and their actual practices, and the coherence between discourses and practices is only partial. In addition, midwives must adjust their follow-ups to what is considered suitable by their community of practice, as interprofessional collaboration requires some level of pragmatism (ibid. 2016).

Giving birth out of the hospital to safeguard breastfeeding

Even long after starting their independent practices, midwives remain imbued with a risk-oriented institutional model of birth management informed by the question "What if things go wrong?" (Scamell 2011). Isabelle was an experienced independent midwife. She graduated in the late 1980s and opened her birth centre in the 1990s. She assisted countless out-of-hospital births at home or in her birth centre. However, when a delivery did not happen as expected, she still imagined the way it would be managed at the maternity ward.

> Sofia was in her mid-thirties. She mainly worked freelance in the applied arts field and was also a part-time employee in publishing. Her spouse, Pascal, was in his forties and was employed in an IT company. They lived in a small town with their two older children. I first met Sofia during her pregnancy to discuss her two previous breastfeeding experiences. This meeting allowed me to better contextualise Sofia's feelings and expectations regarding this new breastfeeding experience.
>
> Sofia and Pascal gave birth to their daughter, Lou, at home. The next day, I joined their midwife for the first postpartum visit. This was their fourth home birth, all assisted by Isabelle.[4] Pascal welcomed me and told me to go upstairs to join Sofia in their bedroom. Night had almost fallen, and I could barely distinguish Sofia in the dim light of her bedside lamp, on which she had put a scarf so as not to dazzle Lou. She sat on the side of the bed eating pizza. Lou was sleeping in her crib. Sofia greeted me and offered me a slice of pizza. We discussed Lou's birth and first feed while waiting for Isabelle. Sofia was very reassured by Lou's suckling abilities, as her second child had never been able to latch and suckle efficiently.
>
> When she arrived, Isabelle first asked some questions about Sofia's health and recovery, then got back to the events of the day before. Sofia's water broke before labour began, so Isabelle gave her the "magic potion" to induce labour.[5] Contractions started right away; they were very strong and very close together. Cervical dilatation was quick, but the baby became stuck in Sofia's pelvis, making expulsion tricky. Labour was particularly quick and intense, but it ended well: Lou was born healthy at home, as expected, and Sofia was fine. Isabelle recounted how she coached Sofia during the expulsion stage. She explained being caught between her willingness to transmit "power and trust to the woman" and "the traumatic images of what would happen in the hospital and saying to oneself, 'No, we are not in the hospital. We must do otherwise'".

In the extract above, Isabelle suggested that the delivery would not have ended as well in the maternity ward. The baby might have been removed with forceps or a ventouse, or perhaps via caesarean section. Despite her strong experience of out-of-hospital deliveries, Isabelle still struggled to control her fear and focus on the situation to analyse it efficiently and assist Sofia. As "an emotional expression of risk culture" (Perrenoud 2014: 146), fear interferes with clinical practices, and midwives must learn how to handle it to not let it drive their decisions and actions.

During delivery, Isabelle encouraged Sofia to stand and keep moving her pelvis. From Isabelle's perspective, the lack of technical devices at home facilitates the avoidance of unnecessary and potentially harmful interventions but also requires her to be inventive and not to rely on the devices institutions use to manage labour. Moreover, in midwives' and parents' discourses, hospital care and routines are perceived as a risk factor regarding breastfeeding initiation and the smooth course of breastfeeding in the long term.

> Jeanne was an employee in the health sector. She was in her early thirties. She had planned to give birth to her first baby at home with Odile, her midwife. Her partner lived in Colombia and was not able to come to Switzerland for the birth. Jeanne planned to join him a few months after their son's birth. She was transferred to the hospital during childbirth because of labour stagnation, which led to her exhaustion. She underwent a caesarean section under general anaesthesia because the epidural did not work properly. Before my first meeting with Jeanne, Odile told me on the phone that since leaving the maternity ward a week earlier, Jeanne's son, Nils, had "lost quite a lot of weight". Jeanne felt quite distressed during the immediate postpartum period and preferred to be alone with Odile at the time of the first visits after her return home. I met her ten days after Nils's birth, at her home, during one of Odile's postnatal visits. Jeanne told us to sit on her bed, like her. Nils was calm and relaxed in her arms. She and Odile began discussing the unforeseen and undesirable birth circumstances.

> Jeanne regretted not having been sufficiently prepared for her four-day postpartum hospital stay: "The only regret I have is that I was not prepared for it. For me, a caesarean section was impossible. If I had to do it again, I am sure that I would do as I want with this breastfeeding. I did not have enough confidence in myself. I had not thought enough about it. Even at the prenatal [service], I would have said, 'Ask a midwife to come. I do not want him to have a syringe [of formula], but my colostrum'". During their hospital stay, Nils reached a weight loss of 7 percent. One night, a midwife asked Jeanne to give Nils a syringe of formula milk. Jeanne declined at first, so the midwife called a paediatrician to support her advice. Jeanne said, "I had the feeling that I was seen as a bad mother who thinks more about her breastfeeding than about her baby's needs". Odile asked, given the undesired circumstances, "What could have been helpful during [birth] preparation for breastfeeding?" She explained that when she was trying to address the possibility of a transfer to the hospital—and even a caesarean section—parents who had prepared themselves for natural delivery had a hard time listening. She wondered how this could be brought into the discussion without being too stressful for the parents. Jeanne had no answer, but told her, "It made me feel so good when you came [to the maternity ward]!" She also observed that "it is true that I was very confident, in fact. I trusted my body".

The strong distrust of the hospital institution and the need to be prepared at best to avoid the pitfalls of medical interventions and hospital protocols highlighted in the section above were recurring elements in my fieldwork. My observations thus join those of other researchers, in Switzerland (Gouilhers-Hertig 2014, 2017), other European countries (Cheyney 2008; Fage-Butler 2017; Sjöblom, Nordström & Edberg 2006), and the United States (Boucher et al. 2009), who found that home birth parents attempt to protect themselves and their baby from iatrogenic risks caused by hospital birth management and medical interventionism. By choosing to give birth out of the hospital, they aim to prevent interventions perceived as potentially harmful and threatening to the integrity of the maternal and infant bodies, such as episiotomies, epidurals, instrumental births, or caesarean sections. These procedures, especially caesarean section, were also thought to be impediments to breastfeeding initiation. Caesarean section usually involves a delay in the first physical contact between the mother and the baby, and therefore the first latching at the mother's breast, hindering the initiation of breastfeeding.[6] Home birth parents identify their midwives as allies who can help them navigate the "traps" of hospital protocols. Moreover, they have faith in their midwives' commitment to the physiology of birth and trust their judgement if they consider it necessary to intervene medically or to transfer a parturient to the maternity ward.

Midwives also agree and reinforce the conception of the home—or birth centre—as a safer environment for a physiological birth and the postpartum period. For midwives and parents, giving birth out of the hospital allows for "a passive protective effect consisting in avoiding any exposure to a risk environment" (Gouilhers-Hertig 2017: 354). Moreover, Gouilhers-Hertig (2014) identified "a process of risks subjectification", by which home birth mothers "prioritise their values and lived experience, which, according to them, are little integrated in the dominant patterns for risk classification" (2011). From this perspective, hospital management of birth focuses on medical and physical risks but increases emotional risks to the mother and the newborn.

Maud, a new mother, explained her choice to give birth in a birth centre: "I'm afraid of hospitals. I do not really trust their methods. Women are not actresses. Women are ripped from their deliveries by making them passive". During her pregnancy, reading out-of-hospital birth stories reinforced her decision. "At last", she said, "I had positive feedback on delivery because everyone tells you only negative things. It was good to read nice stories. It gave me courage". Jelena also reported that she was told she was courageous for giving birth out of the hospital. However, she said, "I don't think I'm brave. I think they are brave to go to the hospital and have a hospital stay". More specifically, several women told me that they had chosen out-of-hospital birth to ensure safe, effective breastfeeding initiation. In their minds, giving birth out of the maternity ward was a way to avoid interventions perceived as potentially damaging, such as supplementing newborns with formula.

Catherine felt very frustrated with her two previous breastfeeding experiences, which ended much earlier than she had planned. She attributed these failures to poor management of breastfeeding initiation at the maternity ward, and she chose to give birth to her third child at home. In particular, she hoped for a more satisfying breastfeeding experience. Two days after her son's birth, Catherine was anxious. She had a crack on her nipple, and latching was quite painful. She worried about the long-term success of breastfeeding and had already asked her midwife if she would be able to see a lactation consultant after the end of her postpartum follow-up if breastfeeding remained problematic. Her midwife reassured her that it was only the third day after birth, and the postpartum follow-up would last as long as Catherine needed it. For this consultation, she did not find it necessary to weigh the baby. Catherine expressed her relief: "I am very happy not to be at the maternity ward. There, he would already be completed with syringes of formula".

Other women had mixed feelings about their postpartum hospital experiences, especially regarding breastfeeding initiation. Lauriane had planned to give birth to her first child in a birth centre, but she eventually had to be transferred to the maternity ward due to labour stagnation and exhaustion. She described the first latch right after delivery as "traumatic, constrained by force". She deplored poor breastfeeding support: "[The midwives] were very nice at the maternity ward, but for breastfeeding ... I'm lucky I had no problem". Lisa had gestational diabetes and was forced to abandon her out-of-hospital birth project. Despite her abundant colostrum supply, she was under pressure from hospital staff to supplement her newborn with formula, which she refused: "He never had hypoglycaemia, but it's very guilt-inducing. I told them what I thought anyway. If you follow their protocols, it messes up your breastfeeding. Even knowing what I wanted, they are ultra-guilt-inducing". According to Inès, "hospital standards mean that natural breastfeeding does not seem to fit the norm at all because you must have milk two hours after giving birth. Midwives all have different discourses, and as a woman who has just given birth, you are a little weakened. If you have not thought about it, it's hard to keep some consistency after that". Christophe, her spouse, added, "At home, the midwife can do individualised work".

If midwives and parents perceived the hospital as a hazardous environment for delivery that threatened the mothers' and babies' physical and emotional integrity, they applied the same logic to breastfeeding initiation. Reciprocally, holistic care was considered a way to promote and protect breastfeeding. This protective effect was attributed not only to the avoidance of hospital protocols but also to the midwife's guidance and reassurance, which could be maintained even in case of hospital birth. For example, in both situations of gestational diabetes I followed, the midwives had suggested the mothers express some colostrum before birth and bring a syringe to the hospital. As a result, the newborns did not receive any maltodextrin solution,[7] which the parents appreciated very much.

Depending on the place of birth, midwives and parents confronted two opposing logics regarding breastfeeding and weight gain management. On the one hand, the institutional logic, based on a biomedical risk management model framed by rigid protocols, calls for the supplementation of newborns as soon as they approach a 10 per cent weight loss. On the other hand, the holistic care logic prioritises breastfeeding and its good initiation. This tension was expressed in the above extract when Jeanne, during her hospital stay, felt that hospital staff perceived her "as a bad mother who thinks more about her breastfeeding than about her baby's needs". Here, the mother's commitment to breastfeeding success is perceived as in competition with her baby's health and needs, whereas breastfeeding is presented by public health agencies as well as nutrition and child health experts as the most appropriate infant feeding mode. Some critical authors point out that the biomedical model establishes a separation between the mother and the newborn, whose needs and interests are not necessarily compatible, and might even be antagonistic (Davis-Floyd 1992; Katz Rothman 2007b; Martin 1987). At home, midwives care for mother and child as "an interdependent unit" whose needs are seen as complementary (Katz Rothman 2007b: 73). In my fieldwork, midwives constantly tried to reassure mothers about their breastfeeding success and their newborn's well-being, which was mainly expressed through a non-weight-centred evaluation of breastfeeding.

Assessing breastfeeding "success"

Even though breastfeeding is recognised as the best choice for feeding babies, it also generates specific concerns, especially because accurately quantifying the amount of milk babies ingest is difficult, leading to a perceived lack of control over their weight gain. Contemporary biomedical culture values seeing more than feeling, especially in the area of perinatal care. During pregnancy and childbirth, women are already used to feeling dependent on the "visual check", which validates their incorporated experience. In the context of breastfeeding, these checks translate into a careful monitoring of infants' weight gain (Dykes 2006). Regular weighing of the baby appears as the only way to determine the amount of milk ingested; in other words, the child's weight gain is considered objective evidence of good health and of the nursing's success (Dykes 2005; Maher 1992). From this perspective, the infant's body and growth become evidence of maternal skills, whereas lower weight gain is interpreted as a failure of breastfeeding and a sign of maternal incompetence (Lupton 1996 in Dykes & Williams 1999). Because parents are rarely equipped with a suitable scale, infants are most often weighed by professionals. Although it can be perceived as reassuring for parents to know their child's precise weight, the excessive promotion of this indicator, to the detriment of other qualitative indicators such as the child's behaviour, reinforces mothers' feelings of incompetence. Rather than learning to trust their feelings, they rely on experts' evaluations (Dykes & Williams 1999; Marshall, Godfrey & Renfrew 2007).

At the maternity ward, protocols require daily weighing of the baby. At home, depending on the midwives' preference, the newborn might not be weighed systematically. Weighing practices varied from one midwife to another. Some preferred to stick to hospital protocols, as Odile explained to me: "I start on the basis of the protocols, I follow the protocols as much as possible so that I won't get blamed [by the parents or by the paediatrician]". She weighed babies systematically if they were awake at the time of the midwife's visit and noted, "It also allows me to see them naked and to check their colour, and it is not annoying if, the next day, they are asleep". Odile affirmed that she allowed weight loss "up to 10 percent without worries" and stopped weighing babies every day once their weight began to rise. Odile was aware that some of her colleagues took more freedom regarding protocols and observed that "everyone has their own limits". However, she admitted that she was becoming increasingly flexible with experience. When Odile started midwifery school, she already planned to attend home births and practise holistic care. After graduation, as she did not have the opportunity to work as an assistant to an established independent midwife. Instead, she completed two years of hospital practice before starting her independent practice. She described this period in the hospital as a constraining time, during which she often felt frustrated by institutional rules and management. However, rather than her hospital experience, Odile attributed her very cautious attitude regarding infant weight gain to her personality and described herself as not very self-confident. Moreover, beyond each midwife's judgement and sensitivity, weighing frequency was also related to the baby's age. Weighing was more frequent during the first ten days after birth, which fitted into a formal logic based on a risks objectification.

A postpartum consultation usually included a feed. While feeding, midwives invited mothers to engage in clinical observation by making them attentive to the movements of the baby's temple indicating full jaw engagement, to the muscular relaxation that occurs as the feeling of satiety settles or to the sounds indicating swallowing or contentment. For example, Anne, a midwife, said to a mother, "Do you hear that sound? That's all good, all done!" In addition to this careful observation, midwives referred to other indicators, such as babies' alternating sleep and "calm awakening" phases[8] or the fact that they urinated regularly. For Capucine, another midwife, referring to these qualitative indicators gave mothers a sense of control and competence: "If you only refer to the scale, it can be destabilising because control comes from the outside". According to her perspective, "weight is just the last piece of information, just curiosity", as well as a matter of parent empowerment: "I do not want them to keep the idea that we doubt ourselves as long as we do not have the scale weight". In her postpartum follow-up, Adeline also sought to put the weight information into perspective. She dissuaded parents from using the scale, saying, "You must not enter into the cycle of fear", and she assured them that it is normal for a healthy baby to have weight gain plateau.

All of my interlocutors were very critical of the practice of daily, systematic newborn weighing. "We are not frantic about babies who only gain ten grams per day", said Chantal on the behalf of her and her colleagues. However, what was considered a "beautiful weight gain" would always be emphasised by exclamations and encouragement from the midwives. Chantal explained to me that she "says something when there is a nice weight gain and nothing when it's not really good" to protect the breastfeeding mother, who may feel directly responsible.

A qualitative assessment of breastfeeding also included considering it as a relational and reciprocal process between mother and child. Midwives encouraged mothers to "trust" their children. For example, Capucine said, "We do not see what we give, and we cannot quantify. One of the breastfeeding rules is a blind trust of your baby. They adjust when they need to eat, how much and how". This idea breaks with the dominant biomedical approach, which considers breastfeeding primarily as a transfer of milk, targeting a rapid weight gain and linear growth curve.

> When I first met Carole and Michael, Gaspard, their son, had been born a few days before in the maternity ward. They had chosen to be followed by an independent midwife during pregnancy, but they did not feel comfortable giving birth out of the hospital. Both were in their early thirties. Carole was an HR professional. Michael was an employee in the construction sector. They lived in a small village in the countryside. Carole's delivery unfolded quickly and smoothly. Nevertheless, they were disturbed by advice received in the maternity ward, recommending that they "stimulate" Gaspard during feeding to prevent him from falling asleep and to put him at the breast for fifteen minutes every four hours. Once home, Carole and Michael were glad to get back to Capucine, their midwife, for the postpartum follow-up. When we arrived, Carole was feeding Gaspard in the living room. Capucine made her attentive to the swallowing noises, saying, "He suckles very well. That's a more important sign than watching the clock and saying, 'It's good. He's been suckling for fifteen minutes'". Carole was not convinced: "I tell myself, 'We'll see the scale. It will tell'". When Gaspard finished his feed, Capucine observed, "There, you see how he suckled? He withdraws from the breast. He's fine, he's a happy baby". To weigh Gaspard, we moved to the parental bedroom, which also served as Gaspard's bedroom, where the changing table was set with diapers and clothes. He had not gained weight since the last weighing three days before. Capucine reassured Carole, "We see lots of very reassuring signs with Gaspard. [...] He's fine. He's not starving. He's well hydrated". She referred to "the more or less demanding nature of each child" to justify the weight stagnation.

Capucine reminded the parents that each individual is unique and proposed adjusting to Gaspard's demands: "I don't want to tell you to wake him up to eat". She instead suggested giving him "the possibility of wanting more easily" by favouring moments when he was "near the breasts" and offering them to him when he seemed interested.

A few days later, Capucine weighed Gaspard again and found that he had regained weight. She commented, "He's gaining weight; it rises harmoniously. There are standards, and then there is each individual". Carole, visibly relieved, congratulated Gaspard, "Good job!" Capucine showed her satisfaction, too, but added, "I'm glad to see that he gained weight, but we will not stick to weight curves".

For midwives, a critical stance regarding weight control was also a way to distance themselves from hospital practices and affirm the specificity of the holistic care they provided. On this topic, Pauline commented, "Risk is part of a global vision and is not related to protocols, like in a situation where you don't know people's path". Indeed, midwives supported an individualistic and contextualised evaluation of each child's development.

Milo was born at home with a low birth weight—under three kilograms—and lacked coordination during feeds, a behaviour identified by Anne, the midwife, as "disorganised". Milo's inability to suckle effectively resulted in a weight loss approaching the 10 percent limit, followed by weight stagnation. After ten days of close collaboration between Anne and the parents, the baby's weight increased, and his ability to suckle improved. Anne insisted on the specificity of the postpartum follow-up outside the hospital, adding, "With a weight like that, in the hospital, we'd be immediately trapped by the protocols". For a fortnight, Milo, who was not very demanding, was fed every three hours at the breast, then with a syringe of breast milk or a supplemental nursing system fixed on the finger. In the end, he was never supplemented with formula, but with a little "sweet water" (maltodextrin solution) during his first days of life to avoid hypoglycaemia. "It takes a lot of patience", concluded Anne.

As mentioned above, in many Swiss hospitals and in accordance with the Swiss Society of Neonatology recommendations (2007), all full-term newborns with a birth weight of less than three kilograms are systematically subjected to a protocol intended for newborns at risk for hypoglycaemia. In the situation described above, Anne did not push the baby's parents to supplement him with formula, but she subscribed to the hospital protocol of giving him maltodextrin solution. In an institutional context, the application of protocols responds to a logic of risk management that, to Anne's regret, results in care standardisation to the detriment of clinical examination that considers the uniqueness of each individual. Here, Anne found a happy medium by abandoning certain aspects of the protocol but retaining others. This example is a good illustration of midwives' endeavouring to find their own risk management methods by compromising between their desire to act as keepers of normal birth and institutional points of reference from which they cannot easily distance themselves.

Emotional weighing, indifference and reassurance

Sachs (2005, 2013) conducted an ethnographic study in the United Kingdom in a child health clinic that included longitudinal interviews with breastfeeding mothers. She observed that baby weighing was at the heart of both mothers' and professionals' expectations:

> The measure of baby well-being appears to have been reduced to a recorded weight gain trajectory which follows a centile on the chart, with the fiftieth centile seen as the most desirable. Women appear to value the reassurance of seeing the plotted weight and to be prepared to sacrifice breastfeeding in order to maintain the line.
>
> (Sachs 2005: 214)

In my fieldwork, home birth parents and independent midwives developed a critical stance regarding systematic weighing resulting from their unshakable trust in the physiological birth process. Léa felt very confident about her milk supply and her daughter's weight gain, whereas her midwife proposed weighing her daughter on her first visit after Léa returned home from a caesarean section birth. Léa observed, "It doesn't make me stressed at all. I see that she suckles very well. I am super confident". As a baby, her mother breastfed her. "She said to me, 'You'll see; you'll have a lot of milk'. I have a lot of milk". For some mothers, this confidence translated into an obvious indifference towards their baby's weight. Céline explained to me, "I have no interest in knowing the weight of my baby. I'm not asking you how much you weigh; why should I know how much your baby weighs?" Another mother, Sarah, criticised the prevalence of quantitative assessment over parents' feelings: "I have little interest in weight. I don't realise what it means. I trust what we feel. We are not barometers. We are not machines". Laurence emphasised her observations to assess her daughter's well-being:

> Whenever people ask me, I say, "I don't know. I can't tell you how much she weighs". I do not care. I see in her if she is well or not, and that is enough for me. I don't know, maybe it's stupid that I think that, and it's unfounded, but I tell myself that as long as she is at the breast, I do not have to worry that she does not receive enough or that she receives too much. I've never said that to myself, and I am very much in tune with my feelings. I feel that she is well, that she is thriving.
>
> (interview with Laurence, transcription)

Laurence's thoughts are in line with the midwives' holistic care approach. During pregnancy follow-up, only two ultrasounds are usually prescribed (a dating ultrasound during the first trimester and a morphology ultrasound during the second trimester) and paid for by health insurance, whereas obstetricians generally perform an ultrasound at each consultation. During prenatal consultations, uterine height is gauged using a tape measure, which facilitates estimation of the foetus' growth, and specific palpation manoeuvres make it possible to determine its position. This limited use of technology makes it possible to detach oneself from the culture of seeing and the logic of systematic controls aimed at producing numerical data, and to rehabilitate clinical examination and midwives' experiential knowledge, as well as parents' observations and feelings.

The trust demonstrated by home birth parents in the physiology of birth and the capacity of women's bodies to give birth without medical intervention (Sjöblom, Nordström & Eldberg 2006) extends to postpartum processes and to newborns' bodies. Some parents refused to give any supplements to their newborns, such as the widely used vitamin K.[9] For example, Daniela and her spouse did not agree to give vitamins K and D to their baby. They thought there must be a reason for newborns to have very low vitamin K levels, and they were opposed to the urge of "always wanting to normalise them to adult values". Daniela wondered, "Why do we have to interfere all the time?"

As Broderick (2016) notes, giving birth at home is a "subversive act" that is part of a broader thought system: "Home birth is wedded into a much larger stratum of intentionality and resistance that attempts to disrupt the conventional social imaginary" (380). Through home birthing, parents "tried to disrupt the modern-technical temporal rhythm that reduces everything into isolated parts" (ibid. 2016: 380). They refused the fragmented biomedical perspective on the birth process and did not consider the newborn an unfinished human being who requires medical intervention and surveillance to function adequately.

Midwives encouraged parents to assess their child's well-being based on their observations and feelings and to detach themselves not only from the scale but also from shared representations of healthy babies. During a consultation, Odile and Lucie, a new mother, took a critical look at "the ideal of the chubby baby, who sleeps systematically after each feed". Odile regretted that this kind of stereotype could lead mothers to question whether their situation seems too far from this ideal. Four months after Gaspard's birth, Carole and Michael were still "always a little worried about his weight", said Michael. According to him, this might have been related to the fact that their friends would "rather have Michelin men",[10] whereas Gaspard was thinner. Again, the ideal of the chubby baby distorted their perception. Carole said, "It is very disturbing to situate him on a curve. It's very easy for people to make us lose confidence in our child. I was glad to hear Capucine repeatedly say that insufficiently nourishing breast milk is a myth". She concluded, "Fortunately, Capucine was there, because otherwise we would have been totally anxious. Capucine emphasises notions of self-confidence and trust in your child and in their ability to not starve to death".

When parents seemed too eager to know their baby's weight, midwives interpreted this as a sign of unusual anxiety, which alarmed them and prompted them to investigate the cause of this concern.

> Lisa, a social worker, was married to Alexis, who worked as a teacher. Both were in their early thirties. After a first traumatic hospital delivery that was heavy on medical intervention, they planned to give birth to their second child at a birth centre. However, this project fell through when Lisa was diagnosed with gestational diabetes. Her labour began at home with their midwife, Eva, before moving to the hospital. Eva was allowed to stay with Lisa, thanks to the flexibility and comprehension of the staff. Lisa was pleased with the way her delivery took place due to Eva's unexpected presence. She said, "We slipped through the protocols net".
>
> Two days later, Lisa was back at home. Eva and I arrived together for the first postpartum visit, which took place in the parental room while Alexis was taking care of their eldest daughter in another room. Eva asked Lisa if she agreed to an examination of her breasts in my presence. Lisa gave her consent. Eva carefully observed her breasts' coloration and palpated them to verify their suppleness. Some milk was immediately expressed, and she commented in a humorous tone, "It flows very easily; you'll be able to feed your baby!" Eva was aware that Lisa's first breastfeeding's experience was a bitter disappointment and tried to reassure her. Because Lisa's daughter, Angèle, never managed to properly latch and suckle, Lisa expressed her milk and administered it using a bottle. "After a month, I stopped because it was too depressing", said Lisa. She told us that she dreaded her son Paul's first latch: "In fact, he immediately took it. It really relieved me. Then he suckled for an hour after going back to the room, so I thought it would not be the same, but I had a profound fear".
>
> Three weeks after Paul's birth, Eva was still following up with this family. Before our arrival at Lisa's home, Eva confided her feeling of disempowerment. She regretted that Lisa did not openly express her feelings. As a result, Eva feared that she could not support her efficiently. During Eva's previous visit, Lisa had told her that Alexis was "very little invested" in caring for Paul. Lisa welcomed us without Alexis. She was still very insecure about her breastfeeding, despite her son's regular weight gain. After discussing on the frequency of feeds, which worried Lisa because she interpreted it as a sign of Paul's hunger and dissatisfaction, Eva proposed to weigh Paul.

Eva: "Regarding the weight gain level, he's perfect, really. At three point eight kilograms, we can't ask any more of him".

Lisa: "So how should I do to do better? I know that I'm stressed for nothing ..."

Eva: "Not for nothing, but now it's up to you to say how you feel if you want to change things. Breastfeeding is about always asking yourself questions like 'Do I give enough? Is it the right rhythm?' Is this something you can discuss with Alexis?"

Lisa: (Crying) "I don't dare to talk to anyone anymore because I do not want to annoy people".

Eva: "For me, it's important that I adapt to your project because breastfeeding is also about sharing a pleasure".

Lisa: "I'm always worried about my supply ... but it does not bother me that he suckles every two hours if he's happy that way".

Eva: "My help is limited if you don't express your desires more clearly, aside from coming with the scale, but it does not answer everything ..."

In the situation described here, Eva felt helpless because of Lisa's reservations. She did not know how to help her. From my observations, a significant part of the independent midwives' follow-up involved listening to mothers' feelings and reassuring them. For example, one midwife, Chantal, told me that holistic care was "very much about feelings". In the event of a breastfeeding problem, she asked the mother, "How do you feel about that?" She also reported that she relied heavily on mothers' empirical observations, which she considered "generally very accurate". For her, concerning the use of interventions in the newborn's growth monitoring, "it's a matter of synergy between the mother and the midwife that pushes in one direction or another".

Despite this emphasis on mothers' feelings and perceptions of their child's well-being, weighing babies remained a mandatory part of midwives' jobs during the postpartum follow-ups, and part of their role was to ensure the baby's health. As Capucine explained, "the moment you set foot in a situation, you have to refer to something". From this perspective, she said, "completely neglecting the weight would be a mistake".

"Weighing" risks in holistic care

In some cases of breastfed babies' failure to thrive, midwives had to question their position and challenge their comprehensive and individual approach to babies' weight gain. These "grey zone" areas allowed me to highlight the negotiation between midwives and parents.

Céline was a stay-at-home mother. Julien, her spouse, was an employee in the transportation sector. Both were in their mid-thirties. They lived in a small city apartment. I met Céline at a La Leche League meeting when she was pregnant with her second child.[11] Her midwife, Odile, had already told her about my research and asked if she was willing to participate. Before becoming pregnant with Yvonne, their first daughter, Céline had been treated for endometriosis. Regarding this process, Julien observed, "We waited for Yvonne for five years and we had time to get ready, so we did some work on ourselves". They designed a home birth project and developed specific thoughts about infant care practices, including breastfeeding and bed-sharing.

Céline and Julien welcomed their second daughter, Morgane, at home in the evening with Odile, their doula, and Yvonne. Céline sent me a message early in the morning inviting me to join Odile's first postpartum visit a few hours later. When I arrived at their home, Céline and Julien were thrilled after their smooth and peaceful home birth. They had also planned a home birth for Yvonne but eventually had to be transferred to the hospital because of a very long labour stage during which Céline developed exhaustion. Céline and Julien reflected on the events of the previous evening with me. Julien said to Céline, "What amazed me compared to the first time is that you gave me the impression of having gone through hell, and a second later, you were radiant, happy, available". Céline smiled and said, "At eleven o'clock, we were all together on the bed eating chocolate cake". She concluded, "It was so logical, so natural". Julien added three weeks off to his two weeks of paid paternal leave so he would be with Céline for the first five weeks of Morgane's life. Breastfeeding their eldest, Yvonne, went very smoothly. It was a positive experience, so Céline felt very confident. Even if she had noticed that her supply eventually dried up at some time during her pregnancy, she had never stopped breastfeeding Yvonne. For Morgane's breastfeeding, she had not planned to do anything special to stimulate the lactation process. "I am confident", she affirmed.

Two days after birth, Morgane was sleeping at the time of Odile's visit. She saw no need to weigh Morgane "given how she suckles and what you told me ..." A few days later, the scale indicated that she was losing weight. Odile and the parents stayed confident because she had just eliminated and had not yet eaten. Céline affirmed, "I'm not worried". Odile proposed, "We have two options: either I weigh her again tomorrow, or on Thursday". "It does not matter to me", Céline answered. "I'm not afraid". However, Julien disagreed: "I would not be against your coming tomorrow". Morgane continued to lose weight in the following days. First, Odile suggested putting her at the breast more often, then pumping and giving her the pumped milk in addition to each feed. Worried about preserving her baby's suckling skills, Céline refused to use a bottle and chose to give her the extra milk with a supplemental nursing system attached to the breast. As Morgane's weight still did not increase, Odile phoned the paediatrician to ask his opinion. He advised immediate supplementation with formula. Céline was now worried, too, but she was not yet resigned to giving Morgane formula.

When I meet with Céline and Julien two weeks later, the baby was receiving formula in addition to pumped breast milk and breastfeeding sessions. Her weight had increased. Céline commented on the paediatrician's reaction, "When he learned the tandem breastfeeding, he freaked out. He is pro-breastfeeding, but he doesn't get a bloody thing".[12] "The phone call to the paediatrician is also a way to not be alone in this situation to make a decision", observed Julien, justifying Odile's decision to involve the paediatrician. Céline was still shocked by her daughter's failure to gain weight: "It annoyed me, especially since breastfeeding is something I happened to know!" She found support from her La Leche League group, where her local leader lent her the supplemental nursing system. Julien was confused by the incompatibility of the various advice they received and said, "It is completely contradictory, what is proposed on one side and on the other". He was surprised that their anthroposophic paediatrician, who approved their non-vaccination stance, opposed tandem nursing and advised breastfeeding Morgane on schedule. The local La Leche League leader approved of tandem nursing because it stimulated Céline's lactation and recommended feeding Morgane on demand. Odile's position was between the two, but she aligned with the paediatrician's advice to supplement Morgane with formula until her weight stabilised.

A few months later, I met Céline and Julien again, and we reflected on these events and the underlying decision-making process. Morgane was now back to exclusive breastfeeding, and Céline was still astonished: "I gave formula, the thing I never thought I would do. To give this first feed of formula was very hard. Once it's done, you get used to it, I saw that it was okay, that it did not change her behaviour, but it was out of the question to give formula with a bottle!" Céline and Julien remembered conversations they had with Odile. Julien explained, "Initially, she really let us decide [...] what do you want to do? What period do we set?" After ten days without weight gain, she insisted on supplementation with formula. The parents explained that dialogue was constant at every stage, and Odile came every day. They first negotiated to delay the introduction of formula, then the amount: "We were involved in everything that was done", said Julien. During this troubled time, they also relied on their doula's support. Céline reported, "She's more inclined to let go. I think that, in my place, she wouldn't have got worked up like I did, but she was a good support, very good moral support" adding, "She reminded me 'Your milk is what it is, and it is perfectly adapted to your baby' ". Céline and Julien went to see the paediatrician for the four-month consultation the day before our meeting. Céline commented, "I think he forgot that she had weight issues. I did not want to bring it back up, not with him. He does not know enough about [breastfeeding]".

I also revisited this situation with Odile, who admitted, "When it matters so much to them, it's complicated to manage". She explained that it is important to her to give parents time to change their perspective on the situation. They often end up realising the problem by themselves, based on their baby's behaviour. She concluded, "Some people need to make their own way, so we walk with them as long as it takes".

This extract reveals a risk management method specific to the holistic care model: midwives and parents attempting, simultaneously, to maintain breastfeeding and to avoid any danger to the baby. In addition, midwives have to manage risks to their career: if the weight issue is detrimental to a baby's health, they must be able to justify their actions. Because they practise outside the institutional context of the hospital, midwives are on their own to define the limits of non-intervention and the level of risk that is acceptable. By giving parents time and negotiating with them at every step, midwives restore their position as full actors in the decision-making process concerning the management of unsatisfactory baby weight gain. Odile's involvement is reflected in her words. Even if she knew early on which action she would eventually like to implement, she agreed to "walk with them as long as it takes", accompanying the parents in their daily reflections and practices. This approach meets Mol's definition of care:

Caring does not mean intervening on bodies to treat diseases or to choose not to intervene. In contrast, caring means taking charge of day-to-day life. It is an activity that, one way or another, is shared. It does not depend on a single choice, but on the contrary on persistent efforts. Caring means tenacity, inventiveness and solicitude.

(Mol 2009: 11)

Mol (2009) criticised the individual choice ideal that dominates neoliberal societies, including biomedicine, and opposed this logic of choice with a "logic of care". In the logic of choice, choices are made at specific times, whereas the "logic of care" allows for continuous adjustments between daily concrete exigencies and care interventions. For midwives, committing themselves to caring for a family during the perinatal period is a matter of tinkering and requires permanent readjustments to follow parents' wishes and projects without compromising their work ethic and agenda.

Sachs (2005) pointed out that body techniques aimed at improving the effectiveness of breastfeeding were rarely implemented by health professionals during her fieldwork in cases of failure to thrive. The most common interventions were breast milk expression to give it to the child using a bottle or supplementation with formula milk. These interventions aim to objectify the milk quantity absorbed, but they do not address why the baby is failing to thrive.

In Sachs' study, the professionals' and mothers' objective was the baby's weight gain; the maintenance of breastfeeding was secondary. In my field-work, weight loss or weight stagnation was perceived as a symptom of a breastfeeding issue rather than as a problem in itself. Thus, the proposed solution was not to supplement the baby but to observe latching and act on breastfeeding practices to optimise the baby's breast milk supply. Pauline enumerated the measures she set up in cases of weight stagnation as follows: "First, on-demand breastfeeding, a good latch, observing the baby's dynamics at the breast, breast compression, putting the baby at the same breast at the next feed to start with the fat.[13] Afterwards, breast-pumping and supplementing the child with the pumped milk, once it is found that the child cannot stimulate enough". The situation below illustrates Pauline's commitment to "give breastfeeding a chance", which implied taking a step back from protocols.

> In a situation of weight stagnation, Aurore, a new mother, asked Pauline, "How serious is it?" Her two-week-old daughter, Margaux, had not gained any weight since birth. Pauline reassured her, "The reason is right in front of us [Margaux's short tongue frenulum, which caused poor stimulation and inefficient milk transfer]. There is no other serious reason". She said again to the parents, "For me, it's okay that she only regains her birth weight at three weeks". She suggested, "Give breastfeeding a chance. Find a balance between what might be suitable for breastfeeding, for you, for Margaux".

Inadequate weight gain also forces midwives to face the limits of the model of care they defend. One of them, Capucine, told me she felt "betrayed" when she first faced a situation of failure to thrive. The underlying belief was that if a physiological childbirth project succeeds, lactation and breast-feeding should succeed physiologically as well. She said, "It's the situation that betrayed me, which showed me that I have to remain vigilant beyond observation". Capucine felt she could trust her observations and the parents' feelings to some extent, "but the scale remains a necessary confirmation".

> I have hoped that this would not be the case, but it is. For me, it's hor-rible to imagine that you cannot have absolute confidence in your body. The more you trust yourself, the more difficult it is to enter this grey area, and it is even more difficult for [midwives] to come to a diagnosis and introduce interventions.
>
> (interview with Capucine, notes)

Each experience leads midwives to reposition themselves regarding the advice they give and to revaluate their practices. A few months after our last visit to Céline, Julien and Morgane, I accompanied Odile for the follow-up of another family experiencing newborn weight stagnation. She confided to me, "This [previous] situation made me review the advice I give", and she added, "In this case, we have to move on", implying that after this follow-up, she would be more prompt to implement actions to accelerate a baby's weight gain.

Well-versed parents negotiating boundaries

Critical reflection on biomedical birth and postpartum management leads parents to choose holistic care, following their engagement in "work on themselves", as described above by Julien. Their birth project is the subject of reflection and a particular elaboration, and they consider breastfeeding part of this continuity. Consequently, home birth parents actively seek information, and they do not necessarily regard their midwives as their first resources on breastfeeding.

Several mothers I met found answers to their questions through a Facebook group formed by breastfeeding mothers around concerns related to breastfeeding.[14] A number of the moderators and most of the group's active members were La Leche League leaders or participants. Christine, a mother breastfeeding her third baby, would have liked to participate in local La Leche League meetings, but the meeting schedule was inconvenient:

> So the Facebook group was much easier for me because I posted my question, and I had a lot of opinions, you see. I did not only have one view from one person. Sometimes, I had several opinions or several assumptions. [...] You say, 'I have this and that as symptoms. What can it be? Well, it can be this, it can be that, it could also be that, you see, for example ... I had a mother who tested this. Give it a go; it seems to work well!' Well, that's what I liked a lot, and these moms are really ... ultra-well-versed, really, at a level ... (laughs) Frankly, they only rely on ... they are always reading things related to lactation. That's it.
>
> (interview with Christine, transcription)

Medical publications on specific topics such as galactogenic drugs or the link between toddlers' dental cavities and breastfeeding were uploaded regularly in a section of this Facebook group. For mothers, this space constituted a virtual breastfeeding support platform. Apart from this group, mothers often read specific literature on breastfeeding on their own initiative.[15] With this background, mothers could appreciate their midwives' advice, but they also had the ability to question it when it appeared at odds with their own knowledge.

When I returned with Céline and Julien to Morgane's failure to thrive and the way they negotiated with Odile, Julien informed me that "a similar situation" had already occurred when Yvonne, their eldest daughter, was born: "She gave us advice, and we did not follow it". Céline explained that she had to say no to Odile because she knew she had better knowledge about breastfeeding and the physiology of lactation. Although Yvonne was slow to gain weight after birth, Odile advised allowing at least two hours between feeds. Yvonne cried for about forty-five minutes during this imposed delay. At the next consultation, as Yvonne had still not gained weight, Odile suggested three-hour intervals. Céline refused and decided to breastfeed on demand again and noted that "she was plugged twenty-four–seven". She explained to me that "a baby that suckles more often has more fat milk than if they have a big feed every three hours". Yvonne's weight indeed increased, and Odile took note for future situations.

However, in the case of this new postpartum follow-up, at some point, Odile estimated that it was necessary that Céline and Julien give Morgane a formula supplement. "After ten days without weight gain, when she saw that my way was not working, she told me that she would not allow any more waiting", said Céline. Julien added, "We wanted to push back as much as possible".

The well-established relationship between the midwife and the parents also enables them to discuss and express doubts if something is not right for the parents or for the midwife. During consultations, the midwife leaves room for questioning and encourages parents to follow their ideas based on their in-depth knowledge and observation of their baby, as well as their experiential knowledge.

"Do what you feel is right for you. You are the ones who know best!" was a statement that recurred regularly in the midwives' speech. In this way, parents' feelings were considered valuable sources of non-intellectual, embodied knowledge, as demonstrated by other studies regarding out-of-hospital birth (Cheyney 2008, Sjöblom et al. 2012). The notion of experiential knowledge thus also extended to parents, as some of them had acquired a solid appreciation of newborns' behaviour through their parenting experience, as well as through other personal or professional experiences. In particular, this sensory knowledge was developed through the interaction between their child's body and their own body. From birth, constant exposure to their newborn's gestures, sounds, expressions, and smells sharpened their perception of their babies' unease or well-being.

In other situations, midwives encouraged parents to keep trying—"to give breastfeeding a chance", as Pauline said—instead of feeding the baby with formula. In the case of Margaux's weight stagnation, Pauline did not push the parents to supplement with formula, despite the father's suggestion. On her previous visit, she had advised the parents, Aurore and David, to breastfeed Margaux every three hours, and then give her a supplement of pumped breast milk. I did not attend this consultation, but I joined Pauline for the next one three days later.

> After our arrival, Pauline proposed sitting and reviewing the situation. She asked Aurore and David about their morale. Aurore was tired, and she had slept poorly. She said, "I was upset because Margaux did not want to go back to sleep". She did not consider herself a "good mother", as she got angry with her daughter. David had slept in the living room on the sofa, and he regretted that Aurore had not woken him up: "That's not how a team works!" Aurore said, "The fact that there is a failure of weight gain puts even more pressure to succeed". Pauline pointed out that there is a "great deal of psychological pressure on women who feed with their milk". Aurore was afraid she might not hear the alarm clock that she set to wake up and feed Margaux so that she could respect the three-hour interval between feeds. Pauline refuted this worry: "It's okay. It's perfect just as you are doing it". David was more optimistic. He thought that the three-hour interval between feeds suited Margaux's needs better than the two-hour interval Pauline had proposed initially. After each feed, David gave Margaux the pumped milk with a bottle. He said, "I give the bottle very slowly. I try to get closer to the experience at the breast. She takes breaks like at the breast". David observed that she wanted to suckle more often, but he tempered his optimism: "The verdict will be the scale". He also evoked the possibility of giving Margaux formula: "I say if we have to give her dietary supplements, so what? You've got to be cool. It is useless to be completely extremist, purist. What matters is the intention". Pauline did not agree with this idea of "extremism". She said, "Sometimes we have to use a lifebelt and give formula supplements to get her weight back up, but it's a temporary lifebelt", implying that, eventually, the goal was to feed the baby exclusively with breast milk.

Aurore, for her part, was firmly opposed to giving Margaux formula. As she told me a few times over our meetings, "Formula is poison!" She agreed with Pauline's proposal for how to deal with Margaux's weight stagnation. Although it might take more time to increase her weight, it served a greater purpose in that it ensured the continuity of exclusive breastfeeding. In other situations, I found that midwives took a stance for breastfeeding by making parents aware of certain risky practices regarding breastfeeding initiation. Eva, for example, brought to the attention of her clients, Inès and Christophe, that "it's a little early to give a pacifier. To not disturb his sucking reflex, it is necessary to wait ten days. It's better to give the finger because it does not disturb the sucking reflex". Inès and Christophe had given Romuald, their son, a pacifier the night before, so they could get some sleep after feeding him "from 9 pm to 3 am". Inès explained that she wasn't aware that it could disrupt his sucking reflex. Eva put things into perspective:

"At 3 am, you're clueless! It will not jeopardise your breastfeeding. It's your third breastfeeding. You have experience!" When I met again with Inès and Christophe a few months later, we revisited this episode. Inès explained that she had given Romuald the pacifier anyway because "he wanted to suckle, but wasn't hungry". She elaborated, "I was fully confident; I knew it was going to work well. I said to myself, 'I don't care, I am way more confident, and I can transgress rules'". Inès's confidence, based on her experience, led her to trust her experiential knowledge more than her midwife's medical and theoretical knowledge. This statement put her in a posture of resistance, while complying with midwives' care approach of telling parents to "do what feels right for them".

The paediatrician: a ubiquitous absent negotiator

In Switzerland, a paediatrician takes part in two postpartum follow-ups along with the midwife. The first occurs within 48 hours after birth, and the second is the one-month check-up.[16] In between, in the absence of specific reasons, parents do not see their paediatrician. Even though paediatricians were largely absent from the follow-ups I attended, they remained very present in the midwives' minds in cases of difficulties related to the child's weight gain, with the one-month check-up appearing as an ultimatum. Capucine explained to me that in each situation, she takes advantage of the "amount of time before a third person [the paediatrician, in addition to the mother] gets involved". Her follow-up resulted from a compromise between her vision and the paediatrician's expected vision, as she conceived it, to "prevent a messy situation" in case of a mismatch between the baby's weight curve and the standards expected at the time of the check-up. For her, this was about protecting parents against a critical discourse, which could undermine their self-confidence. As Carole said, "Luckily, she was there because otherwise, we would have been overwhelmed" when facing the paediatrician's speech. During the postpartum follow-up, Capucine insisted on the notions of "confidence in the child" and his "skills, including his ability to not starve to death". During a visit, she said to Carole, "If I alone were to follow you throughout the whole breastfeeding duration, I would only look at what happens between the two of you", implying that she would not pay attention to the baby's weight.

Odile also recognised that she anticipated visits to the paediatrician with her clients: "Sometimes we saw each other just before to anticipate. I want them to go to the next check-up without her or him saying they need to give formula". Depending on the paediatrician and how well Odile knew them, she worried "differently". Together, we reflected on her phone conversation with the paediatrician in the situation of Morgane's lack of weight gain, which his father interpreted as "a way to not be alone in this situation when making a decision". Odile evoked another motive for calling the paediatrician: "I have the impression that if we warn them [paediatricians], their reaction is different". She advocated for more frequent communication and closer collaboration between paediatricians and independent midwives. Odile was pleased to report to me that, following a close collaboration with another paediatrician in a situation of a baby's weight stagnation, the involved paediatrician now contacted her directly in case of difficult breastfeeding situations. Odile regretted a feeling of mistrust shared by midwives regarding paediatricians and said, "It's up to us to let go of our own belief that we never do well and that paediatricians will reproach us for something".

Nevertheless, paediatricians' consultations were most often thought of as an event to be anticipated and a source of worry, even if the nature and intensity of this worry depended on the specific paediatrician involved. Eva shared this perspective and told me that, in case of a weight loss approaching the 10 per cent limit, her reaction depended on the paediatrician and her past experiences with her or him. Concerning the midwife–paediatrician collaboration issue, she gave me a concrete example from Lisa's follow-up regarding Paul's umbilical cord. Like all the midwives I observed, Eva recommended taking care of the umbilical cord by applying some cicatrising powder from an organic cosmetics brand instead of a local antiseptic or soap and water. Before the paediatrician's check-up, Eva had warned Lisa that "on the third day, it may be less pretty, and she may say something". The paediatrician was indeed dissatisfied with the cord and prescribed antibiotics, which Lisa decided not to use. Eva emphasised that she had warned Lisa "to preserve my credibility with her. I know my cords well. I know how they evolve". In such a case, Eva also deemed it necessary to anticipate the paediatrician's check-up. As Gouilhers-Hertig (2010) pointed out, in Switzerland, midwives' prerogatives are restrained; they do not formally have specific skills or a monopoly over obstetricians or paediatricians. Their prerogatives are at the interface of those of obstetricians and paediatricians, without official recognition of a specialisation of their own by medical authorities. As a result, rivalries and tensions persist between these professions. Perrenoud (2016) also noticed the sometimes confrontational nature of relations between independent midwives and paediatricians: "the construction of the relation to risk is the subject of frequent negotiations between ideals and a certain pragmatism necessary for interprofessional collaboration" (292).

Midwives sometimes took a stance against paediatricians' advice on issues such as vaccination, bed-sharing, or the use of antibiotics. Léa, whose child Simone was five months old at the time of our discussion, told me how she managed Simone's treatment when she had an ear infection. The paediatrician, after confirming the diagnosis, prescribed antibiotics. Léa tried to negotiate the treatment, saying, "How will she build her immune system if you treat her first ear infection right away?" The paediatrician stood firm on his position, warning Léa that she would endanger Simone's brain development if she did not give her antibiotics. She said, "They take you by fear, but he immediately understood that I was not receptive". Léa called Mireille, her midwife, and "she gave me different advice: 'Wait a little and see how she's doing'". When Simone's fever spiked, Guillaume, her father, wanted to give her the antibiotics, but Léa still did not want to. They finally tried to give Simone the antibiotics, but she refused to swallow them. Simone ended up recovering without complication, but Léa and Guillaume did not tell anyone that Simone did not take the antibiotics. Léa commented, "Fortunately, there was Mireille. Otherwise, there would have been no one to support me". Mireille advised her to learn how to recognise healthy and infected ears by herself. "She told me, 'Buy yourself an otoscope!'". Léa felt deeply disappointed by her paediatrician's reaction regarding Simone's ear infection. So far, Simone only had standard check-ups and had not received any vaccines. They had selected their paediatrician precisely on the basis of his reputation for flexibility and openness regarding vaccination. In Switzerland, vaccinations are indeed non-mandatory. Parents remain free to take their own decisions on this topic, regardless of their paediatrician's advice.

Well after the end of the postpartum follow-up period, even if they stopped having contact, midwives often remained reference persons for parents. Unlike the paediatrician, the midwife is a figure of chosen medical authority. In contrast, paediatricians are close to a default choice, often recommended by midwives for their supposed openness concerning vaccination or medicine prescription. From this perspective, "good paediatricians" stand out because of their self-effacement. Inès, for example, was very pleased with her paediatrician and said, "He never worries about anything! He gives the fewest possible drugs". Jelena was more cautious: "I would classify her as an average paediatrician, but there's no pressure about vaccines. I don't know why I'm going there". She was, however, annoyed by the prospect of the next check-up because "I will have to hear her speech on vaccines all over again and she will have to hear mine. I keep her in case there is a real emergency". Parents often did not give their paediatricians much credit. Laura, the mother of Maëli and Arwen, said, "I don't see what the paediatrician check-up brings me. I do it to be a good mom in the eyes of society. It's like a car inspection. I have no questions because I'm not interested in the answers he provides".

This disregard for the paediatricians' approach was even more acute on topics related to breastfeeding. Parents openly perceived their paediatricians as ignorant and often avoided bringing the matter up with them, as in the case of Inès: "He never broaches the subject. He does not give his opinion at all". Confident in her own knowledge, Céline evoked "regular clashes with the paediatrician concerning breastfeeding", during which she "put him back in his place", and she remarked, "I correct him when he makes mistakes about breastfeeding". She was, for example, very surprised that he had never heard about the supplemental nursing system, and when he affirmed that babies take 95 per cent of what they need within the first five minutes, implying that there is no need to leave them at the breast any longer. "He certainly ruins plenty of breastfeedings!" commented Céline.

All the parents I met nevertheless brought their babies to each stand- ard check-up recommended by the Swiss Society of Paediatrics (2011), no matter what they thought of their paediatricians' care approach. When I pointed out the discrepancy between their critical discourse regarding their paediatrician and their diligence concerning paediatric check-ups, parents generally evoked anticipative guilt in the event that they might overlook something going wrong with their child. As Julien explained, "I think it's reassuring … he could see something we would not see", imply- ing something that they were unable to see. Lisa explained why she con- tinued with regular visits to her paediatrician, who was "very allopathic medicine oriented and not open at all", despite significant differences in views about health and childcare: "You are accountable. Even if you don't care, you don't know what can happen. It's hard to take responsibility. I don't want [my son] to suffer from stunted growth". For her, this defer- ence to the paediatrician was specific to children's first months of life, and she observed that "with time, it changes. When they get bigger, they're a little stronger".

These parents' obedience to their paediatricians called into question the limits of their self-confidence regarding their own empirical and theo- retical knowledge. As part of a risk-centric approach to health, the logic of risk anticipation guided my interlocutors' parenting style. In addition, regular check-ups during pregnancy and the immediate postpartum period accustomed them to relying on medical controls to ensure their baby's health and well-being. After their midwife's follow-ups ended, most of the parents I met did not contact her again. Even if they continued to refer to her discourse and recommendations frequently to explain and legitimate their childcare practices and choices, the paediatrician remained the only medical reference person with whom they continued meeting in the long term.

Parents admitted their vulnerability towards the paediatrician, who embodied the biomedical authority. Despite their critical stance, especially when their baby's weight was at stake, they submitted to the paediatrician's authority.

Clara and Rémy were both in their early thirties and employed part- time in the health and social sectors, respectively. They lived in a small urban apartment. They were parents of Jade, age three years, and Léon, age one day, when I first met them. Both pregnancies were followed up by Eva, their midwife. Clara told me about their health journey, which started when they found out she was pregnant with Jade and led them to an out-of-hospital birth project. Regarding vaccination, she explained that they have "learned a lot, through discussions with Eva, readings … We tried to build our own point of view".

Léon was born in a birth centre, two weeks before his due date, with a low birth weight—that is, under three kilograms. He was back to his birth weight at ten days, and during Eva's postpartum visits I attended, there was no mention of his weight. Eva's postpartum follow-up ended up after a fortnight.

Almost two months later, I met with Clara. The family had just moved into a larger apartment. Clara looked worried and told me immediately, "Breastfeeding is not that easy. He does not gain much weight". She feared that the move made her too tired and had been detrimental to her lactation. At the two months' paediatric check-up, Léon had only gained seven hundred grams since birth. The paediatrician proposed supplementing each feed with pumped breast milk or formula. Clara said, "I do not want to give formula, but I'm afraid I do not have enough milk to supplement with pumped milk". Clara felt exhausted by pumping in addition to feeding: "In the end, you only do that: feeding Léon, pumping your milk". She had also done some acupuncture sessions to boost her lactation. Clara and Rémy agreed that Clara would take a "breastfeeding holiday" during which she would only be resting and breastfeeding while Rémy took sole charge of Jade's care and the housework. On their own initiative, Clara and Rémy had rented a baby scale "to weigh him before and after each feed, to see if I have enough milk. Considering the energy that it requires, I do not want to do it for nothing". Clara, Rémy, and the paediatrician had agreed to allow another fortnight without introducing formula to see if Léon's weight would increase. Clara said, "The paediatrician trusts me anyway, but she is afraid that it will be necessary to supplement. We have a very good paediatrician. We can really discuss, exchange views, but it's clear … for vaccines, we have a very different opinion. She sees that we are not out of control, and she respects us. I think there is a good bond of trust. We feel her sensibilities, but she respects those of others. It's really an honest exchange".

Five months later, I met with Clara again. She summarised her journey where we had left off: the fortnight of the "breastfeeding holiday". She was confident before the paediatrician check-up and said, "For me, we had really put this breastfeeding back on track", but Léon had only gained fifteen grams. Eva called the next day and proposed visiting them "to catch up on Léon's news", as "the paediatrician had already called her. I was happy that they communicated with each other". However, "Eva was very embarrassed, as the paediatrician seemed very worried on the phone. The paediatrician talked about hospitalising Léon. Eva told us she was badly caught between trusting parents and a very worried paediatrician. She suggested that Léon was maybe not able to express his need to eat anymore, and that is why he remained smiling". Clara explained, "We were not founding our evaluation on his weight curve, but on his general condition" when assessing his health and well-being. For her, "it was unbearable to hear that", especially because he had long moments of calm awakening and was smiling. "The next day", she said, "I had no milk anymore, and I had my periods back. Léon yelled, and I saw that my son was telling me he was hungry", implying that this was not the case before. Clara was too tired and discouraged, and observed that "it was not possible to redo the last month process to revive my lactation". She stopped breastfeeding at Léon's fourth month, far sooner than she imagined. Clara and Rémy went to the paediatrician together to discuss this incident. "I understand what happened in her mind. She wanted to hospitalise him to do a battery of exams, and if nothing had emerged, she would have accepted the idea that it was his growth curve and that we did not have to worry. She used Eva as an intermediary to make us hear that it was alarming".

At the end of her story, Clara was crying, and so was I. She told me that she had not answered my call immediately because she knew that it would be hard to tell me. She confided when we left each other that she had hoped this meeting would comfort her and that it would allow her to reach closure because I was there from the beginning.

In this situation, the paediatrician seemed aware that Eva had a greater influence over Clara and Rémy's decisions than she did. I did not have the opportunity to discuss the matter with Eva. When I met Clara, she was still dealing painfully with "breastfeeding grief" (Tomori, Palmquist & Dowling 2016) and was, in a way, mourning the motherhood model she favoured and identified with. Clara and Rémy tried to base their judgement on their experiential knowledge and resist the paediatrician's recommendation, but they eventually gave their son formula milk as the paediatrician primarily suggested, allowing for an accurate calculation of food intake so that Léon's weight was no longer a concern.

Babies' weight gain difficulties allow paediatricians to regain authoritative knowledge, even with well-informed, sceptical parents. By agreeing to subject their child to paediatricians' supervision and regular check-ups, parents also accept the paediatricians' intervention in the child's care and preferred food intake, especially after the midwife's follow-ups have ended. For example, parents generally agree to bring their babies for an additional check-up, in the absence of any illness or signs of discomfort, if their paediatrician requests it, to keep a close watch on the baby's weight gain or to do additional exams.

At the two-month check-up, Jeanne's paediatrician told her that Nils was not gaining enough weight. She gave Jeanne an ultimatum, telling her that if Nils had not gained 250 grams by the next appointment a week later, he would have to be supplemented with formula. Jeanne explained, "I felt that it was the paediatrician, positioned as the baby's defender, who focused mainly on weight gain and the growth curve evolution. Here, in this case, she did not take into account the benefits of breastfeeding, the mother–child relationship, etc. It was like, 'Okay, there, if he does not gain more, well, it will be necessary to review his diet. It will be necessary to supplement him'". She was very upset: "It shook me up, and the next day, I had no milk anymore. Nils was getting upset and everything, and I was like, 'What's going on?' I wanted to pump my milk to see, but I could not do it". Jeanne tried various strategies to revive her lactation. She also rented a baby scale to weigh Nils before and after each feed, against her midwife's advice, who encouraged her "to not focus on Nils's weight gain". Jeanne, however, was very worried. She said, "It's really … a baby who lacks food intake can have serious consequences … so you tell yourself, 'Damn!' You feel guilty, too. You just doubt your skills as a mom who can breastfeed". One week later, Nils had gained the weight required by the paediatrician: "He was at the breast twenty-four–seven that week!"

Like Clara, Jeanne decided to conduct test weighing—weighing a baby before and after each feed—a practice implemented at the beginning of the twentieth century (Apple 1987, Sachs 2013) and currently perceived as retrograde by most medical authorities and highly condemned by the holistic midwives I observed, even though it is still applied in some maternity wards.

> It helped me understand. Understanding his reactions, his behaviour, from times when he takes well and times when he takes less, I could make connections. How did he behave during the feed? Yeah, I could understand him better, too. After that, I stopped with this baby scale, because I said to myself, "I have to let go, too".
>
> (interview with Jeanne, notes)

In contrast with a qualitative and feeling-based assessment of their breastfeeding as taught by their midwives, the accurate quantification of their baby's breast milk intake allowed some mothers to reclaim their breastfeeding. From this perspective, test weighing can be understood as an act of resistance. Mothers resist their paediatricians' authority and suggestion to supplement their children with formula, but they also resist their midwives' teachings. Midwives indeed mostly discourage parents from weighing their babies by themselves at all, and they disapprove even more of test weighing.

Despite their critical posture regarding weighing, the scale remains an important symbol of midwife care and represents a gesture that midwives identify with. As Pauline said, "I would never have the idea of leaving a scale [at a family's home]. I somehow identify with the idea that it's my job as a midwife [to weigh the baby]. My role is to make sure the baby is healthy, including the baby's weight gain progression". Pauline also referred to the parents' curiosity: "I think there is also a certain pride that results from this. The weight is a numeric result that supports their pride". She finally suggested that fathers sometimes get more involved during this part of her consultations, for example, by taking pictures.[17] Indeed, on many occasions, I observed parents using their cameras to capture the moment when the midwife weighed their baby. The scale itself is a simple fabric hammock attached to a weighing probe that is preferred at home because of its lightness and small volume and it is not used in hospitals. Associated with the gesture of lifting the baby and swinging in the hammock, the act of weighing epitomises the independent midwifery practice. I also noticed during my fieldwork that, among all the parents, only one father had become accustomed to lifting the hammock himself.[18]

In this context, parents who rented a baby scale adopted a posture of resistance, as highlighted by Bobel (2002) in her study on "natural mothers":

> Natural mothers rail against systems of control in the form of institutions and so-called experts. Tiny acts of rebellion fill their days. When a mother treats her child's ear infection with garlic oil instead of doctor-recommended antibiotics, she resists. She resists when she breastfeeds her three-year-old in the public library in spite of the disapproving gaze of those around her. When she ignores another school enrolment period or state-mandated vaccination date, she challenges the generally accepted norms of "good parenting".
>
> (Bobel 2002: 105)

Parents who rented a baby scale with the aim of weighing their baby themselves resisted medical authorities by not submitting to the norm, as professionals are exclusively in charge of weighing babies. Simultaneously, they also embraced a weight-centric assessment of their child's health and well-being.

Parents and midwives' emotions as a source of authoritative knowledge

In birth management, biomedicine and resulting protocols represent authoritative knowledge. Independent midwives embody and reproduce authoritative knowledge, but they also question its normative protocols. According to Davis-Floyd and Davis (1996), during a home birth, independent midwives "do not consider such protocols authoritative per se" (251). By acting on the basis of their experiential knowledge, they object to the "cultural consensus on what constitutes authoritative knowledge in birth" (ibid. 1996: 258). In this way, "they are becoming experts at balancing the protocols and demands of technologically obtained information with their intuitive acceptance of women's uniqueness during labor and birth" (ibid. 1996: 260). In my fieldwork, this resulted in the intuitive acceptance of the uniqueness of each breastfeeding dynamic between a mother and her baby, as well as each baby's distinctive growth. For example, in the case of Gaspard's weight stagnation described above, along with other positive indicators, Capucine reassured the parents, "This is not a baby that worries me [...] There are standards, and then there is each individual". Capucine relied on her experiential knowledge to analyse the situation and evaluate Gaspard's health status based on past follow-up experiences.

By focusing on clinical examinations and relying not only on their experiential knowledge and intuition but also on parents' feelings and observations, midwives convey an alternative and competitive source of authoritative knowledge that differs from the dominant technocratic approach. Parents choose this authoritative knowledge, embodied by their midwife, but they also question it. Arguably, they may choose this model of authority precisely because they can question it. Sarah explained why she preferred to rely on her own observations and feelings concerning her daughter, rather than soliciting her midwife, like this:

> If I only ask questions, I do not feel any more. I do not feel. If I gave birth with an independent midwife, it is because I am pro-independence in general: having the freedom to treat yourself, looking for information by yourself.
>
> (interview with Sarah, notes)

In parents' speeches, choosing to give birth out of the hospital with an independent midwife was also a choice for autonomy and was underpinned by the idea that making autonomous decisions within the framework of biomedical risk management is difficult, if not impossible (Cheyney 2008). In this regard, Malacrida and Boulton (2014) noted a shift in holistic care from the promotion of autonomy and self-determination to a normative injunction to embrace these values, sometimes against the parents' desires.

Cécile regretted that her midwife was "not comforting" during the postpartum period and that her follow-up remained "fairly basic", and she stated, "She also said that she did not like mothering her clients". Parents were invited to position themselves towards all decisions related to their child's health. For example, midwives left information leaflets about the Guthrie test,[19] asking parents to read them and proposing to discuss it so that parents could decide whether or not they wanted their babies to be tested. I observed that parents, often overwhelmed by emotions and their newborn's care in the early days after birth, could not find the time or were not interested in reading the leaflet. These circumstances made it difficult to exercise informed choice, which is typically highly favoured by parents who, in this specific context, would rather rely solely on their midwife's opinion.

Beyond weight gain and towards a personalised risk culture

Most parents I met had engaged in a deep and documented reflection on their birth plan, as well as their child's health and care—breastfeeding included.

Fabien, Milo's father, was keen on infant nutrition. He was very critical of the paediatrician's information leaflet presenting a timetable for babies' food diversification, particularly the prescription of a certain quantity of breast milk or formula until the end of the first year of life (Swiss Society of Paediatrics 2017). Fabien hoped that his son would be breastfed until at least 12 months, but he strongly opposed feeding Milo with formula and preferred to feed him other foods if necessary. In his opinion, parents who followed the paediatricians' recommendations were not well informed: "If we are not informed, we reproduce errors without knowing it". Maud and Jonathan, for their part, were thoroughly informed on vaccination. Maud said, "We had long discussions with Jonathan about vaccines. We went to conferences, we read books, we double-checked information each time". Parents who were familiar with the results of scientific research on nutrition or vaccinology lamented a gap between scientific research and biomedical protocols. Regarding breastfeeding, many mothers aimed to never give formula and to ensure a gradual transition to solid foods without using milk substitute. From their point of view, giving formula was a risky practice, and it was sometimes seen as riskier than weight stagnation. As Aurore said repeatedly, "Formula is poison!" In the same vein, Lisa compared her two experiences of infant feeding: "When you give your milk, you think it's the best thing for him, and with Angèle, I felt like I was giving some crap!"

In contrast, parents perceived breast milk as providing protection against external threats and perturbations. For instance, Maud said, "I have the feeling that my milk protects [my daughter], despite day care, etc. She develops her immune system. I think my milk is the best for her". Tamara and Jérome, the parents of Camille, shared this point of view. According to Tamara, while ingesting breast milk, Camille "has everything she needs for her immune system, so she is never sick". Jérome added, "Since we're made that way, it's not necessarily for nothing. Not everyone can breastfeed, but it is possible that in the long term, [the health of] a non-breastfed child is not like that of a breastfed child". Parents also perceived the outside world as a threat to their child's body, whereas they considered breast milk a form of protection against environmental menaces such as viruses and allergens, as well as emotional threats, since breastfeeding was also used as a comforting practice.

From this perspective, infants' bodies are vulnerable and permeable. According to Brownlie and Sheach Leith (2011: 203), "Bodies of infants, like those of women, are experienced as disturbing exactly because '[They do] not respect borders, positions, rules' (Kristeva, 1982: 4)". In the context of vaccination, this so-called permeability leads to the fear of a "transformation" of the baby's body by the vaccine. In parents' minds, breastfeeding, coupled with other carefully selected care practices and remedies, acted as a natural substitute for vaccines, protecting their children against viruses and illness. When I met with Maud nine months after her daughter's birth, she was very upset. One week earlier, Rose, her daughter, had an ear infection with perforated eardrums. "We were so disappointed!" she said, enumerating the precautions she and her spouse took to prevent this, including on-demand breastfeeding, pumped breast milk during day care, probiotics, and grapefruit seed extract every day for Maud and Rose. She added, "I don't understand how she could catch an ear infection. You cannot imagine our guilt as a couple, the total failure of our vision! After that, you have to let go. You cannot control everything". As mentioned above, Rose was not vaccinated, but "when you see a baby with a 40°C fever, you ask yourself, 'Are we doing the right thing or not?'"

Based on her research with mothers in Switzerland who chose to give birth outside the hospital, Gouilhers-Hertig (2014) suggested that an out-of-hospital birth choice corresponds to the construction of a "personalised risk culture" (116). From my observations, it appears that this "personalisation" of the "risk culture" continues beyond birth, through babies' care practices and choices affecting their health and nutrition. These choices are often perceived as risk-inducing factors from a biomedical perspective, but parents justified them based on a logic of risk prevention. For example, they justified the choice to not vaccinate their children to allow them to "build their immunity", a process supported by breastfeeding. From this perspective, the breastfeeding project induced a specific form of risk perception and management.

This "personalised risk culture" resulted from the information process on which parents' holistic health approaches were based. In addition, midwives encouraged parents to develop a critical stance towards authoritative knowledge and the dominant risk culture. They fostered this process of building a personalised risk model by supporting practices perceived as risk factors from a biomedical perspective. For example, Odile openly discussed bed-sharing practices with parents, deploring the dominant idea of the danger associated with this practice: "There are ongoing discussions between midwives, paediatricians, nurse visitors". She also said with humour, "I am convinced that no baby ever happened to fall out of bed!" She elaborated on her stance on bed-sharing during a one-on-one discussion with me: "I give them information. Then it's the parents' decision. If there is a great deal of fear, they should not do it. We are here to strengthen certain decisions, to allow people to strengthen themselves with their decisions. The goal is not to convince, but to be there for people who want that". Midwives' approval on my fieldwork differed from Tomori, Palmquist and Dowling's (2016) observations regarding breast milk sharing, night-time breastfeeding, and long-term breastfeeding. In these authors' paper, combining three studies conducted in the United States and the United Kingdom, parents felt stigmatised by the disapproving gaze of health professionals regarding their unconventional breastfeeding practices. This internalised stigma led parents to keep quiet about these practices, preventing discussion opportunities with health professionals. In these studies, parents had not planned to engage in these practices. On the contrary, in my study, parents had planned to share their beds with their newborns, sometimes on their mid-wives' suggestion. In some cases, parents had initially adopted this practice but felt inadequate and then later felt approved of and legitimatised after telling their midwife.

Despite paediatricians' disapproval, midwives, who also represent authoritative knowledge, can validate and reinforce parents in their choices. Again, risk management revolves around feelings, and midwives suggest emotional risk management approaches. Concerning vaccination, having recommended some readings to allow parents to deepen their reflection, Mireille explained the difference between a simple vaccine and a combined vaccine: "With a combined vaccine, the child only gets the mercury once!" Because "the baby cannot make antibodies before three months", she also disapproved of vaccination before this age. For Mireille, the parents' reasoning went beyond a balance between the risks of disease in the case of non-vaccination and the harmful effects intrinsic to vaccines. According to her, the decision was ultimately about feelings and emotions: "You have to vaccinate against diseases that scare you". In this way, she agreed with Odile, who said of bed-sharing, "I give them information, and then it's the parents' decision. If there is a great deal of fear, they should not do it".

Lupton (2013) highlighted the links between emotions, risk perception, and behaviours. Both emotions and risks are "ways of making sense of situations, naming responses, part of the diverse cultural meaning systems that we use to try and understand the world" as "embodied features of emotional experience" (Lupton 2013: 638).

> These embodied/material dimensions are always interpreted via a social and cultural lens, predicated on individual past experiences as well as collective memories. We name certain embodied sensations as "emotions" based on our interpretations of them. So too, we name certain phenomena as "risks" based on our interpretation.
>
> (Lupton 2013: 638)

Lupton (2013) also proposed the notion of "emotion-risk assemblage" to refer to this intersubjectivity between emotions and risk perception,[20] and she addressed "the shifting dynamics that are inherent in the embodied nature of risk understandings" (640). By using the notion of the emotion-risk assemblage, she emphasised that "both emotion and risk interact with each other and in the process, configure each other. Emotions create risks and risks create emotions" (Lupton 2013: 640-641).

In a situation of failure to thrive, parents' and midwives' emotions are at stake, induced by their respective interpretations of what is risky or not, leading to emotional risk management. Midwives demonstrate reflexivity regarding this process, as Pauline observed regarding vaccination: "Practices, risk prevention measures, are based on fear. They are used by professionals to negotiate, to impose things on parents, but people who do not vaccinate also do so out of fear". She argued that parents must also "choose the information that suits them", not on the basis of "ratiocinative" risk management (Davis-Floyd & Davis 1996), but on the basis of emotional risk management.

> I'm not someone driven by fear as a midwife. But there is a form of stress that catches me and acts as a call to order, saying, "The risk exists. You must also pay attention. Nature is not always tender; it makes its law. We imagine that we accept, but in our society, we do not want to accept death. [...] Along with the collaboration with parents, day after day, we negotiate the deadlines, until the day comes when the mother feels that she has reached her limits of risk tolerance".
>
> (interview with Pauline, notes)

Pauline's words show that she used her experiential knowledge and emotions, as well as the parent's observations and affects, as information on which to base her judgement and implemented actions. Sometimes, the various protagonists' feelings conflict, leading to more confusion. In the situation of Margaux's failure to thrive described above, her parents, Aurore and David, did not share the same feelings regarding their daughter's weight. Aurore was both worried and eager to persevere with breastfeeding, whereas David was relaxed and not opposed to the possibility of giving formula.

Pauline, for her part, was also affected by the situation. When we met in front of the couple's apartment, she confided that the day before—I was not there—she had heard David telling Aurore they should not listen to her too much, because his brother had told him that "professionals" were always the same and insisted on weight. Pauline was hurt "to be in the 'professionals' category, depersonalised, now that there were complications". The following night, she had a nightmare about Margaux's weight stagnation, dreaming that she was in the maternity ward. She entered Aurore and Margaux's room and was confused about how to feed Margaux, as there was an abundance of breasts and formula bottles. During the consultation, just before weighing Margaux, Pauline told the parents there were three possible scenarios: weight loss, weight stagnation, or weight gain. She announced that in the case of weight loss, "it will be necessary to put more drastic things in place". However, the question did not arise: Margaux had finally gained weight. Pauline held Aurore in her arms and congratulated her, visibly relieved. Aurore commented happily, "I was saying to myself, 'Filling something up must have had an effect!'" David also showed his relief and observed, "It's stupid that [breastfeeding] is not something you can share. It would be more practical!" In this messy situation, the tangled feelings of the midwife and the parents served as an action lever for achieving a common goal: getting out of a potentially "risky" situation and back to the norm. Pauline's unusual anxiety strengthened her decision to act though the baby had still not gained any weight. She had "reached her limits", as she said herself about mothers. Aurore's worry pushed her to actively make her daughter eat, whereas David's apparent collectedness favoured his calm commitment to the breastfeeding process by cleaning the pump after each use and giving his daughter the pumped breast milk slowly using a bottle.

Conclusion

If breastfeeding has become the standard of good motherhood (Wall 2001), this is even truer in the context of holistic care. As Pauline pointed, "breastfeeding is a goal in itself". Therefore, mothers and midwives were committed to maintaining breastfeeding and ensuring proper lactation even in cases of weight stagnation. To achieve this goal, an intensive programme was established, constituting an "extreme form of body management" (Avishai 2007: 146). The involvement of midwives, who devoted two hours per visit if needed, was consistent with the maternal commitment.

Independent midwives favoured and supported breastfeeding, sometimes even taking liberties with protocols to serve this purpose. They took advantage of their independent status, which allowed them to enjoy a high degree of autonomy. Hospital protocols were nevertheless present in their practice and served as landmarks to guide them. As health professionals, independent midwives are subject to biomedical standards and protocols regarding their birth and postpartum management. Davis-Floyd and Davis (1996) highlighted the tension between these biomedical guidelines and independent midwifery holistic care:

> Midwives must attempt to meet these cultural imperatives. Such attempts place midwives in conflict with their own holistic paradigm and the patience and trust in birth and the female body that it charters. Contemporary midwives cannot fail to be aware of this dilemma—it is a central defining theme of their practices and their lives, ensuring that for them, every homebirth that is not textbook perfect will pose ethical, moral and legal dilemmas that might end them up in a courtroom in danger of losing the right to practise. The level of tension between the technocratic and holistic paradigms with which homebirth midwives must constantly cope makes their occasional willingness to rely solely on intuition—sanctioned by the holistic model and condemned by the technocratic model—a strong marker of their commitment to holism and its underlying principle of connection.
>
> (Davis-Floyd & Davis 1996: 239)

Similarly, by acting on the basis of parents' feelings and experiential knowledge, as well as their own experiential knowledge regarding the management of newborns' failure to thrive, midwives take a hard stance against the biomedical model of risk management. However, the postpartum period, unlike delivery, is not defined by medical authorities as a "fateful moment" (Scamell & Alaszewski 2012). In the case of a baby's weight stagnation, the urgency of birth is over, and the situation can be handled more flexibly. In this context, midwives concentrate on the paediatrician's one-month check-up, which acts as a normative "call to order". For this only institutionalised marker involving "a third person", as Capucine said, during the postpartum follow-up, midwives are held accountable for the baby's health. Midwives are torn between their commitment to their holistic care practices and their projections of paediatricians' expectations, as they must maintain their credibility and authority with paediatricians and parents.

In parallel, midwives establish themselves as the defenders of a range of controversial infant care practices, such as bed-sharing and non-vaccination, creating a personalised model of risk management that they share with parents. Bed-sharing, for example, is perceived in this model as a protective practice that supports breastsleeping (McKenna & Gettler 2016). In the same vein, non-vaccination is connected to breastfeeding practices because breast milk allows infants to build immunity resistance, whereas vaccination prevents babies from "building their immunity". From this perspective, commitment to breastfeeding leads parents and midwives to a custom model of risk perception and management.

Midwives expressed a strong critical stance against the weight-centric evaluation of breastfeeding success and newborns' health, defending the specificity of independent midwifery care. Midwives also perceived a qualitative approach as part of an empowerment process for parents. Parents tended, for their part, to embrace their midwives' committed position, often showing an obvious disinterest in their child's weight. At the same time, although midwives claimed that weighing babies was not the highlight of their visit, the act is part of midwives' consultation accountability and has become, in a certain way, emblematic of the independent midwife practice, as opposed to other less action-oriented moments.

However, in cases of failure to thrive, the baby's weight remains essential, focusing parents' and midwives' expectations. As Odile said, "You need to see if what you put in place actually works". The actions implemented to improve infants' weight gain were nevertheless discussed and negotiated at length with parents, engaging midwives in a tinkering care process involving constant readjustments intended to respect parents' wishes as part of a "logic of care" (Mol 2009).

Controversial but unavoidable, the weighing of babies remains a symbolic ritual of the postpartum home follow-up. As the only quantified, "objectified" data from a follow-up based on observing, listening, and feeling, the baby's weight highlights a breaking point between the midwives' care model, their professional responsibility to ensure babies' health and the parents, the informed and "enlightened" interlocutors with whom they negotiate.

Notes

1 McKenna and Gettler (2016) coined this neologism to describe night-time breast-feeding practices including bed-sharing, the baby falling asleep at the mother's breast, and feeding during the night.

2 On the contrary, studies showed that breastfeeding and bed-sharing contribute to reducing SIDS rates (Gettler & McKenna 2010, in Tomori 2015). There is no evidence that bed-sharing, "in the absence of smoking, alcohol, and other drugs, on a firm surface, and with care in avoiding the use of soft bedding, results in increase of SIDS" (Tomori 2015: 72). Biological anthropologists have also highlighted that intercorporeality between mothers' and babies' bodies at night takes part in the regulation of both sleep and breastfeeding (ibid. 2015). In addition, the Swiss Society of Paediatrics recognises room sharing as the safest option for decreasing the risk of SIDS, but it dissuades parents from bed-sharing (Jenni et al. 2013).

3 As mentioned above, most independent midwives attending home postpartum consultations with families discharged from a hospital do not offer holistic care. As a result, some of them stick strictly to hospital protocols during their postpartum follow-ups, and their risk management can differ tremendously from the model I describe in this chapter.

4 Their first child died two days after birth from SIDS.

5 Some independent midwives use this "potion" to induce labour, for example, in cases of overdue term. The potion prepared by midwives always contains castor oil, and the other ingredients vary from one midwife to another. It usually includes something sweet to improve the taste, such as ice cream or fruit juice, and sometimes sparkling wine.

6 See, for example, Pérez-Rios, Ramos-Valencia and Ortiz (2008); Rowe-Murray and Fisher (2002); Zanardo et al. (2010).

7 According to the Swiss Society of Neonatology, a specific protocol is intended for various newborn categories, including, among others, born after thirty-four to thirty-six pregnancy weeks, with a birth weight over four and a half kilograms or from a mother with gestational diabetes (Société Suisse de Néonatologie 2007). This protocol prescribes the systematic administration of a dietary supplement to the baby after each breastfeeding session, which must take place every three or four hours. This "complement" can be either a maltodextrin solution or formula milk.

8 Midwives use this term to describe waking moments during which the baby shows no signs of discomfort or nervousness.

9 The Swiss Society of Neonatology recommends giving a dose of vitamin K to all newborns at birth, on the fourth day of life, and after four weeks of life (2002).

10 The Michelin man, or Bibendum, is the mascot of the Michelin tyre company. Made of white tyres, he has a round body and many "love handles", both of which are expected characteristics of a healthy baby in the collective imagination.

11 During the exploratory phase of my research, I attended some La Leche Legue meetings. Later, when I started focusing on home birth parents and their breastfeeding journey, I stopped attending these meetings. I noticed a lack of connection between home birth mothers and La Leche League. Only Céline regularly attended La Leche League meetings, while two other mothers called the La Leche League hotline a few times to have some telephone support regarding specific concerns when their baby was older and they were no longer in contact with their midwife.

12 Tandem breastfeeding or tandem nursing refers to the simultaneous breastfeeding of two children.

13 Breast milk evolves during a single feed: it is first rich in water, and it becomes fattier later on.

14 Even if the group is not formally a women-only space, none of the fathers I met was active in it.

15 The most frequently cited books were *The Womanly Art of Breastfeeding* from La Leche League (first edition 1958) and *L'allaitement. De la naissance au sevrage* from Marie Thirion (first edition 1994).

16 The paediatric check-ups are usually scheduled at birth, at one month of life, at two months, four months, six months, nine months, twelve months, eighteen months, twenty-four months, then once a year until the child's sixth year of life (Swiss Society of Paediatrics 2011). Aside from the check-up that occurs during the first hours or days after the child's birth, the other paediatric check-ups are non-mandatory and depend on the parents' will.

17 In this instance, Pauline did not refer to home birth parents in particular but also to hospital birth parents. According to my observations, home birth fathers usually participated during the midwife's entire visit.

18 In previously described situations, Clara and Jeanne conducted test weighing using standard baby scales rented from the pharmacy, not hammock scales.

19 The Guthrie test detects the presence of rare metabolic and hormonal diseases. It is performed on the fourth day of the newborn's life and requires a pinprick in the newborn's one of the heels to collect six drops of blood on a blotting paper, which is sent by mail to a laboratory in Zurich that centralises all analyses for Switzerland.

20 Lupton borrowed the concept of assemblage from the actor network theory, which refers to a constellation of interconnected elements: affects, place, space, human and non-human, and living and non-living engaged in a social situation (Marcus & Saka 2006).

4   Building the lactating body

Avishai (2007) highlighted the "breastfeeding project" of middle class white American mothers, involving readings, consultations with experts, and goal setting in terms of produced breast milk quantity and breastfeeding duration. Similarly, in my fieldwork, home birth parents were generally strongly committed to breastfeeding, resulting in a "breastfeeding project" established before birth and entailing "self-assessment and surveillance" (Avishai 2007: 139). This project defines breastfeeding modalities and duration inspired by the WHO recommendations (2001, 2003): parents had planned to breastfeed their child exclusively and on demand during the first six months of life, and then to pursue breastfeeding in combination with other solid and liquid intakes, often until at least the end of the first year of life. I noticed that parents especially emphasised the six months of exclusive breastfeeding, which frequently appeared as an important milestone to reach. Comparatively, the total duration of breastfeeding, as well as the on-demand modality, were more flexibly addressed.

In the first part of this chapter, I discuss home breastfeeding initiation in the early postpartum days, involving a co-construction of the lactating maternal body accomplished by mothers and midwives. As a "dyadic bodily encounter" (Stearns 2013: 364), breastfeeding requires the joint efforts of both the mother and the baby, whose body and behaviour are also disciplined by the parents and the midwife's interventions to comply with breastfeeding. In addition, I develop how fathers get involved in this process, supporting their spouse in lactation management.

In the second part, I elaborate on the means and strategies put in place by parents to maintain breastfeeding and achieve their objectives in terms of duration. As developed by Stearns (2013), I adopt an embodied perspective on breastfeeding, centring my analysis on "the doing of breastfeeding: how mothers go about and think about breastfeeding within the immediate social context and structural constraints of their lives" (361).

Body work to achieve a maternal body

Anthropologists have shown that bodies are socially contextualised and shaped by cultural practices (Conklin & Morgan 1996; Csordas 1990; Lock

DOI: 10.4324/9781003124108-4

1993; Scheper-Hughes & Lock 1987). Csordas (1990) suggested substituting the Bourdieusian notion of "habitus", first introduced by Mauss (1936) as "a means to organize an otherwise miscellaneous domain of culturally patterned behaviour", with "embodiment" (11). In Csordas's opinion, the notion of embodiment allows one to overcome the dualistic Cartesian assumption which underlies the notion of habitus developed by Bourdieu (1972) as unconscious bodily inscription of dispositions and skills. Csordas's (1990) thought is based on a "postulate that the body is not an object to be studied in relation to culture, but is to be considered as the subject of culture, or in other words as the existential ground of culture" (5). He argued for the emergence of a "new body" under the anthropologist's gaze which can no longer be reduced to a fact of nature (Csordas 1994). Csordas (1994) highlighted stimulating perspectives for the discipline: "if indeed the body is passing through a critical historical moment, this moment also offers a critical methodological opportunity to reformulate theories of culture, self, and experience, with the body at the center of the analysis" (4).

On this topic, Davis (2007) regretted postmodern feminism's disregard for women's bodies and embodied experience. She argued for linking "individual women's subjective accounts of their experiences and how these affect their everyday practices, with an analysis of the cultural discourses, institutional arrangements, and geopolitical contexts in which these accounts are embedded and which give meaning to them" (2007: 57). More particularly, subjective accounts relating to women's bodies' reproductive functions—the "reproductive burden" (Hausman 2004)—reveal resulting gender inequalities and bypass strategies set up by couples to avoid them. Moreover, women's bodies are especially trained for birth and postpartum management, regardless of the chosen model of care. As highlighted by Pasveer and Akrich (2001):

> [Women's bodies] are not given and ready to be discovered, but are constituted by and constitutive of the trajectories and apparatus that mark them. Bodies are trained, or educated, and during that process they become "loaded" with experiences and competencies which match the trajectories designed for them. They "learned to be affected"
>
> (Pasveer & Akrich 2001: 232)

Breastfeeding has been identified by socio-anthropological research as a socially and culturally constructed biological phenomenon (Maher 1992). However, it is also a biological process, a bodily experience, and a "body technique" in the Maussian sense (1936) that requires a learning process. Therefore, professionals can help teach or optimise the breastfeeding "technique". New mothers often experience a feeling of incompetence in the postpartum period regarding their ability to breastfeed. They feel the need to be guided by birth professionals to ensure that they care for their baby "the right way" (Dykes & Williams 1999). Nevertheless, as highlighted by

Tomori, "breastfeeding expands upon Mauss's concept because it requires that two bodies unite in a coordinated manner—it is an intercorporeal body technique" (2018: 56). Consequently, even if the focus remains on the mother's body, techniques, and habits, the professionals' gaze also affects the baby's body and sucking technique, sometimes justifying a medical intervention, such as in the case of a tight lingual frenulum.

Under their midwives' supervision, mothers engage in the bodily and emotional work necessary to build their maternal bodies as required to perform breastfeeding. "Body work", as defined by Gimlin (2007), refers to "the work that individuals undertake on their own bodies and to the paid work performed on the bodies of others" (365). Stearns (2009) proposed to apply this notion to breastfeeding as it involves both dimensions mentioned above: the work that mothers undertake on their own bodies and the unpaid work performed on the body of their children. Moreover, my fieldwork observations revealed that maternal identity is significantly built through the accomplishment of this body work. After pregnancy and delivery, breastfeeding acts as a final body transformation, an accomplishment of the maternal body and identity. But unlike these time-limited processes, setting up breastfeeding and maintaining it over time requires continuous and demanding work—both physical and emotional—from mothers.

As demonstrated by Dykes (2006), breastfeeding initiation in hospital responds to a logic of rigid temporal controls imposed by institutional protocols. In a context dominated by notions of linear time and efficiency, breastfeeding is primarily considered as a transfer of milk from mother to child. Thus, breastfeeding success is evaluated on the basis of quantitative criteria and based on a productivist logic. Through techniques targeting the optimisation of milk transfer and assessment tools such as daily weighing of the infant, breastfeeding is rationalised by professionals. In opposition to the technocratic model described by Dykes (2006), home birth parents have conceived their own model of care together with their midwives. Nevertheless, I noticed that even if the content of the recommendations differs, the project of lactating body production remains. First under their midwife's supervision during the postpartum follow-up, then autonomously in the long term, mothers engage in a work of production of their lactating bodies.

This process reflects Darmon's (2003) observations in her research on the self-transformation work at stake in an "anorexic career" (84).[1] She identified a first phase of voluntary "taking in hand",[2] corresponding to the career entry, followed by a phase of "commitment continuation", during which the commitment continues and reinforces in the form of different practices. Through a "systematic process of dispositions transformation", this second phase allows the incorporation of new dispositions, becoming "second nature" (ibid. 2003: 340).

In the situations I observed, the "taking in hand" phase corresponded to the postpartum follow-up and was implemented collaboratively with the midwife; the "commitment confirmation" expanded individually over the long term through mechanisms set up to maintain "work upon oneself" over time (Darmon 2003: 341). As in the case described by Darmon, this was a voluntary commitment, since the mothers were convinced of breastfeeding's virtues and had for the most part established a breastfeeding project before birth. Nevertheless, as Darmon (2003) emphasises, "the voluntarist modality of this transformation work must not, however, lead us to consider it as a 'life choice'" (342). This work fits into a specific context of "social and structural conditions for opportunities" (ibid., 2003: 342). Breastfeeding promotion occupies an important space in the Swiss perinatal landscape, especially within the care model chosen by the mothers I met. These mothers not only committed themselves voluntarily and individually to breastfeeding but also built structural and material settings to achieve their projects: the choice of a midwife in line with their conception of birth, a supporting partner, the practice of bed-sharing to facilitate night-time breastfeeding, or for some of them, an extended maternity leave.

Alongside these structural and environmental arrangements, breastfeeding brings women to pay a new attention to their bodies, which becomes the instrument to achieve their project. This relationship to and the dependency on the body to achieve one's goals can be linked with the way professional athletes perceive and rely on their bodies. In an ethnography conducted with professional boxers, Wacquant (1995) showed how their relationship to the body is deeply reshaped by the practice of boxing:

As Joyce Carol Oates (1987:5) perceptively noted, "Like a dancer, a boxer 'is' his body and is totally identified with it". Fighters feel and know this equation well for their organism is indeed the template and epicentre of their life, at once the site, the instrument and the object of their daily work.

(Wacquant 1995: 66)

The new mothers I met, who were not professional sportswomen, had to consider their bodies and their—good—functioning with a new perspective to perform breastfeeding. This reframing profoundly changed the way they lived in their bodies, their breasts becoming the epicentre of their transition to motherhood. Like boxers, mothers had to "learn to decipher [their bodies] in order better to enhance and protect [them]" (Wacquant 1995: 67), as their lactating bodies required adequate management to optimise their performance. Breastfeeding affects not only the physical appearance and physiology of a woman's body but also "[her] 'body-sense', the consciousness [she] has of [her] organism and, through this changed body, of the world about [her]" (ibid. 1995: 73).

Young (2005) highlighted the sensory dimension of breasts, "the simple daily feeling of being in the world with these breasts" (95) thus prevailing for women on their visual aspect. The breasts indeed act as a barometer of bodily changes related to the processes of motherhood. A change of sensation in the breasts is often the first indicator of pregnancy. But it is usually during breastfeeding, which activates new sensations in the breasts, that women are particularly attentive to them: for example, to identify the beginnings of the milk ejection reflex or to recognise the early signs of breast congestion. As part of their postpartum follow-up, midwives teach mothers to decipher these new sensations, to "read" and take care of their newly lactating breasts.

Supporting breastfeeding initiation: a co-construction of the lactating body

The choice of holistic care by an independent midwife is associated with specific parenting practices derived from the ideological and practical principles of attachment parenting. Breastfeeding, considered the "natural" continuity of childbirth without medical or technical intervention, is central to these practices. Beyond arguments related to the positive impact of breastfeeding on infants' health, midwives highlight the "made-to-measure" nature of breast milk, specially created for children and ideally adapted to their needs in terms of both quantity and composition. Capucine, for example, explained to a new mother the sustained rhythm of night-time feedings: "At night you secrete more hormones to make milk, and [the child] knows it. If she wants to grow well, she will suckle during the night". In this way, midwives valued the synergy between the newborn's behaviour and the production/composition of breast milk, thus encouraging a productivist reading of breastfeeding. Capucine continued, describing breastfeeding initiation in these terms: "[The child] is born with an innate knowledge of nutrition, just as you are born with an innate knowledge of breastfeeding, and it is the meeting of the two". Breastfeeding is presented as an "innate" process related to physiology to a "normal" postpartum course. In this perspective, breastfeeding "failure" can be experienced by mothers as sorely difficult, as it can be interpreted as a transgression of the chosen birth model. After the visit, I asked Capucine to develop this naturalistic analysis of breastfeeding. She explained that from her point of view, biological determinism "offers tools, gives strength to mothers". She mobilised biological determinism in a perspective of mothers' empowerment and in order to reinforce their sense of maternal competence: "you can do it because you are built to do it". She evoked a "breastfeeding instinct", however disturbed it may be by "social roles and influences", and conceded that the technical act of breastfeeding may require learning. She finally estimated that breastfeeding was "50 percent innate, 50 percent acquired".

This naturalist explanation of breastfeeding as an innate skill was challenged by feminist science studies that question the categorisation of bodies in two sexes and reveal the "naturalness" of biological sex as a scientific question (Gardey & Löwy 2000; Laqueur 1990; Oudshoorn 1994). Since the early twentieth century, the locus of sexual difference in biological and medical discourses has moved from bones or organs to sex hormones: "the new field of sex endocrinology introduced the concept of 'female' and 'male' sex hormones as chemical messengers of femininity and masculinity" (Oudshoorn 1994: 8). This hormone-based conception of the sexual body quickly became a dominant way of thinking about the biological origins of sexual difference:

> Many types of behavior, roles, functions and characteristics considered as typically male or female in Western culture have been ascribed to hormones. In this process, the female body, but not the male body, has become increasingly portrayed as a body completely controlled by hormones.
>
> (Oudshoorn 1994: 8-9)

Midwives' as well as parents' discourses reflected this postulate and relied heavily on sex hormones to explain women's feelings and behaviours during the perinatal period. Sex hormones, or more precisely "breastfeeding hormones", were randomly conjured to justify a quick let-down reflex ("a great hormonal answer!"), the safety of bed-sharing (thanks to them, the mother would stay "alert" even during her sleep), or even an easy overcome of sleep deprivation (as said by Jelena, a new mother: "It's so magical, this impression that you sleep two hours and you have the feeling that you slept four hours"). Moreover, the hormone-based discourse extends to newborns, described as highly sensitive to "breastfeeding hormones", and thereby "knowing" or "feeling" when to feed—that is, when the milk comes in.

Compliant body, conformity of experience

During their postpartum follow-up, beyond maternal and child health monitoring or the knowledge transmission about breastfeeding and infant care, a central aspect of midwives' role was to reassure parents both on their skills and about the intense events they experienced in the beginnings of their cohabitation with a newborn. Even though I met primiparous and multiparous couples, it occurred to me that breastfeeding a second or even a third child sometimes raised as many questions as in the case of a first experience. Each breastfeeding is experienced differently, parents' feelings being influenced by multiple factors.

Supporting parents when the milk first comes in, for example, includes giving meaning to the newborns' behaviour and their intense solicitations to access their mothers' breasts. Often disconcerted by this behaviour, mothers tended to interpret their child's agitation as hunger and doubt the adequacy of their milk production with the child's needs. Midwives encouraged, on the contrary, a positive reading: according to their terms, the baby "stimulates" milk production. In this perspective, midwives' productivist reading of breastfeeding aimed to reassure mothers about the "normality" of their experience and the conformity of their child's behaviour with respect to the expected characteristics of a healthy newborn.

In midwives' discourse, breastfeeding was perceived as the "natural" continuity of childbirth without medical or technical intervention, as part of the physiological birth process: if delivery unfolded "naturally", so would breastfeeding. A discordance between the midwife's prenatal theoretical speech about breastfeeding and women's embodied experiences could make mothers feel betrayed by the chosen model of care or by their midwife, but also by their own body which was able to give birth but struggled to perform breastfeeding. Aurore, a mother, felt a strong discrepancy between her midwife's presentation during birth preparation courses and her own experience of breastfeeding initiation: "Pauline introduced it, I heard, like, 'breastfeeding, it works systematically'". Her spouse David added, "We stayed on that thing. a woman who doesn't have enough milk does not exist". Aurore continued, "There was a moment when I got angry with her because I told myself, 'that's not how she sold it to me'. I had the idea that once the childbirth passed, it was alright". In this situation, there was a misunderstanding between the midwife—who made an effort to present breastfeeding in a positive and encouraging way, fighting against false prejudices such as insufficient milk syndrome—and the parents, who deduced that it was not possible to be confronted with difficulties during breastfeeding initiation. Another mother, Maud, shared this feeling of betrayal, in her case regarding her own body rather than her midwife:

> I really didn't think it was going to be such a pain for me. When she was sleeping, I loved it, but as soon as she opened an eye, I was afraid. I had so much pain that I took her off the breast. In hindsight, I don't think about it anymore: I love to breastfeed! I couldn't understand that you couldn't "empty" a breast. I had a hard time accepting that you had to let go to make it flow. I didn't understand that when there was a breast congestion, Rose couldn't suckle. I didn't understand why it wasn't easy when the pregnancy and the delivery had gone so well. It seemed to me an insurmountable mountain to climb. Thankfully, Pauline came to motivate me, to encourage me. She always had the same line of thought.
>
> (interview with Maud, notes)

According to Maud, Pauline played a fundamental role in her breastfeeding success, as she felt very insecure regarding her ability to fulfil Rose's needs: "Having Pauline who regularly said, 'She does her job, that's all good how she's doing'. She made me trust my baby. I said to myself, "Trust her, she knows what she's doing". Other parents regularly mentioned the importance of care continuity, specific to the holistic practice of independent midwives: "The importance of being with one person whom you come to know, with whom you share a certain vision", as Corinne said. Tamara, another mother, compared the holistic care model with the dominant technocratic model: "What I found great is the relationship of trust that we created. Compared to ultrasound consultations, where you have the impression of being only a number ... When the midwife is as interested in the mother as in the baby, you can feel that it's important for her. For the delivery, I knew I had confidence in her. [My spouse and I] were alone, we were the both of us, it was our moment". Jérome, her spouse, completed, "In hindsight, we are happy that we did not receive contradictory opinions. From the beginning of the pregnancy to Camille's arrival, it was the same person [who advised us]".

Depending on their prior representations, mothers had varying expectations regarding their experiences. For example, having milk come in was badly experienced if it turned out to be "too" intense, causing pain, and constraining management, but it was also poorly lived if it did not manifest strongly enough with respect to the mother's anticipation. Carole explained how unsettled she was when her milk came in. She perceived it as not "intense enough", whereas she had anticipated it by equipping herself with natural remedies aiming to relieve the aches, as advised by her midwife: "It does not help, you ask yourself a lot of questions". More broadly, when their experience deviated too much from their initial project, mothers had a feeling of transgression regarding the holistic care script, but also regarding their midwives as representatives of this care approach. In Giddens's (1991) perspective, this deviation from the initial script causes a rupture in the coherence of the self-narrative, which needs to be restored through a new construction of meaning.

Lucie was a trained seamstress and unemployed at the time we met. Antoine, her spouse, worked as an independent in the entertainment sector. Both were in their mid-thirties. They lived in a small apartment in the city with their three-year-old daughter, Élise. I visited them a few days after the home birth of their second daughter, Emma. While waiting for Odile, their midwife, Lucie and I discussed her first breast-feeding experience, also attended by Odile. Lucie explained to me that after the postpartum follow-up was over, she had not dared to contact Odile again when she encountered breastfeeding difficulties: "It's also a question of pride, because it does not correspond to the ideal of home birth". After having a "very violent" experience when the milk came in and a worry-free breastfeeding initiation, her milk supply had suddenly dried up, and Élise had not gained any weight for two weeks. In hindsight, Lucie attributed this drop in her milk supply to a lack of motivation to breastfeed and a "small" postpartum depression.

Odile arrived at Lucie's place. They came back together on these difficulties and Lucie's silence: "You, you were the one to whom I could not talk about it," explained Lucie. A joint decision to extend the post-partum follow-up was taken to anticipate this situation. This second breastfeeding ended after two months. This time, Lucie felt supported by Odile, with whom she had already talked at length about breastfeeding during her pregnancy follow-up.

When I met with Lucie three months after weaning, she went back to this second experience, lived more serenely and highlighted Odile's role: "It was not peaceful, but at the same time it was fine because Odile was always there to discuss in the most critical moments". She especially enjoyed having only one reference person. During her first breastfeeding experience, Lucie felt "at the same time alone, and confronted to too many different opinions" from people around her as well as from early childhood nurses on duty at the local community centre where Lucie regularly went to weigh Élise. She developed on her feelings: "Odile never said that I had to breastfeed. She said, 'We try, and if it's not working for you, we stop'. It was important for me to have this dialogue and that a reference person told me that it was okay". She continued, "For me, breastfeeding is not central, maybe because it's not working well. [...] it becomes a source of anxiety very quickly". Lucie found it difficult to be completely responsible for feeding her child: "If it does not go well, it's very stressful all the time". She admitted that "it was already the case during pregnancy, but there is nothing to do!" Quite the opposite, for Lucie, breastfeeding required self-investment and restrictive body management, "a whole business!" She regretted having to keep her bra on "all the time, even at night to handle the lactation. [...] The fatty stuff you put on the nipples, frequent laundries because of milk leaks, et cetera. It gives a rhythm, things to do. I want my body for myself, and also during sexual intercourse. It takes a lot of space in daily life, you have it in mind all the time. I was palpating my breasts all the time". Joining a naturalistic conception, Lucie finally emphasised with humour that breastfeeding seems "naturally" not to work for her, which provided a justification "by nature" to her reluctance to breastfeed. Nevertheless, she conceded that she "still wanted to make it work, so the first milk received by Emma was mine. I didn't want it to be industrial food".

As highlighted in Lucie's discourse, breastfeeding requires heavy management to make women's bodies suitable. In midwives' and new mothers' discourse, the maternal body appears as "compliant" or "non-compliant". The nipples' shape, for example, was not left to chance. Desirable nipples "come out well"—unlike so-called "flat" or "inverted" nipples—and are "hard" so as to facilitate the newborn's latching on. In cases of non-compliance, strategies were put in place by mothers on their midwives' advice. During pregnancy, nipples identified as "too flat" could be "pulled" outwards daily using a syringe. For less problematic situations, no treatment was required before birth, but before each feeding, the nipples were massaged to "shape" them. The maternal body was thus remodelled to give it the desired shape for breastfeeding. The adherence to a non-interventionist approach and a commitment to the respect of physiology does not mean a lack of interventions around breastfeeding but rather the selection of specific tools and techniques in line with the birth model selected.

During pregnancy, an out-of-hospital birth project requires significant involvement and self-discipline from the mother, including bodily preparation for delivery to support the process physiologically. This preparation involves the practice of specific physical activities such as swimming or prenatal yoga, initiation to relaxation techniques, stretching of the perineum with the help of dedicated tools, and the consumption of herbal teas supporting uterine activity, to name a few (Chautems 2011; Gouilhers-Hertig 2017). However, this management can be experienced by mothers as heavily constraining and time-consuming. For example, Sandra, a new mother, was struck by the requirements and the time investment that are necessary to carry out the birth preparation as advised by midwives and admitted that she did not follow all the recommendations, saying, "There are so many things to do in the last weeks!" Alongside these delivery-focused measures, Marion, a midwife, recognised that she systematically recommended an elaborate breast training programme before birth, including breast massage and nipple stretching: "I really associate it with sports preparation. We can't know how the skin will react and it is not too invasive; there is no impact". Bodily preparation for birth thus also includes specific breast training. At the time of breastfeeding, the required body work is part of a continuity, in line with bodily practices mothers have already implemented in their daily lives since they found out they were pregnant and engaged in their out-of-hospital birth projects.

Shaping infants' bodies

Babies' bodies are also trained and reshaped to be suitable for an effective breastfeeding process. The parents I met frequently asked an osteopath to check their newborn shortly after birth in order to detect possible body tensions after birth. Midwives also frequently advised parents to get an osteopathic check-up to correct newborns' sucking. Maud, who encountered some difficulties in properly latching her daughter to her breasts, followed this suggestion and entrusted an osteopath with manipulations on her newborn daughter. The day after, she talked to her midwife about it, stating, "I think it's better. I really saw a big change in Rose's palate. It helps for latching". Aurore and David also brought their daughter to an osteopath a few days after birth. Aurore commented to her midwife, "She made Margaux go through her birth again. She reharmonised the sucking".

Some babies were diagnosed with a "tongue tie" by midwives, which may, according to them, hinder their sucking abilities.

Aurore and David had given birth to their daughter, Margaux, in a birth centre. I met them the next day for their midwife's first postpartum consultation. Aurore was a 40-year-old employee in the health sector. David, in his mid-thirties, had just resigned from his job as a social worker. They were living in a small city apartment. The delivery had been smooth, but when I arrived with their midwife, Pauline, they seemed in great distress. They invited us to sit in their living room, while Margaux was sleeping in their bedroom. Aurore described Margaux's behaviour at the breast: "She gets angry; she eats her hands". David added, "As soon as she cries, I am on alert. Aurore can't handle it, because she's exhausted and because it's not working [intended breastfeeding]". They both complained that Margaux had whined the whole night through, preventing them to get any sleep. "I have the feeling that I was feeding her and that it was useless since everything came out immediately", said Aurore. Pauline encouraged them: "In everything you describe, nothing is abnormal". Aurore still had the feeling that Margaux was "out of control" at the breast, suspecting a sucking inability. Pauline had previously examined Margaux's mouth and affirmed there was nothing wrong with her frenulum.

A few days later, the situation had not improved. Pauline observed Margaux's lingual frenulum again, observing, "The frenulum is posterior; it does not prevent Margaux from taking out her tongue, but could rather have an influence on the amplitude". Pauline proposed to ask a co-worker trained as a lactation consultant to examine Margaux. Pauline later informed me that the lactation consultant confirmed the tongue tie but did not see the need to intervene. According to her, Margaux could still get enough milk and her sucking abilities were quite satisfying. She suggested to Aurore to "set herself on hyperlactation mode" to offset Margaux's poor stimulation.

When Margaux later encountered some weight gain issues, Pauline finally suggested cutting her tongue tie and gave Aurore and David the contact information of a dentist [who is] able to perform the intervention.

Three months later, I met with Aurore and David. Margaux had undergone the surgery after all. Aurore found the process gruelling and preferred to look away during the intervention, while David handled Margaux to allow the dentist to cut her tongue tie. Nevertheless, they were now very happy. "She had to relearn how to suckle; it got better and better. Now, I have forgotten how she suckled before cutting the tongue tie" said Aurore.

This extract highlights the difficult and sinuous decision process to intervene on Margaux's body, even for the greater good of breastfeeding success. As in the case of parents' perspectives on vaccination (Brownlie & Leith, 2011), cutting a baby's tongue tie raises concerns about "the boundaries between 'the natural' and 'the cultural' in relation to infants" regarding medical interventions on infants' bodies (202). The "physicality of the intervention" upsets parents, who are expected to immobilise their baby and allow the professional to perform the medical act (ibid. 2011: 202). More broadly, parents are responsible for agreeing to perform a painful act on their child. When breastfeeding is presented by midwives as "natural" and part of a newborn's "innate knowledge", the necessity to alter infants' bodies is difficult to conceive for parents.

If mothers have to "learn" from experts how to have a "natural childbirth" (Mansfield 2008; Pasveer & Akrich 2001) or how to be "natural" mothers (Büskens 2010; Wolf 2011), newborns as well require the guidance of health professionals to unveil their supposedly "innate knowledge" of breastfeeding. For example, midwives sometimes rectified a baby's position at the breast to let her or him "knead the breast like a kitten". In the situation with Margaux's tongue tie, Pauline, the midwife, proposed to "give biological nurturing a try".[3] She asked Aurore to lie on her back on her bed with Margaux on her chest. The baby was expected to find the breast alone, without help from her parents. "The idea is that we promote the baby's nutrition reflexes, and the suction quality would be better. There is also more contact area between the mother and the baby, which promotes hormone production", explained Pauline, again using a hormone-based argumentation. In opposition to techniques routinely used by midwives and lactation consultants and perceived as more interventionist, with "biological nurturing", "the aim is to find a natural stimulation, to let the baby's instinct express itself without intervening", concluded Pauline. Margaux successfully found her mother's nipple by herself and started suckling, which was greatly appreciated by Aurore: "I like the sensations, and I can see her chin moving very well". More broadly, a newborn's sucking skills were always emphasised: "She has a mind-blowing sucking force", said one midwife. A new mother and her midwife also commented, "She catches it very well!" "Yeah, she's great!". These remarks contrast with the idea of a "breastfeeding instinct", since a newborn's "innate" sucking skills generally appeared as a good surprise, arousing midwives' as well as parents' admiration. For less "gifted" babies, however, a range of body techniques was applied to help them ensure efficient milk collection.

Tools and body techniques

Through their postpartum follow-up and the promotion of specific tools and practices, independent midwives engage with mothers in a process of co-construction of the maternal identity and body. Tension sets in between the potentially prescriptive character of knowledge transmission and the enhancement of maternal skills by inviting mothers to rely on their own feelings and desires.

During their visits, midwives observed feeding sessions. They provided advice on the respective positions of the mother and the baby, sometimes correcting them, and were particularly attentive to the child's latching. An inadequate latch can lead to a nipple injury or hinder the child's sucking efficiency. Ensuring a "good" latch was the parents' responsibility, but the baby was also guided by the midwife in case of an imperfect latch. Midwives frequently suggested that mothers open their children's lips wider with their fingers, commenting, "She takes the breast with a vacuum cleaner effect". If a baby was sleepy while feeding, midwives suggested undressing them in order to put the baby in "skin-to-skin" contact with the mother or by rubbing their feet ("it stimulates him"). If the stimulation was not vigorous enough, the midwife corrected the mother: "That's not stimulation! You really have to bother her!"

Midwives also suggested diversifying positions, by trying, for example, a face-to-face position, which was more stimulating in Eva's opinion. During a visit, she encouraged a newborn at her mother's breast: "You're all right against mom's breast. You've already suckled well, but you can take a little more". For her part, Capucine frequently recommended the "sandwich technique". This consisted of performing a breast compression, causing a milk influx to "stimulate" the baby's active suckling.

> We were in Aurore and David's bedroom for Pauline's third postpartum consultation. Margaux was three days old and had difficulties to suckle efficiently. Aurore was sitting bare-chested on her bed. Her milk had come in violently the day before. Her breasts were hard and tense. She was in pain. "It's completely beyond me to have such a body—that it has changed so much in such a short time. What stresses me is the size of these things [pointing to her breasts]; I don't feel at home anymore", said Aurore. Pauline suggested to try the "she-wolf position", using gravity to better drain her breast. She said to Margaux, "You know what? Mum needs a big helping hand from you. You'll be able to enjoy yourself!" Margaux was on her back on the bed. Aurore presented her breast from above. Pauline and David were lying on each side to closely observe the latch. We could distinctly hear Margaux's swallowing noises. Pauline commented, "She enjoys it! It sprinkles her palate!" Pauline nevertheless remained unsatisfied with Margaux's latch: "There is in all likelihood something that prevents her from having an optimal position".

As explained above, a lactation consultant later confirmed the diagnosis of a tongue tie, and Aurore and David eventually had the frenulum cut by a dentist.

In addition to positional advice, midwives provided mothers with techniques and tools to facilitate the breastfeeding initiation period and to alleviate sensitivities and pain when the milk came in or when nipples were subjected to intense and unusual solicitation. Midwives, for example, taught mothers massage and drainage techniques to avoid breast congestion or offered to fix silver shells on nipples to soothe and heal cracks. Along with breast management measures, midwives also suggested galactogenic remedies such as herbal teas, homoeopathy, aromatherapy, and increased intake of beverages. Breastfeeding also required the acquisition of more or less expensive goods, which took on a "fetish value" (Avishai 2007: 147) for mothers and midwives, who relied on these tools for smooth initiation and the continuation of breastfeeding in the longer term. In Giddens's (1991) perspective, these tools act as "reflective devices" meant to support a reflexive project. Consumption choices are the material translation of a selected lifestyle. In the frame of holistic care, the specific tools assisting breastfeeding initiation and lactation are "not only about how to act, but who to be" (Giddens 1991: 81). They are the material pillar of new mothers' routines and support the construction of maternal identity as elements of the holistic care script.

Midwives' recommendations sometimes also included basic nutrition advice. For example, Mireille systematically asked mothers about their meals' schedule and composition, correcting them if their answer did not satisfy her: "You don't eat enough, you have to eat six times a day! With breastfeeding, you're melting like snow in the sun, be careful not to lose too much, too fast! You have to take small meals; it allows the milk to be more stable".

In addition to initial biomedical training, midwives often also learned complementary therapies on their own initiative, leading to specific proposals to parents. Nevertheless, according to my observations, the same remedies—except for a few minor nuances—were proposed by each midwife, as if there was an effect of standardisation beyond their specific training in accordance with the idea of a "community of practice" (Jordan 2014).

On the other hand, some specific tools were not approved by midwives, or were at least perceived as such by mothers.

> Maud and Jonathan were in their late thirties. Maud was an employee in the early childhood sector. Jonathan was self-employed as a sport coach. When I first met them, they had given birth two days earlier to their daughter, Rose, in a birth centre. The delivery had been quick and smooth—Maud would tell me about it a few weeks later, saying, "I loved my delivery". Yet she was very anxious and stressed. The milk had come in brutally the day before, and her breasts had greatly increased in volume. "It's really impressive!" Maud exclaimed. She already had severe and painful cracks on both nipples despite a preventive use of the silver shells. Her breasts were very sore and hard.

After welcoming us and participating in the first fifteen minutes of the visit, Jonathan left to get breastfeeding support material. Maud was in their bedroom. She invited her midwife, Pauline, and I to sit with her on the bed. Rose was sleeping in her arms. Maud laid her gently to show her nipples to Pauline. "Yesterday, as she had regurgitated and she had taken three breasts, I told myself 'my goodness, it's going to be a nightmare'". Pauline told her about the need to massage the breasts to drain them. Maud explained not being "enthusiastic" to this idea of adding a supplementary step to her already intensive breast management, saying, "I have the impression that they will never be in peace!" She showed her second, less cracked nipple to Pauline. "But I think that now she has also screwed up this nipple a little. I have the feeling that she would never stop to suckle if she could". Pauline observed, "She also spends time doing herself good, at her mom's breast. With a breast in her mouth, she is in heaven".

Maud hesitantly evoked the possibility of using a nipple shield—a soft plastic shell fixed on the nipple during feedings—to enable her nipples to heal, saying to Pauline, "I'll tell you, it will not please you, but the nipple shield ..." Although they had never discussed it, Maud was well aware that the tool she wanted to use, largely administered in hospitals, deviated from the frame of reference of the care model she had chosen. The perceived risk is that the child may become used to the nipple shield, so that it can become difficult to remove, and an "instrumented" breastfeeding which reduces stimulation is set in long term. Indeed, Pauline did not seem enthusiastic, but validated the suggestion.

Jonathan came back from the pharmacy with compresses and clay in order to make a poultice and relieve Maud's breasts. He immediately returned to the pharmacy to buy nipple shields. Ten minutes later, he was back with the nipple shields. He asked Pauline if he could perform a breast massage to relieve Maud's breasts. Rose woke up and rapidly manifested her hunger. Her mouth was open, she turned her head on one side then the other, she waved her arms and brought her hands to her mouth. She was "searching", as midwives often said. Maud took homoeopathic arnica capsules in anticipation of the pain of feeding. She fixed the nipple shield on her nipple and asked Pauline for advice on how to bring Rose to the breast. Pauline pulled Rose's chin slightly to retract her lip. Maud was visibly in pain despite the nipple shield, but the feeding continued until Rose was satiated.

Through elected and non-elected advice and tools, midwives contribute to the construction of a "good maternal body": a body that performs breast-feeding successfully in terms of milk production—neither too much nor too little—as well as the nipples' shape, which should be easy for the child to grasp. The "good maternal body" is an available body which produces easily accessible milk for the newborn.

Beyond physical availability, from the midwives' perspective, it was also a matter for mothers to make themselves "emotionally available" to produce milk. During a visit, Odile, Lucie's midwife, commented on the sudden drop in lactation Lucie had experienced when her first child was born. She considered that the lack of milk was mainly related to an "unfavourable psychological state" and linked it to Lucie's lack of motivation to continue breastfeeding. In this regard, midwives also suggested practices to ensure that mothers were in a favourable mood for milk production. The practice of skin-to-skin contact, perceived as a means to reinforce the emotional bond between mothers and their children, was widely encouraged. Christine, a mother breastfeeding her third baby, told me about how she used this practice to prevent a possible drop in lactation:

> What I do a lot is skin-to-skin, I do it a lot for milk production. In the evening, like, it's skin-to-skin. I get him bare-skinned, I get myself bare-skinned, I have a skin-to-skin thing. I slip him in so he does not get cold, and I do it all night long.
>
> (interview with Christine, transcription)

In the same vein, Capucine proposed to a mother, "Don't hesitate to sniff his scalp before putting him at the breast". According to this approach, to produce milk, it was necessary to find a more affective and sensory dimension to breastfeeding, one beyond the rational and technical management of lactating breasts. Enjoying it would be a necessary condition for successful breastfeeding.

To help mothers connect with pleasurable physical sensations, midwives invited them to "settle" in their bodies and not "overthink" the breastfeeding process. Adeline systematically proposed a postpartum massage to mothers to "envelop, close up, reconnect with your body". She believed that "there is often a great mismatch" between mothers' thoughts and their embodied feelings. As a holistic practitioner, her role would be to help fix this mind–body gap. The mind–body interconnection was greatly emphasised by midwives, especially in the context of breastfeeding and oriented lactation management strategies.

Chantal was aware of the emotional dimension of breastfeeding support tools. For example, she advised a mother to continue using galactogenic phytotherapy "if it makes you happy to take it". In her perspective, the effectiveness of the product was not the most relevant requirement to continue or stop the treatment. She observed that women often told her family birth and breastfeeding stories and that it was useful to "work upon it":

> When women of the family say that they could not breastfeed, that they did not have milk, it permeates the representations around one's own breastfeeding. In holistic care, we know all that. They tell us spontaneously about family, et cetera. It's the same for delivery: If a woman has

in mind that her mother has a small pelvis, she may doubt her own ability to give birth vaginally.

(interview with Chantal, notes)

Chantal was especially attentive to her clients' familial backgrounds and the resulting representations they had developed regarding their own physiological bodily functions, including breastfeeding. Spending time listening and talking about these prior representations fit in midwives' holistic care approach and in their commitment to a contextualised understanding of each family.

Parental breastfeeding and paternal commitment

If fathers often have a hard time finding their place in the maternity ward (Reed 2005, Truc 2006), their involvement in birth preparation and during delivery is a constituent component of the natural childbirth model (Pruvost 2016; Quagliariello 2017a). At the beginning of the natural childbirth movement, Dick-Read already stressed the parturient's need for emotional support, ideally provided by her spouse, thereby reinforcing marital ties among middle-class families (Wertz & Wertz 1989 [1977]). In the context of an out-of-hospital birth project, the father's active participation is an unquestioned requirement. Home birth parents, for example, have to prepare for the possibility of giving birth on their own if labour is progressing quickly and their midwife cannot arrive on time to assist the delivery, as happened to one of the couples participating in my research. Midwives teach parents how to manage this situation during their birth preparation classes. More broadly, during the pregnancy follow-up, specific massages and technical gestures are taught to fathers to support their spouses during childbirth, so that at the time of delivery, fathers often act as midwives' partners (Pruvost 2016). According to Mireille, "couples completely unveil themselves during delivery".

At her first postpartum consultation with Corinne, Mireille discussed the course of delivery a few days before and the role played by her spouse. Their baby's body was held back by his umbilical cord, and the father had to help Mireille perform a manipulation to release him. Mireille emphasised his confident gesture: "I found him very calm, very helpful". Corinne confirmed his diligent involvement in the out-of-hospital birth project. In another postpartum follow-up, Isabelle told Sofia how she felt as though she were intruding when she had joined Sofia and her spouse the day before for the delivery: "You were great, just the two of you, when I arrived. It's really hard to find out which choreography we should create". After two hospital deliveries, Ines was finally able to give birth at home, a plan she had for her previous deliveries but which could not be achieved. In her opinion, this home birth had a positive impact on her relationship with her spouse.

For me, Romuald is the only baby we really gave birth to together, in a common effort. From the beginning, he is a baby who connects us. Everything we had projected, we could put into practice at the moment of birth. We welcomed him knowing where the other was, where everyone was, as if we had established a strong trust bond regarding our role as parents.

(interview with Ines, notes)

In these birth narratives, the father's role is presented as central in the discourse of midwives as well as of mothers. In the situations described above, the fathers' attitudes during childbirth were enhanced by midwives. In contrast, midwives sometimes told me privately of their disapproval of a father's attitude during childbirth, for example, that "he was constantly on his smartphone!" Fathers' performance was evaluated by midwives according to the unspoken standards adopted by the community of practice (Jordan 2014). As also highlighted by Perrenoud (2016), midwives position themselves as women's defenders, promoting a caring, supporting attitude from fathers. Consistent with other researchers' findings in Italy, the United States, and France, a compliant paternal behaviour emerges from these narratives: committed, cooperative, and calm (Quagliariello 2017a; Reed 2005; Truc 2006).

One of my interlocutors, Jeanne, was living alone at the time of her son's birth: her partner was abroad and was not able to come to Switzerland. She had planned to give birth at home with her midwife and a close friend but eventually underwent a caesarean section (her friend was allowed to stay with her at the maternity ward). She joined her partner three months after birth and had regular contact with him by phone in the meantime. In this unusual setting, she precisely justified her choice of holistic care in relation to her partner's absence at the end of the pregnancy and for the delivery. In this context, her close relationship with her midwife, enabled by the holistic care model and especially the continuity of care, allowed her to feel supported and taken care of. The midwife's support was perceived as a substitution for the absent spouse's involvement.

Apple (1987) and Kukla (2005) demonstrated that mothers are the main targets of health professionals' attention. However, at the time of the postpartum, fathers are often absent from midwives' discourses, which focus on the mother–child duo and on the maternal body. As highlighted by Miller (2011), "Discourses which frame men's experiences of transition to fatherhood do not invoke biological predisposition or the need for medical surveillance" (1096). Fathers thus escape normative injunctions issued to mothers concerning their newly maternal body and its lactating management. In Miller's study on transition to first-time fatherhood in the United Kingdom, breastfeeding was described as an obstacle hindering fathers' involvement in childcare. Quite the opposite, I observed that breastfeeding initiation and the related management of the lactating body was often a privileged moment of fathers' involvement. According to my discussions with parents, fathers' involvement was also suggested by midwives during birth preparation classes. Midwives emphasised the spouse's supporting role, for example, that they could prepare a galactogenic herbal tea or provide water or food to the breastfeeding mother. This supports the thesis of "fatherhood in the service of motherhood" (Truc 2006: 343), in which fathers take care of their children by taking care of their mother. As a result, fathers' involvement and commitment to breastfeeding often resulted in the desire to produce a favourable material environment by taking care of housework (groceries, cooking, cleaning, laundry, et cetera) and some aspects of the newborn's care, such as diaper changing or soothing the baby. To create suitable conditions, fathers also assisted mothers and babies by helping them settle in comfortably at feeding time. "It was as though he was part of the process. He settled us both comfortably. It was not like I was breastfeeding. It was a three-part organisation. It's really the three of us", said Léa when speaking about the first days of breastfeeding and her spouse's involvement. Fathers also engaged in hands-on breastfeeding support by helping their spouses handle lactation when the milk came in or by providing practical and emotional support, including sharing wakefulness during night-time breastfeeding or listening to their spouses' concerns regarding the suitability of their lactation.

Couples facing midwives' matricentric approach

If the feeling of being out of place is dominant in fathers' experience of their spouses' postpartum stay at the maternity ward (Truc 2006), at home, fathers feel mostly integrated into their midwives' postpartum consultations. David, for example, greatly appreciated the discussions with his midwife, Pauline. "It allowed debriefing beyond just breastfeeding. It felt good to tell myself, 'She will come, we will be able to chat together'". Nevertheless, midwives' postpartum follow-ups remained "matricentric"—that is, fathers' role was primarily defined by their ability to meet their spouses' needs (Goody 2001 in Truc 2006). Unlike David, Emmanuel told me that he considered Eva to be Sandra's midwife rather than the couple's midwife:

> We don't know what to expect during the first weeks. You imagine that it will be a lot more natural, but no—Breastfeeding is hard to settle. Also from a psychological point of view, when the baby arrives, we know that we put ourselves in danger: The baby is completely dependent. It would help to have someone to rely on during the first weeks. I could not talk to the midwife: I saw that Eva was mostly focused on the baby/mother logistics.
>
> (interview with Emmanuel, notes)

This matricentric approach is underpinned by midwives' integration of gender norms concerning parental roles and responsibilities. Through a gendered approach, they also contributed to the reproduction of those norms. For example, during one of Capucine's postpartum consultations, Jérome undressed Camille, his daughter, to weigh her. Capucine commented, "he is doing well, your daddy! You're comfortable, it's cool". During her previous visits to the couple, but also more broadly during the consultations I attended with her, I never heard Capucine congratulate a mother for her baby-undressing skills. Later during the same visit, Camille lost a sock. Jérome immediately noticed it, picked up the sock, and put it back on Camille's foot. Nevertheless, Capucine turned to Tamara to inform her of the existence of socks with an integrated elastic band, preventing babies from losing them. Despite Jérome's attentive attitude towards Camille's dressing, Capucine had the reflex to talk to Tamara, as if Jérome could not be responsible for the purchase and choice of Camille's clothes.

This understanding reflects the shift that has occurred in the fatherhood model since the eighteenth century, when industrialisation and men's paid work changed gendered parental roles. Since fathers were working away from home during the daytime, rearing infants progressively became mothers' rather than fathers' responsibility (Lupton & Barclay 1997 in Faircloth 2014b). The spread of Ainsworth and Bowlby's work on attachment and "maternal deprivation", which presented mothers as central attachment figures for their children, strengthened assertions that "men and women had different but complementary roles within the family as well as society more broadly" (Faircloth 2014b: 187).

As the consultation described above marked the end of Capucine's home follow-up, she scheduled the last appointment with Tamara at her practice for the six weeks' consultation.[4] Jérome then let Capucine know that he might not be able to come. Capucine complimented him: "It's true that you're here each time I come—well done! There are dads I never see". The father's presence was valued by midwives but not expected at each consultation. However, an attitude of avoidance towards the midwife was identified as a deviant behaviour. In Lisa's situation, Alexis, the father, was "very little invested" (in Lisa's words) in caring for Paul, his son. After her first postpartum visit, their midwife, Eva, commented on his attitude when we were alone. "He is absent. Even when he's present, he's little involved". Alexis had spent the entire duration of Eva's visit playing with Angèle, their oldest child. He had barely greeted us at our arrival or said goodbye when we left. I have never seen him again afterwards. Two weeks later, after another visit, Eva again condemned Alexis's absence from postpartum consultations, as well as from Paul's hands-on care: "She's a boss lady, she handles all the daily life. For me, he's a big selfish baby". In this situation, Eva did not directly address Alexis's absence with Lisa until Lisa openly complained about it, crying. Eva just listened to Lisa, without giving any advice.

Reed (2005) conducted an ethnography of American middle-class men's transitions to fatherhood. He observed that childbirth preparation classes socialise parents into gendered parental roles. Fathers are expected by professionals to embrace the role of protectors during the birth process, while also complying with professionals' authority. My findings conform with those of Tomori (2015), suggesting that this role also applies to breast-feeding. As "women's defenders", midwives do their best to involve fathers in their efforts to support their spouses. At the time of delivery, they set up a collaboration with fathers to make labour smoother and facilitate the birth process. During breastfeeding initiation, fathers continue to act as midwives' partners to ease their spouses' experience.

Sofia's second child was not able to suckle properly. As a result, her breasts were not adequately drained and she spent the first month sick, having one breast infection after another. Her milk production was so abundant and out of control that Isabelle, her midwife, and Pascal, her spouse, once "milked" her. "I was on all fours, Pascal on one breast, Isabelle on the other one, in total confidence. It wasn't funny at the time, but now the three of us laugh about it" commented Sofia. At the time I met her, she had just given birth to Lou, her fourth child, again with Isabelle's help. She and Pascal were well trained to handle the feeling of pain when the milk comes in.

> The day after Lou's birth, Isabelle and Sofia tried to assess whether the milk was coming in. "And the breasts, are they supple?" asked Isabelle. "They started hardening this afternoon", answered Sofia. Pascal had gone out to buy cabbage to relieve Sofia's breast congestion. When he joined us later in the room, he had already prepared some sage herbal tea and offered Sofia cabbage leaves with a spread of fresh cheese to put on her breasts.

> Two days later, Sofia was worried. The milk came in "very intensely", and she dreaded breast engorgement: "They are really like big stones, I have enough for eight babies!" She explained to Isabelle her lacta-tion management strategy in detail: milk pumping after each feeding, sage herbal tea to counter her hyperlactation, cabbage and fresh cheese poultices. Isabelle approved and asked Sofia whether she wanted her to weigh Lou. Sofia said "yes!" I joined Isabelle as she brought Lou to Pascal, who was preparing poultices in the bathroom so they would be ready to apply directly after Lou's feeding. Pascal undressed Lou to allow Isabelle to weigh her. When we returned to the bedroom, Sofia mentioned that she had not changed a single diaper yet: Pascal had already started elimination communication and was solely in charge of this aspect of Lou's care. Pascal joined us and explained what he had prepared for Sofia and where he had put it. He asked Sofia, "Dare I take a quick shower?" obviously waiting for her consent.

When I met with Sofia a few months after the end of Isabelle's follow-up, we caught up on the developments of her lactation management. She was disappointed with Isabelle's guidance, with the fact that she had stopped visiting after only three postpartum consultations despite her still-stressful lactation management. As with her previous breast-feedings, she had fever spikes and breast infections. She could only talk about it to Isabelle on the phone, as she did not offer to come and see her: "She left me kind of abandoned". Sofia felt discouraged "It's a little exhausting, this milk business. I'm not the biggest fan of breastfeeding, but I find it important to do". During this period, she considered her greatest support to be Pascal. "We really managed to control the thing [her hyperlactation]". She developed the many ways Pascal participated in the breastfeeding process:

"He's always the one who makes the breastfeeding herbal tea. He asks me 'where do you want to breastfeed?' and brings the baby to me. At night, it's always him who sleeps on Lou's side because I'm more tired. He gets up to take her and brings me a glass of water. During the night, it's his role, so we can breastfeed together. These small gestures are settled automatically. He's good at taking care".

In this situation, the midwife's withdrawal was overcome by the father's high degree of commitment, forming a "breastfeeding team" with the mother (Rempel & Rempel 2011). Like Pascal, other fathers embraced the role of protector of the breastfeeding process, sometimes also substituting for the midwife if she was not involved adequately with respect to the couple's expectations or if they felt that she did not consider a breastfeeding issue seriously enough. Some fathers even positioned themselves as their spouses' spokespersons.

Tamara and Jérome were both in their early twenties. She was working as an employee in the early childhood care sector. Jérome was an entre-preneur in agriculture. They had given birth at home to their daughter, Camille, in a small village in the countryside. When their midwife Capucine told me about the delivery, she was thrilled: "It was really great, very fast! Tamara caught the baby by herself. Her gestures were very instinctive and spontaneous". When I first met them, two days after Camille's birth, they were indeed very pleased. Tamara felt fine, and Camille suckled well and often.

One week later, during Capucine's consultation, Tamara and Jérome seemed unsettled for the first time. Camille had cried a lot the past two evenings. Tamara's right nipple was sore. Capucine examined it, saying, "Yes, there is a small crack". She advised Tamara to let some breast milk dry on the nipple after each feeding and to change breastfeeding positions. Precisely at that moment, Camille was hungry. Capucine suggested a new position to breastfeed her and change the stress on the nipple. She helped position Camille at the breast, crossing her legs and placing her against Tamara's stomach, facing her. After a few attempts to latch Camille,

Tamara admitted that she was in pain. Capucine stayed confident: "We'll see with these measures if it's enough to heal this little wound". Tamara had thought about temporarily pumping her milk and giving it to Camille with a bottle to relieve her wounded nipple. Capucine discouraged her: "There are several aspects: you face what you've pumped, some women can only pump very little. And when you put her back at the breast, the wound comes back". Tamara did not insist. Jérome, on the other hand, was not satisfied with Capucine's advice. He seemed afraid that Tamara's wound was more painful than she would express.

At Capucine's next visit, a week later, the wound on the right nipple was not healed yet, and there was an additional crack on the other nipple. We sat in the living room. This time, Tamara immediately addressed her cracked nipples. As suggested by Capucine, she had let a drop of breast milk dry on her nipple after each feed and then had fixed a silver shell on top. Again, Capucine advised to keep Camille pressed against her stomach during feeding. Jérome rapidly intervened: "Yeah, it really hurts! I said to myself, 'my God, I don't know how it will go'",expressing his worries more openly than Tamara. Camille was awake in her mother's arms and eager to eat. Tamara asked Capucine if she "dared" to put her at the right breast, which was still the most painful. "Do you want me to look?" said Capucine. "Yes, you have to look at it!" Jérome answered immediately. Tamara obviously dreaded to offer Camille her wounded nipple. Capucine crouched beside Tamara, sitting on a couch. She recommended to try the sandwich technique to allow Camille to get some milk without sucking too hard on the nipple. Tamara moved Camille closer to her breast. Capucine indicated to Tamara how to position her: "Don't be in a hurry; you can really caress her mouth from top to bottom. Here, I think that it's not too bad, I really saw her lip retract". Jérome also kneeled beside Capucine to look closer at Camille's latch while listening to Capucine's explanations.

In this extract, Jérome spoke many times on behalf of Tamara, judging that she was not complaining loudly enough regarding her nipples' cracks. In this way, Jérome took on the role of spokesperson and protector of his spouse's interests and well-being. In this protector role, as analysed by Tomori (2015), "men's support for breastfeeding both reinforced and renegotiated gendered expectations for their role as fathers" (167). On the one hand, this role falls within a traditional approach of parental roles and responsibilities, assigning the father as the family's protector. On the other hand, the father's structural and emotional support towards breast-feeding and lactation management leads to a new model of an emotion-ally involved father, suggesting that the model of intensive motherhood (Faircloth 2014b) extends to men.

Breastfeeding as teamwork

The literature emphasises gender inequalities regarding intensive parenting culture, with mothers remaining primarily responsible for hands-on childcare (Le Goff & Levy 2016; Shirani, Henwood & Coltart 2012). My fieldwork observations, focused on the marginal population of home birth parents, nuance these results: most fathers engaged in all aspects of childcare, including hands-on lactation care. Beyond their motivation, fathers' involvement depended on practical conditions, especially their paternity leave—or lack thereof—and other work arrangements. At the time of my fieldwork, Swiss federal law did not include any paternity leave so that paid leave for new fathers depended on employers. In practice, fathers were granted anywhere from one day to three weeks off. In the private sector, it was usually restricted to a few days. Fathers generally added paid or unpaid days off to this very limited leave. Pascal, for example, had five days of paternity leave provided by his employer. Since Lou was born just before Easter, the bank holidays coupled with additional days off allowed him to stay home for two weeks after his daughter's birth. In my research, eight fathers were self-employed, enabling some of them to do little or no work in the first weeks after birth. This was the case for Jérome, whom the midwife congratulated for being present at each consultation.

Moreover, studies show that an important part of fatherhood responsibilities and involvement towards their family rests upon their identity as breadwinners, in fathers' as well as in their spouses' minds (Shirani, Henwood & Coltart 2012; Williams 2008). This conjecture is underpinned by the idea that men's primary commitment is work, compromising their involvement in hands-on childcare and housework. This idea contrasts with the work organisation of most fathers I met on my fieldwork, who worked part-time, embracing a "downshifting" strategy in order to spend more time taking hands-on care of their families. Nevertheless, Pascal and Sofia's narrative indicated that a full-time job did not preclude Pascal's commitment to childcare.

Rempel and Rempel's (2011) research showed different involvement modalities for fathers that influence mothers' experiences and practices, including handling household tasks, enquiring about breastfeeding, offering emotional support, and valuing and encouraging their spouses. Even if midwives did not directly address this topic (at least not during the postpartum consultations I attended), some of them seemed aware of the impact of the spouse's gaze on a breastfeeding mother. Capucine, for example, recognised that "the assessment of the breastfeeding performance also rests upon the partner's gaze", beyond mothers' own feelings and their infants' response, including their weight gain. In Carole and Michael's situation, Gaspard's weight stagnation brought Carole to doubt her ability to successfully breastfeed her son. When we met a few months after the end of the postpartum follow-up, we came back to this topic. Carole identified Michael's support as a key element in maintaining trust and motivation regarding breastfeeding. Michael claimed, "I didn't do much". Carole corrected him, "Yes, you did—you were there; you were very understanding; you never said that I might not have enough milk".

As suggested by Carole, besides hands-on support, a father's kind and positive gaze on his spouse's breastfeeding process plays a crucial part in breastfeeding initiation as well as its long-term course. Tomori (2015) suggests that spousal support for breastfeeding contributes to building "kin ties" within the family unit:

> Through defending/protecting the birth/breastfeeding process, and providing emotional and instrumental support, [fathers] enacted the paternal personhoods that they began to craft during childbirth education courses. Through these processes of kin work they actively constructed kin ties with their wives and children and forged an emotionally engaged model of fatherhood.
>
> (Tomori 2015: 155-156)

From a "breastfeeding team's" perspective (Rempel & Rempel 2011), parents engage in a teamwork effort to successfully initiate and maintain breastfeeding. As asserted by Mélody, "it's really something we do together".

Mélody and Simon were both in their mid-thirties. They lived in the countryside and were both self-employed in retail. They were planning a home birth until Mélody was diagnosed with gestational diabetes. Even though it had to happen in a hospital, they were still able to give birth to their baby under their midwife Adeline's guidance, in a delivery room at the disposal of independent registered midwives. However, Mélody's obstetrician found it necessary to medically induce labour at thirty-nine weeks. As the inducement did not work (no cervical dilatation), Mélody eventually underwent a caesarean section.

I met Mélody and Simon with Adeline for their first postpartum visit after returning home. They were shocked by their hospital postpartum stay—more precisely, by the lack of consideration regarding fathers. "No one offers food to the father! They arrive with meal trolleys; there is nothing for him! It's normal that fathers are present, but nothing is done to make space for them, especially at the logistics level", observed Mélody. Before birth, Simon and Mélody had established different strategies for Simon to feel as involved as possible during the pregnancy. They had regularly practised haptonomy so that Simon could "bond" with the foetus. Simon studied the Bonapace method,[5] which prepares fathers to optimally accompany their spouses during delivery. It was crucial for Simon to concretely support Mélody at each step of the birth process: "At least we can do something!" The unexpected childbirth issue made him feel particularly powerless. After the caesarean section, Simon managed to collect the placenta and bring it home. He followed a Chinese medicine recipe provided by Mélody's acupuncturist: first emptying the blood vessels, then steaming the placenta above spice-infused water, cutting in thin slices, dehydrating, grinding into powder with a coffee grinder, and finally, filling small capsules with the powder. Mélody took two of these capsules every day to recover faster and to support her lactation.

It was hard for Simon to be forced into passivity at the time of his son's birth. Throughout the long preparation, he had found a way to feel involved and supportive of his spouse and son. During the hospital stay, he managed to spend each night at the maternity ward with Mélody and Ilias, their son. He slept on a chair next to their bed. Since Ilias's birth, Simon took charge of all aspects of hands-on childcare except for nursing. Nevertheless, as told by Mélody a few months after Ilias's birth, Simon was also proactive during breastfeeding sessions: "Whenever I breastfeed Ilias, Simon is active. Even in the middle of the night, he wakes up and accompanies us. His role is to burp Ilias between the two breasts. He also helps to position him. As soon as Ilias has finished feeding, Simon changes his diaper. He is an integral part of breastfeeding, of the meal cycle".

Through these support strategies and practices, Simon managed to be involved in each aspect of his newborn's care, including nursing. He and Mélody developed a way to equally share the learning process of Ilias's hands-on care. In this process, Simon also learned to "undo" traditional gendered patterns that identify mothers as having primary responsibility for newborns' care (Miller 2011: 1102).[6] This gender "transgression" was incidentally emphasised by Mélody, who said about Simon, "Sometimes I find that Simon is almost more maternal than me". A few months later, she had resumed work and told me about their organisation regarding Ilias's care: "I would almost say that Simon cares more for Ilias than me. He supervises all his diet, for example". Ilias was not breastfed anymore; Simon alone would wake up at night to feed him. Interestingly, Mélody established a connection between the distribution of their parental tasks and the fact that she earned more money than Simon: "It's a combination of the fact that Simon has a very maternal side on the one hand, and contributes little financially on the other hand. Taking care of Ilias is what he can do to provide for the family". Despite their shared efforts to "undo" gendered parental patterns, Mélody still struggled to take a step back from the traditional male breadwinner/female carer parenting approach.

Long-term breastfeeding: keeping lactation afloat

The holistic care model emerged from a desire to respect the physiological course of birth and the postpartum period, in which breastfeeding plays a central role. Based on my observations, mothers I met tended to breastfeed for a longer time than most mothers in Switzerland, where the total median duration is 31 weeks. In the Swiss context, breastfeeding beyond the child's first year can thus be experienced as a marginalised practice undertaken by concerned parents. Based on an emic typology, I chose to define long-term breastfeeding as breastfeeding maintained for one year or more, which was the case for half of the mothers in my fieldwork. In long-term breastfeeding, the act becomes a lasting part of the daily lives of concerned families, far exceeding the so-called postpartum period. Mothers often told me that they wanted to breastfeed for as long as they would produce milk, that their child would fancy it, and—to some extent—that they would also enjoy it: "As long as it works and he wants to suckle", as Corinne, a new mother, summarised.

> Aurélie and Fabien lived in a small apartment in the city. They were both in their early thirties and worked part-time. Aurélie was a social worker and Fabien was working as a sports coach. They gave birth to their son, Milo, at home. Aurélie resumed work after six months of maternity leave. Milo did not go to day care afterwards: His parents and grandparents managed to take care of him in turns.
>
> When Milo was fourteen months old, Aurélie said she did not have a "time-related goal" about continuing breastfeeding. Nevertheless, she was not considering weaning at that time, stating, "I'm still very happy to breastfeed, even if it's complicated". She had been back to work for eight months and continued to pump her milk once a day at her workplace. She mentioned a "demanding management" to maintain her milk production. As soon as she would perceive a drop in lactation, she would take homoeopathic granules and increase fluid intake to revive her milk production. She evoked a "feeling of a vicious circle": in her perception, the anxiety generated by a drop in lactation tended to inhibit her milk production. However, she concluded, "Breastfeeding is not complicated once you have thrown yourself into it. It is anchored in our daily lives". She assured me that she never saw it "as a constraint".

As highlighted in the above extract, breastfeeding may require constant vigilance, even when it is established over time. Specific equipment aiming at "disciplining" lactating breasts or relieving pain caused during breast-feeding initiation is nonetheless no longer required in time. A transition takes place from the management of lactating breasts to the management of lactation. Like Aurélie, many mothers I met pumped their milk in order to keep breastfeeding going after resuming work, thereby both maintaining their lactation and ensuring sufficient milk supply to their children during the workday. In this way, pumping at the workplace often embodies the only way for mothers to achieve their breastfeeding projects (Avishai

2004). The breast pump thus becomes a significant part of their breastfeeding experience.

By separating the product—breast milk—from the nursing process, the breast pump allows mothers to separate themselves from their infant, sharing the responsibility of feeding the child with their spouses or other persons. In this perspective, despite a process often described as gruelling, pumping is also positively perceived by mothers as a way to regain some control and autonomy (Dykes 2005). Nevertheless, there is a clear feeling of frustration that dominates mothers' speech. Avishai (2004) noted, "Pumping at the workplace emerges as a labour-intensive, time-consuming, challenging and stressful enterprise" (143). In particular, successfully pumping at work hinges upon access to a range of facilities, including a private and adequately equipped space (with a seat as well as electricity and water supplies), the possibility to pump frequently enough to both maintain lactation and prevent breast congestion, and a refrigerator to store the expressed milk. As a result, viable pumping at work requires a high degree of flexibility and autonomy, making it only realistic for women who enjoy a privileged working environment.

> Olivia and Alain were in their thirties and living in a small village in the countryside. Olivia worked full-time, employed in the public administration. Alain was a part-time social worker. They had planned to give birth in a birth centre but ended up having a caesarean section in the hospital due to labour dystocia. Breastfeeding initiation was smooth and easy, and Olivia very much enjoyed breastfeeding her daughter, Peregrine, during her maternity leave. When she resumed work after five months, she had planned to pump her milk at work to achieve her goal to breastfeed Peregrine exclusively during her first six months of life, and then to continue breastfeeding supplemented by other solid and liquid intakes for an undetermined period. However, she quickly realised that it was difficult to integrate breast pump sessions to her work schedule: "It started to become difficult when I resumed work. I did not want anyone to know what I was doing". In addition, she never felt the urge to pump: "I almost never had hard or painful breasts. It quickly regulated itself. I didn't have any leaks. I did not have a compelling need to pump". Her milk supply dropped shortly after resuming work, and she had a hard time pumping her milk: "It's very frustrating because I feel that what was missing was just for it to click". This made her feel very guilty, telling herself, "It's me—I can't put myself in suitable conditions for it to work". During pumping sessions, she viewed pictures and videos of Peregrine to put herself in a favourable mood: "I had made short films of her suckling. I was pretty sensitive to the sound, when she swallows well". She was able to reach her six-month goal of exclusive breastfeeding, but one month later, Peregrine suddenly declined her breast and never accepted it again. Olivia had noticed that she had to

pump longer for the milk to come and connected this observation to Peregrine's sudden refusal. Olivia did not insist or try to revive her milk supply. She stated, "I was disappointed that it stopped and that I no longer had these moments of intimacy with her, but I didn't have the energy to do anything else".

As highlighted by Olivia's embarrassment, pumping at work emphasises the body and its physiological functions in the workplace, where it is usually excluded. Breastfeeding employees face a paradox: on the one hand, they must adhere to "the standard of the disembodied, unencumbered professional worker" (Avishai 2004: 145); on the other hand, the experience of pregnancy, motherhood, and breastfeeding blurs boundaries between the public and private spheres and challenges the new mothers' professional identities. Even besides the actual pumping sessions, the physiology of lactation requires constant attention to prevent leaks or engorgements. Their lactating bodies remind themselves to mothers permanently. Rather than questioning the standard of the "disembodied" employee, they comply with it by striving to make their pumping sessions and the demonstrations of their lactating bodies invisible (Avishai 2004; Palmer 2009 [1988]). Corinne, another mother, had an experience which reflects how pumping sessions are devaluated. Despite a work environment "very hostile to breastfeeding and new mothers", she managed to pump at work for seven months. She pumped while eating during her lunch break, "in the bathroom or in a windowless meeting room", fearing to be discovered by a co-worker as the door did not lock.

The awkwardness of pumping at work also relates to the stigmatisation of bodily fluids. Perceived as potentially dirty, embarrassing, or contaminating, these secretions evoke the idea of an out-of-control female body (Bramwell 2001). On the perception of breast milk, several authors recalled that from a historical point of view, the fluids emanating from the female body have long been perceived as uncontrollable and impure (Schmied & Lupton 2001; Palmer 2009 [1988]; Gatrell 2011). The female body's ability to let fluids escape involuntarily—to "leak"—thus breaks subversively with a dominant conception of the individual in modern neoliberal societies defined by a fixed and tight body envelope that acts as a separator between individuals (Kukla 2005).

As noticed by Stearns (2010), pumping is not a matter concerning only working mothers but rather acts as a lactation and breastfeeding management technique. For example, in my fieldwork, Sarah, a temporarily unemployed new mother, imposed upon herself a monthly "breast pump weekend" in order to stock up frozen milk, to make up for a lactation drop since the return of her periods. In addition, she would take home-made fennel and malt capsules daily. "There is one thing about which I can take action: having more milk again", she explained. In her perspective, there were some structural and environmental factors that were stressful and therefore detrimental to her milk supply and that she could not control, but her own body management fell within her responsibility. In the early postpartum period, the breast pump can also be added to nursing sessions in case of weight stagnation. The pumped breast milk is then fed to the baby as a supplement if they do not suckle as efficiently as necessary to get enough milk and stimulate lactation. For example, when their daughter Morgane's weight stagnated, Céline and Julien's midwife suggested to pump and give her the pumped milk after each feeding.

> When I met Céline and Julien a few weeks after the end of their midwife's follow-up, we talked about their breastfeeding experience over coffee. As Céline still breastfed their oldest daughter, Yvonne, Julien observed, "There is Morgane, there is Yvonne and there is the device", suggesting that Céline constantly had someone or something stimulating her breasts. As a stay-at-home mother, Céline never had to use a breast pump for Yvonne: "It's difficult, I don't pump much yet. I pump more and more, but it's not great moments of pleasure". Given that Yvonne had asked much more frequently to suckle since Morgane's birth, Céline accepted "to have something hanging on [her] breasts all the time". For his part, Julien did all the household chores so that Céline could completely devote herself to breastfeeding. Very involved in the management of breastfeeding, he often reminded Céline that it was time to pump her milk.

Avishai (2004) described how mothers produce their lactating bodies "as a carefully managed site, and breastfeeding as a 'project'—a task to be researched, planned, implemented and constantly assessed" (136). Once breastfeeding is established, mothers continue to evaluate its success on the basis of different criteria: their child's weight gain, the quantity of milk produced, or their ability to maintain breastfeeding after resuming work (Avishai 2011; Marshall & Godfrey 2011).

> Nine months after Rose's birth, Maud told me that she initially felt discouraged following her gruelling breastfeeding initiation and that she then "pulled herself together", telling herself, "you have to take it on yourself and grit your teeth". Once initial obstacles were overcome, Rose was still breastfed. Maud had adjusted her daily life to optimise breastfeeding. She was convinced that her milk was the best for her daughter and paid particular attention to her own diet: "I know exactly what I eat, so it's the best for her"—implying that with formula, one does not know precisely the diet of the cows producing the milk. She added various supplements, such as probiotics, to an exclusively organic diet. Before Rose's birth, Maud was a vegetarian. However, she "started to eat meat so that there would be some [meat] in [her] milk". She believed that it was in any case very beneficial for her to pay extra

attention to what she was eating, stating, "I feel so much better. I see it in my energy. I feel like I've never been so healthy".

Five months later, we met again. Rose, then fourteen months old, was still breastfed. Maud still did not drink any alcohol, even occasionally, whereas she had previously enjoyed a glass of wine at mealtime. She told me, "I actually like this idea of not drinking alcohol". On the other hand, she kept the habit of drinking a non-alcoholic beer every night, a ritual instituted because of the galactogenic virtues attributed to malt and maintained because she had developed a taste for it.

Like Darmon's (2003) interlocutors, Maud seemed to have worked actively to change her likes and dislikes. This work was undertaken from the beginning of the pregnancy in a voluntarist way and then continued during breastfeeding in order to make it a sustainable and incorporated disposition. The inscription of dietary habits in the body has been identified by Darmon (2003) as "one of the components of confirming commitment during the taking in hand phase" (150). In parallel to a rationalisation of daily life, the voluntary implementation of habits creates the structural conditions necessary to maintain a long-term commitment.

Beyond the technical management of breastfeeding, the mother's relationship to her body and to her identity is also redesigned. For mothers, the limits fade between their own bodies and their children's bodies: Breastfeeding implies the mother's agreement to continue "sharing" her body for an indefinite period of time after delivery. When I met her five months after her daughter's birth to discuss the evolution of her breastfeeding, Léa explained that she felt a big difference between her motherhood experience and that of her friends who did not breastfeed:

> They do not live the same thing in fact. It's as if I gave birth, but I did not return to being a woman. I still have a part of my body for my child. I have a responsibility regarding her diet.
>
> (interview with Léa, notes)

In another discussion, six months later, Léa confirmed her persistent feeling of "not becoming a woman again". For example, she explained that she still paid attention to her clothing in order to facilitate breastfeeding, remarking "I'm a little less put together than before". She also believed that breastfeeding prevented her from losing pregnancy weight. She saw her body as maternal first and had not yet regained the pre-pregnancy sensations of living in her body. Although she seemed to regret it, she was not yet considering weaning: "My priority is breastfeeding. This is not a reason why I would wean sooner".

As highlighted by Sachs (2005), as long as they are breastfeeding, women are stuck in a liminal state—not pregnant anymore, but still not completely separated from their babies, which may seem intolerable for themselves, but also for others. In this perspective, Léa's observations align with the cultural injunction to rapidly resume sexuality during the postpartum period, including working at quickly getting one's postpartum body back in shape, fitting with an ideal of female bodies as slim, smooth, and virtually pubescently young. Since sexuality has been medicalised following the emergence of sexology as a science during the second part of the twentieth century in North America and Europe, and the lack of desire has been problematised as a psychological or medical issue (Bozon 2009; Giami & De Colomby 2002). The lack of women's desire during the postpartum period has been identified as a specific issue requiring medical care since the 1980s (Hirt 2005). Women internalise this medical injunction which is becoming a cultural norm and feel exhorted to quickly resume sexual intercourse after giving birth. In this context, the recovery of one's pre-maternal body is viewed in common sense as a necessary step leading to fulfilling sexuality.

Interestingly, health professionals also advise women against resuming sexual intercourse too quickly after birth. They are encouraged to wait for their obstetrician's green light at the time of the last postpartum consultation six weeks after delivery in order to verify the womb position and the recovery of the perineal and vaginal tissues. This appointment is also the opportunity to discuss contraception and the resumption of sexuality. Midwives can perform the six-week check-up, but depending on women's contraceptive choices, they will not be allowed to prescribe it: in Switzerland, women wanting a hormonal contraceptive or an intrauterine device must visit an obstetrician. In my fieldwork, I did not attend six-week postnatal appointments and do not know precisely how many women chose to do it with their midwives. However, the subject emerged during my conversations with some of the midwives, who positioned themselves very critically regarding this restraining norm and the idea of the professional "allowing" women to resume sexual intercourse.

Breastfeeding involves a change in the breasts' sensations and shape, which can lead to a feeling of "strangeness" and disconnection of women from their own breasts (Schmied & Lupton 2001). Based on a mechanistic perspective on breastfeeding (Dykes 2006), mothers' speech oscillated between objectification and personification of their breasts. "As long as it works", said Corinne, talking about her plans to continue breastfeeding. Meanwhile, Maud evoked her relationship to her lactating breasts:

> I have the feeling that they are alive. I feel the ejection reflex if she has not suckled; I feel them vibrate when she cries. My body is still working for her. Everything I do, everything I eat, I think of her.
>
> (interview with Maud, notes)

In line with the WHO recommendations, Maud had planned to breastfeed Rose exclusively until she reached six months old. However, she voiced some reservations about sharing her body with her daughter: "Sometimes, I think it could be nice to get my body back". "To get her body back" implied not dedicating it primarily to her daughter anymore, but Maud did not specify whether she would reclaim it just for herself or also for her partner. Again, the issue of sexuality shows through this declaration. According to a heteronormative vision, breasts are primarily related to sexuality, and women's bodies must remain available for their partners (Mahon-Daly & Andrews 2002; Young 2005). A "good maternal body"—that is to say, a breastfeeding body—cannot simultaneously be a sexual body, since sexual and maternal functions are thought of as independent (Stearns 1999). Given a cultural preference for "sexual" breasts rather than "nourishing" breasts, sexually active breastfeeding women transgress boundaries both of the good maternal body and of the norm of the female body as a heterosexual object (Young 2005). However, as Campo (2010) points out, in the Euro-American sexual ideal, breasts are constructed as "solid, passive, inert", and available (55). Lactating breasts do not meet these expectations. They seem animated by a life of their own which involves special attention and management that can potentially conflict with their sexual function and the underlying heteronormativity.

> When we discussed her ongoing tandem nursing experience nine months after Morgane's birth, Céline expressed "a need to space out feedings and to have my body for myself", adding, "I don't know if it's breastfeeding or having a baby in my arms all the time". Julien observed, "Still, you used the word 'vampirism'". Céline continued, "I do not have to pay attention to what I eat. I rarely deny myself a glass of wine". She was still speaking very enthusiastically about breastfeeding: "I find it just perfect that my body produces what she needs. I also love to use my milk for care, irritations ... what I like too is that I do not have my periods back". "Do you think you will miss it?" asked Julien. "No, for Yvonne [her eldest], clearly, I can't wait for her to wean herself!" Céline answered without hesitation. She carried on about her clothes always needing adjustment to breastfeeding, particularly the breastfeeding bras she had been wearing for almost three years. She explained that before Yvonne's birth, she had "a very good relationship" to her breasts, which she considered "aesthetically pleasing". Breastfeeding had negatively changed her perception of her breasts: "I find them big and floppy. They do not hold up anymore. I'm no longer comfortable with them". She also regretted that breastfeeding did not make her lose weight, as frequently argued in breastfeeding promotion campaigns. "On the contrary", she said, "it makes me want to eat sugar". Julien concluded, "Without realising it, breastfeeding takes up all your energy".

Céline and Julien were nevertheless still committed to continuing breastfeeding, to allow Yvonne to suckle as long as she wanted to, and to offer the same conditions to Morgane. Other parents aimed to achieve more specific and well-defined goals regarding breastfeeding. Chloé exclusively breastfed Jules for five months and was committed to pursuing breastfeeding until he reached his first year of age. When I met her 11 months after Jules's birth, she was still drinking fennel tea every day to support her lactation. She was breastfeeding Jules in the mornings and evenings but was worried about a potential drop in lactation:

> Only another month to hang on, and I'll allow myself to slowly let go. I realise more and more that it's tiring. It is also a matter of reclaiming my body. More than enjoying my body for myself, I feel utilised, even if I still have a lot of pleasure during nursing. With the number of feedings decreasing, it's better; I'm less like a dairy station.

For mothers, breastfeeding was also a way of reaffirming their commitment to the chosen birth model by making their bodies available for their children in accordance with the guidelines of attachment parenting. Three months after her third child's birth, Catherine looked back with me on her two first breastfeeding experiences, which were interrupted prematurely and had left her with a feeling of failure. She told me, "This aspect of motherhood didn't start well for me". Breastfeeding epitomised the kind of mother she had planned to be: "Physiologically speaking, we are designed to do it. It was a part of the mothering that I had imagined". Despite having faced various obstacles, such as cracks on the nipples and breast candidiasis, which caused her great pain during her first months of breastfeeding, she proudly showed me the scratch marks left by her child on her breasts where he kneaded while feeding: "He really is like a kitten, I adore it. I call him my little mammal". In her eyes, these stigmas showed that her body was performing what it is designed to do well but were also evidence of her commitment to the body work of breastfeeding, regardless of the difficulties encountered.

Some mothers could not realise their initial out-of-hospital birth projects and had to give birth at the maternity ward. Some of them underwent caesarean sections. In these circumstances, it seems that achieving their breastfeeding projects was even more important to console themselves, but also to "repair the harm" done to their babies which they ascribed to highly medicalised births. As strongly expressed by Mélody, who could not give birth at home after being diagnosed with gestational diabetes, "Damn, I couldn't give birth at home; I'd better be able to breastfeed!" Jeanne had undergone an emergency caesarean section under general anaesthetic, which represented the extreme opposite to her home birth project. She faced significant difficulties during the first months of breastfeeding with a painful breast candida followed by weight stagnation of her son. When I met her three months later, we reviewed these hardships and her strong determination to make breastfeeding work.

I could not imagine that I would not breastfeed, as if it wasn't enough that the birth did not at all happen as I would have liked ... breastfeeding ... That's what really made me hold on, because I would have given up much sooner. And what helped me as a support, well, it's Odile [her midwife]. She is the one who allowed me to believe in [breastfeeding] and believe in myself—in my ability to breastfeed and also in Nils's ability to latch on the breast. Because after childbirth, as it had happened, yeah ... You see, if you had a caesarean section, it is because you didn't succeed in giving birth naturally. The feeling that you may have, and that I had, is that you have failed, that your body ... it has not followed. The question for breastfeeding is, will you be able or not?

(interview with Jeanne, transcription)

Mothers' stories, as well as midwives' discourses, reflect a constructivist vision of breastfeeding. Despite an often naturalistic theoretical perspective of breastfeeding, in practice, the holistic care approach provides mothers with a range of body techniques and tools to perform it. This constructivist view, expressed through a range of actions implemented for the body to achieve breastfeeding, mainly relies on mothers' tenacity. At the time of birth, such willpower does not suffice to have the delivery take place in an expected way. The possibility that a birth plan "fails" and that a transfer to a maternity ward is required is always present. In these situations, parents have to mourn their initial project and breastfeeding presents an opportunity to reintegrate the initially planned script. This especially applies to mothers, who often internalise a hospital transfer, and even worse a caesarean section, as a failure on the part of their bodies. To become the mothers they wished to be, they are determined to invest in the required body work—the intensity and workload varying greatly from one situation to another. The "success" of breastfeeding therefore acts as a way to fix the altered coherence of the reflexive project (Giddens 1991).

During the "commitment continuation" phase (Darmon 2003), the midwife's postpartum follow-up has ended. The stakes of the "commitment continuation work" lie in the mother's ability to "train both body and willpower" (Darmon 2003: 146) to pursue the efforts required for breastfeeding, which are maintaining milk production and consenting to extend the "sharing" of her body. To achieve this, mothers were deploying strategies and tools, structuring their daily lives around maintaining their commitment.

Conclusion

In their postpartum follow-ups, midwives work to make sense of newborns' behaviour, of lactation manifestations, and of new sensations associated with breastfeeding, emphasising the physiological synergy between these different elements. Alongside this naturalising discourse, they promote tools and techniques to support lactation and optimise breastfeeding initiation.

This construction of meaning takes place between two antagonistic poles: a naturalising conception of breastfeeding on one side and the body work performed to "make it work" on the other. On the one hand, the hormone-based medical discourse embraced by the midwives I accompanied encouraged mothers to not "overthink" breastfeeding and to do their best to behave as "mammals", following their "breastfeeding instinct", but also to support their newborn's "mammal behaviours"—for example, by inciting the child to "knead the breast like a kitten". On the other hand, through the techniques and tools mobilised, the breasts and their milk production were subjected to rigorous management that was collaboratively implemented by mothers and midwives and actively supported by fathers. In parallel, infants' bodies and behaviours were also submitted to an active control: measures were put in place in order to rectify any issues and ensure their compatibility with breastfeeding.

Beyond technical aspects, the midwives also highlighted an emotional dimension for breastfeeding success: it is not enough to put one's breast at the child's disposal; it is also necessary to take pleasure in doing it in order to be "emotionally available". If there was a discrepancy between the lived experience and the frame of reference proposed by the holistic care model, the moral burden of failing to breastfeed as a standard of "good" motherhood was increased by a feeling of betrayal towards the chosen care model, which was embodied by the midwife. The "good home birth mother" is one who succeeds in breastfeeding, embracing the body work that is involved.

Once the postpartum follow-up was completed and breastfeeding established over time, the mothers I met continued to perform physical and emotional work, aiming to articulate the demands of breastfeeding with those of their professional, social, and family lives: use of a breast pump, galactagogue consumption, and adaptation of their diets and clothing were among their strategies. The body work they deployed fitted with the state of liminality they were experiencing, crystallising a feeling of having not yet fully recovered their individuality. Still sharing their bodies with their babies, they were deeply at odds with the dominant autonomist values in our neoliberal societies.

The confrontation between the initial breastfeeding project and the bodily experience can create dissonances: the "taking in hand" step can be painful, physically as well as emotionally (Darmon 2003). Mothers agree to "grit their teeth" to overcome these ordeals so that their breastfeeding projects can be pursued. This testimony of self-denial and self-discipline is symptomatic of a "delegated biopolitics" at work in modern neoliberal societies (Memmi 2004: 137). Once informed by the authoritative experts in a concerned field, an exercise of self-discipline is expected of individuals. Parental responsibilities are reconfigured in the light of "parental determinism" (Furedi 2002), assigning risk management to parents, who must choose appropriate educational and care practices. Breastfeeding plays a central role in these practices because of the medical consensus about breastfeeding benefits on health risk prevention. Beyond the individual project, the body work performed by mothers is part of a collective logic of risk management and anticipation of the future by changing current attitudes and behaviours (Armstrong 1995).

If breastfeeding support techniques and tools mobilised as part of holistic care diverge from the dominant technocratic model, the underlying project of producing the lactating body remains similar. However, the voluntarist "taking in hand" necessary for a "delegated biopolitics" (Memmi 2004) is even more obvious in the context of out-of-hospital birth and holistic care. Starting from pregnancy follow-up, an out-of-hospital birth project indeed requires significant determination from parents and self-discipline from mothers, in the form of a demanding bodily preparation dedicated to supporting the physiology of the birth process. The investment in initiating and maintaining breastfeeding over the long term is part of a process of mothers' and fathers' accountability, started long before birth and contributing to the determined commitment of mothers to the body work of breastfeeding.

Anchored in the maternal body, breastfeeding crosses borders between biological functions that can only be performed by mothers and children's care, which can be accomplished by everyone. Breastfeeding requires the mother's body—although it fulfils nutritional and emotional needs that can be satiated in other ways—and thus constitutes an extra-uterine extension of the dependency link between a mother and her child. This co-dependency implies control over mothers' lifestyles. "Parental determinism" is thus expressed through the requirement to "build a [maternal] body", in other words, a breastfeeding body. In this perspective, breastfeeding embodies a particularly striking example of gender performativity, which according to Butler (1993) "must be understood not as a singular or deliberate 'act', but, rather, as the reiterative and citational practice by which discourse produces the effects that it names" (2). Through their discourses, midwives produce the maternal lactating body, which is maintained and reaffirmed by everyday practices implemented by mothers and supported by fathers. Relying on Butler's definition, Shaw (2004) applied the notion of gender performativity to the building of the motherhood identity, highlighting "how motherhood itself is materialized through the constant reiteration and assertion of regulatory norms" (109). In the case of breastfeeding, this is revealed through demanding body work. This reiteration allows motherhood to appear as "a solid, static substance" (Shaw 2004: 109) underpinned by an equally static binary categorisation of gender. Similarly, fathers' commitment to breastfeeding and investment in hands-on childcare challenge this stasis and act to "undo" traditional gendered patterns regarding the sharing of parental tasks and responsibilities among the specific marginal population of home birth parents.

Notes

1 Darmon (2003) used the interactionist notion of "career" introduced by Hughes (1958), then reconceptualised and used by Becker (1963) and Goffman (1968). She mobilised it as "an effective tool for taking into account and objectifying the point of view of those who engage in anorexia" (Darmon 2003: 14).
2 My translation of the French expression *prise en main*.
3 The phrase "biological nurturing" was coined by the English midwife Suzanne Colson based on observing breastfeeding mothers and their babies and underpinned by a neurobehavioral approach (Colson 2010).
4 This last consultation ends the postpartum follow-up. It is mainly intended to review the mother's health condition, discuss perineum rehabilitation, and address the issue of contraception.
5 This method was developed by Julie Bonapace, a Canadian family mediator working on the transition to parenthood and founder of the Bonapace Method company. She studied pain management in the Université du Québec en Abitibi-Témiscamingue (UQAT). The method claimed a "team-building" foundation, aiming to turn couples into "the powerhouse team they're meant to be so that pregnancy is easier and the transition to parenthood is smoother" (Bonapace 2016).
6 According to Deutsch's (2007) proposition, "undoing gender" is accomplished through "social interactions that reduce gender difference" (122), such as a parental organisation wherein a father becomes primarily in charge of hands-on infant care. Deutsch developed her reflection on West and Zimmerman's 1987 article "Doing Gender". This article, arguing that gender is "done" through social interactions and highlighting the failure of structural theories basing gender on socialisation, marked a turning point in gender studies.

5 The communicating feed

All societies make efforts to socialise their babies and affiliate them with the human group to which they belong (Boltanski 2004; Bonnet & Pourchez 2007; Conklin & Morgan 1996; Gottlieb 2004; Kaufman & Morgan 2005; Walentowitz 2013). As written by Kaufman and Morgan, the fact "that newborns are considered in many cultural contexts to be unripe, unformed, ungendered, and not fully human is evidence that personhood is not an innate or natural quality but a cultural attribute" (2005: 317). The modalities and temporalities of this affiliation vary depending on social, economic, political, and cultural contexts. In a neoliberal context, parents are expected to resume their work schedules quickly after their child's birth. As a result, the socialisation process is carried out primarily with a purpose of efficiency. The goal is to produce children who develop early qualities of self-sufficiency and self-regulation, including falling asleep virtually on their own, sleeping through the night in a separate room, and playing without their parents' help. This intention to civilise infants was more broadly developed by Elias as an individuation process, reflecting the growing complexity of individuals' relationship with their body and its biological functions (1973 [1969]). According to Elias, self-control over bodily needs and urges, like hunger, acts as a means of accessing an advanced stage of civilisation (1973 [1969]). Scheduled feeding can, therefore, be interpreted as an early lever of the civilisation process.

Consistently with this self-control requirement, the hygienist model, which was extended to childbirth and infant care in Europe during the interwar period (Thébaud 1986), is based on rational knowledge regarding how and when it is appropriate to feed infants or put them to sleep, but it also carries a specific educational philosophy (Boltanski 1977; Delaisi de Parseval & Lallemand 1998). This model requires an anticipative conception of time: the constraints imposed on the child today, such as strict feeding schedules, will ensure a brighter future. In this perspective, the deprived child would rapidly adjust to this unchanging routine and would quickly fit into an adult schedule. The hygienist model condemns physical, sensual contact between mother and child and limit them to strict care functions—including scheduled feeding (Boltanski 1977; Delaisi de Parseval & Lallemand 1998).

DOI: 10.4324/9781003124108-5

During the 1990s, physical contact between mothers and infants was unstigmatised and restored through a range of practices recommended by birth professionals and gradually implemented in maternity wards (Charrier & Clavandier 2013; Le Dû 2017; Memmi 2014). On-demand breastfeeding is part of this rehabilitation of touch in childcare. Legitimised by Bowlby and Ainsworth's attachment theory, practices involving physical closeness are aimed at promoting infants' "secure" attachment to their parents. Therefore, these practices answer a rising concern about developing an early bond between parents and babies, fitting into a wider process of the medicalisation of parenthood and, more specifically, "the medicalization of maternal emotion and mother love itself" (Faircloth 2014a: 147). As highlighted by Apple (1987), during the late nineteenth and early twentieth centuries, maternal childcare practices, but also maternal emotions, were the subject of expert scrutiny, as part of a "scientifisation" of motherhood. In line with a rising medical interest in parent–child "attachment", hospital staff and birth professionals are particularly attentive to the quality of the mother–infant bond and try to detect early signs of disrupted attachment (Le Dû 2017).[1] A mother's so-called failure to bond, therefore, implies heavy clinical judgement, as her child is perceived as potentially being in danger (Scheper-Hughes 1992).

While attachment is conceptualised as body-anchored (Charrier & Clavandier 2013; Memmi 2014), communicating with a baby is inherently non-verbal and is realised through the body and through bodily techniques, like breastfeeding. Furthermore, early communication primarily revolves around babies' primal needs—eating and eliminating—and translates into on-demand breastfeeding and, for some families, elimination communication. These parenting practices are the continuity of a child-centred birth project, based on Leboyer's (1974) precepts. A set of gestures are implemented during childbirth to meet this purpose: delaying cutting and clamping of the umbilical cord, avoiding direct light and noises, and letting the baby crawl to access the mother's breast, rather than imposing a feed in a standardised way directly after birth. Home birth parents and midwives speak of a collaboration with the baby at the moment of delivery, and they perceive the baby as a full-fledged participant in the birth process (Pruvost 2016).

In industrialised countries, breastfeeding initiation in maternity wards mostly follows a clock-centred logic that determines feeding patterns (Dykes 2006, Millard 1990). Indeed, most hospitals promote feeding on demand, based on WHO recommendations, "but only up to a limit" (Millard 1990): newborns are not supposed to be at the breast round the clock. Similarly, hospitals implement some practices related to the attachment parenting philosophy while retaining a weight-centric assessment of breastfeeding (Lee 2008). Despite a recent shift towards a relational-based approach to breastfeeding in the WHO guidelines, which has translated into the notion of "responsive feeding" replacing that of "on-demand breastfeeding"

(Aryeetey & Dykes 2018; World Health Organization 2018), this weight-centric assessment of breastfeeding still prevails in the majority of birth facilities in Switzerland as well as in birth professionals' discourse.

In this final chapter, I discuss breastfeeding practices in the frame of a broader child-centred approach to parenting care, which allows me to develop some topics further that I addressed in the previous chapters. On the one hand, communication-oriented parenting practices revolve around risk management, which is the central theme of Chapter 3. According to attachment parenting theories, on-demand "full-term" breastfeeding, or bed-sharing, foster a child's "secure" attachment, thus favouring optimal psycho-emotional development to ensure long-term wellbeing. Reciprocally, choosing not to engage in these practices would mean risking the future of one's child. On the other hand, in line with Chapter 4, this chapter explores how midwives and parents conceive of bodies and bodily processes like breastfeeding as "natural". Child-centred parenting practices presume discipline in the parents' bodies—for example, learning to sleep while sharing their bed with a baby or making their body constantly available to honour the child's feeding demands. Even in the case of a child-centred parenting model, babies' bodies are disciplined to fit within adults' daily organisation and work requirements. For example, the baby's "natural" rhythm is subjected to a co-construction of meaning based on parents' and midwives' observations and interpretations, but newborns are also expected to adjust to midwives' consultations and parents' schedules.

First, I elaborate on the conception of the communicating child underlying the holistic care model and the approach of home birth parents. Second, I build on time-related aspects of breastfeeding and the modalities of on-demand breastfeeding, including night-time feedings. Finally, I focus on other arrangements and practices set up by parents to reinforce their child's self-confidence and strengthen communication. More particularly, I develop upon elimination communication, thought of as a communication tool, which allows for bonds between parents and babies to be reinforced. Even if they could be implemented independently, in my fieldwork, these practices were always thought of as being related to breastfeeding, sometimes in a direct causal relationship. For example, bed-sharing was presented as a staple to support breastfeeding, especially in the long term, sustaining both mothers' lactation and parents' sleep.

Babies eager to communicate

Scheper-Hughes (1992) studied the expression of maternal attachment and the management of infant deaths in the shanty town of Alto do Cruzeiro in Northeast Brazil. In this context of extreme poverty, where infantile deaths were frequent, mothers here were slower than Euro-American parents "to anthropomorphize their newborns", a process through which parents gradually and steadily attribute human characteristics to their babies such as self-awareness, intentionality, or the ability to suffer (Scheper-Hughes 1992: 413). Alto mothers delayed this "personification" process, often waiting until the end of the first year of life before assigning specific meanings to their child's manifestations, such as screaming and crying or facial expressions. They nevertheless operated a selection based on the signals sent by the infant, favouring children who appeared to be strong. Based on the same logic, they prevented early emotional investment in babies whose survival was uncertain and limited exchanges with them. Scheper-Hughes' (1992) analysis thereby challenged attachment theory, understood as a "universal maternal script" (341).

In Euro-American societies, biological and social births are concomitant, with social birth even predating biological birth, especially with visual technologies like ultrasound. Conklin and Morgan (1996) observed that the Wari Amazonian society distinguished between these two moments: social birth was accomplished by a series of collective and relational acts and ended with babies' first feeding at their mother's breast. From a Wari perspective, the individual is constituted and perpetuated through social relations and the sharing of bodily substances, including milk. Biomedical discourses link the individuality of foetuses or newborns with biological dispositions, attesting to their ability to survive outside the maternal womb. Conklin and Morgan (1996) emphasised the tension between this conception of the individual and the actual modalities of babies' existence, which is entirely dependent on their caregivers. More broadly, this tension is expressed through, on the one hand, the neoliberal ideal of an independent individual and, on the other hand, the strong interdependence between people, especially during the first years of life. The autonomist cultural values thus create the idea of a "natural" body: within a society like the Waris', basing the individual on relationality, the "natural" and "precultural" do not exist (ibid., 1996). Like Alto mothers, Waris base their conception of the individual on communication: the baby is apprehended as a new member of the community through exchanges with the other community members.

Associated with the "child by project" era (Boltanski 2004), the parents I met in my fieldwork reflected on their birthing and childcare practices. Guided by their midwives, they had carefully prepared for their delivery and had developed specific ideas about how they wanted to care for their child, basing their parenthood style on communication. Eager to value their baby's singularity from the moment of birth, parents engaged in an active quest for communication with the baby, whether through breastfeeding or through other vectors such as massage, attention to the baby's elimination needs, or the learning of sign language. Communication was sometimes initiated in utero, using haptonomy, a technique aiming to "get in touch" with the foetus through manipulations of the mother's stomach. Among the range of communication tools implemented by parents, and sometimes introduced by the midwife, breastfeeding—obviously on demand—occupied a central place.

According to this model, babies are always able and willing to communicate. The difficulty for parents lies in needing the sharpness to observe and correctly interpret signals that infants send to indicate their physiological needs. My fieldwork observations show that midwives play a central role in this process, by inviting parents to consider breastfeeding as enabling communication with their child.

Midwives as newborns' interpreters

According to McBride-Henry and Shaw's (2010) observations, an important component in building the breastfeeding relationship is learning how to respond to the baby's behaviour so as to foster a positive response, interpreted as a visible measure of breastfeeding effectiveness. How mothers interpret their child's behaviour impacts their breastfeeding assessment: the baby's perceived satisfaction reassures them of breastfeeding success. In my fieldwork, midwives were involved in this interpretation process by suggesting to mothers a positive reading of their infant's behaviour. They pointed out, for example, a newborn's clenched fist during a feed, as an indicator of relaxation: "She is all right at the breast!" In this way, midwives insisted on the emotional dimension of feedings, comparing, for example, a baby's daily feedings with adults' self-care practices to "feel good, or comfort themselves, such as taking a bath or calling a friend", as Marianne interpreted, for example.

Midwives played a crucial role in how mothers approached breastfeeding and interpreted their baby's behaviour. By bringing the baby's signals to the mothers' attention, the midwives encouraged mothers to respond to the signals but also to identify the infant's positive reactions to breastfeeding, thus reinforcing mothers' self-confidence. Midwives therefore assumed a role as interpreters, making themselves the children's spokespeople and transmitting the children's needs and desires, sometimes at the cost of their own non-judgemental professional posture, as in the following extract.

> During a postpartum consultation with Anne, Milo, a one-month-old, slept during the entire visit. Anne did not consider it necessary to interrupt his sleep to examine him. As the visit ended, Anne and I were about to leave, and Milo woke up and cried. Aurélie told him, "I'll give you some later. I'm making you wait a little". Anne expressed her disapproval: "Why are you making him wait? Here, it's pretty clear!" Aurélie eventually installed Milo at the breast. As we left the building where the family lived, Anne came back to this episode and underlined that if the visit had been shortened, she could not have pleaded in favour of the baby: "Have you seen that? I could not have seen that she wanted to make him wait".

Thus, midwives identified the duration of postpartum visits—usually from one-and-a-half hour to two hours—as a factor allowing an in-depth and contextualised understanding of the relational dynamics around breast-feeding. Beyond the duration of each visit, the continuity of care allowed by holistic care enabled midwives to access a good amount of knowledge of each couple, their upbringing, including family birth and breastfeeding stories, and their own approach to parenthood. However, the extract above suggests that this intimate knowledge could sometimes allow the midwives to adopt an "intrusive" posture, in contradiction with the professional ideal of the "ethos of the slightest footprint" (Perrenoud 2016: 199). Perrenoud (2016) describes this notion as an anti-interventionist attitude adopted by independent midwives during home visits, aimed at "minimising their impact on the family ecology" (199). The holistic care model claims a women-centred approach, as opposed to the technocratic, institution-centred model (Davis-Floyd & St. John 1998, Katz Rothman 1991 [1982]). However, the situation described above shows that injunctions are also addressed to mothers within this model. Underpinned by an "ethic of maternal availability", it urges women to react immediately to their babies' signals (Garcia 2011: 12).

Midwives' deficiencies and competing interpreters

Midwives'' interpreting skills result, on the one hand, from their medical knowledge of newborns and, on the other hand, from their "experience-based knowledge" and their care practices with families (Perrenoud 2016). The parents I met valued both categories of knowledge. However, they were not always convinced by the interpretation proposed by their midwife.

Some of them then got in touch with another "interpreter": a kinesiologist practising the so-called *parole au bébé* ("baby's speech") approach,[2] whose skills are based on a different register of knowledge and legitimacy. This approach was developed by Brigitte Denis (2009), a Canadian perinatal kinesiologist who defined herself as a "baby interpreter". The presence of one parent is necessary to conduct a session, whom the practitioner uses as the baby's intermediary. The practitioner asks closed-ended questions to the baby. The answers are obtained by a "muscle testing" performed on the parent's arm. Depending on the answer, the baby's arm should yield to or resist the pressure exerted by the practitioner.[3]

Like the Beng parents whom Gottlieb (2004) met, the parents in my field-work attributed a high level of agency to their newborn. Bengs believed that understanding and interpreting babies' intentions require specific translation skills and are not within everyone's reach (ibid. 2004). Parents, therefore, resorted to soothsayers who had mastered communication with newborns through spirits living in "the afterlife" where unborn babies were supposed to reside (ibid. 2004). Through the soothsayers, babies expressed their desires, which the parents, in turn, committed themselves to realising. From this perspective, babies are eager to communicate, but adults fail to understand them. The aim for parents is to do their best to interpret and satisfy their babies' desires, and not to decide for their children what these desires should be—for example, when they should be hungry or sleepy.

Several parents facing persistent breastfeeding difficulties despite their midwife's guidance told me they spoke to therapists practising *parole au bébé*. In these configurations, the midwife's interpreting skills were perceived as insufficient: even if she had mastered the biological components of the newborn's behaviour, access to a more spiritual dimension was out of her reach.

> Cécile and Jonas were both in their early thirties. They lived in a small apartment in the city. Cécile worked part-time as an employee in the health sector, alongside her independent practice as a holistic practitioner. Jonas had just completed a degree in IT and was doing his civilian service. He had planned to look for an 80 per cent job afterwards. Their daughter, Gaëlle, was born at home. The delivery progressed smoothly, but Gaëlle had to be transferred to a hospital shortly after birth because of a respiratory issue. She spent a few days in the neonatology service before being released.

> I met Cécile and Jonas five days after Gaëlle's birth, as I joined their midwife, Capucine, for the first postpartum visit at home. Cécile and Jonas greeted us with their eldest daughter, Mélanie, and offered me a seat in their living room. After introducing myself and my research, Cécile and Jonas told me about their first breastfeeding journey with Mélanie. Both were very pleased with this experience, which went off without a hitch, "once the first fortnight passed". A tension was rapidly perceptible when they switched to the topic of Gaëlle's transfer to the hospital and their stay at the neonatology ward. Cécile started crying: "I even said to myself, 'Shit, we lost time'". A misunderstanding between the parents and Capucine had happened regarding the urgency of the situation: Capucine had immediately evoked the necessity of showing Gaëlle to a paediatrician, but Cécile and Jonas did not understand that she had to be transferred promptly and were shocked to see the ambulance called by Capucine. Indeed, Capucine felt embarrassed about brutally interrupting Cécile's and Jonas's happy moment of discovery with their newborn. She recognised that she may have minimised her words in order to avoid panicking them.

> When I later met alone with Cécile, she returned to this incident and told me her experience. Once in the neonatology ward, Gaëlle spent her first twenty-four hours in the intensive care unit with a gastric catheter and an infant Flow® SiPAP system: "She was connected everywhere!"[4] Since she was not able to breastfeed her during this time, Cécile greatly appreciated that she could give Gaëlle her first feed at home, before the transfer. She then pumped her milk and hospital staff gave it to Gaëlle through the catheter. She also received some formula:

"It bothered me that they supplemented her, but I was afraid of undetected gestational diabetes". Indeed, Gaëlle was born with a particularly high birth weight.[5] Cécile was grateful for the help of hospital staff regarding her breastfeeding initiation under these challenging circumstances: "It was adequate. They encouraged me a lot". After the first twenty-four hours, Cécile was able to breastfeed Gaëlle, and they came home a few days later. Gaëlle was fine, and the hypothesis of the undetected gestational diabetes had been rejected. However, Cécile was still angry with Capucine, and their bond of trust was disrupted for the rest of the follow-up.

Gaëlle had lost almost no weight during the immediate postpartum period but gained very little afterwards. Regarding this weight stagnation, Cécile considered Capucine's advice unhelpful and her follow-up to be "little comforting". Cécile was very surprised by midwives' theoretical education on breastfeeding: "In fact, midwives have very little training on breastfeeding. It's really shocking". After unsuccessfully consulting several specialists in breastfeeding and infant nutrition (their paediatrician, a lactation consultant, and a paediatrician specialised in gastroenterology), Cécile and Jonas turned to a *parole au bébé* practitioner. This session of *parole au bébé* was perceived as decisive by Cécile: "I also realised that Gaëlle [her daughter] understands everything". She linked Gaëlle's difficulties gaining weight with "elements of her previous life": "Regarding her birth, it becomes clearer and clearer … We are not only physical. We certainly don't have only one life. There were things in her incarnation that were wrong". Cécile concluded her impressions of the therapist's intervention: "I think she has a gift. She's more like a soothsayer".

Le Dû (2017) conducted an ethnography in France with mothers and traditional infant therapists, called "touchers" (*toucheur* in French). Like *parole au bébé* practitioners, touchers are not recognised by medical insurances. However, unlike touchers, whose skills are based solely on the notion of a "gift", some *parole au bébé* practitioners are trained in kinesiology. Parents must pay for *parole au bébé* consultations, while touchers seemed more flexible in Le Dû's (2017) research. *Parole au bébé* does not refer to any formal religion but includes some spiritual components with new age inspirations. The practitioners, for example, explain that they are talking to the baby's "wisdom" or "soul" or refer to the notions of "light" and "energy". Unlike Le Dû's (2017) interlocutors, who were reluctant to talk to her about their search for assistance from a toucher at first, my interlocutors spontaneously spoke to me about their *parole au bébé* consultations. This difference can be partially explained by the fact that Le Dû wore two hats at the time of her study: she was both a midwife and a researcher. As her interlocutors were also her clients, they might have been reluctant to talk to her about their consultations with other—non-biomedical—practitioners. Because I was a layperson in the medical profession, parents probably were more comfortable with confiding to me about this type of experience without fear of disapproval.

Based on my observations, home birth parents are avid consumers of complementary medicine. On the one hand, parents' mistrust of biomedicine primarily leads them to turn to complementary medicine in case of mild inconveniences during the perinatal period. On the other hand, independent midwives providing holistic care often master one or several complementary medicine disciplines (such as homoeopathy, aromatherapy, or naturopathy) and frequently recommend complementary medicine practitioners from other disciplines (like osteopathy or acupuncture). In a context of medical pluralism, which characterises the therapeutic offerings in Euro-American societies, patients use complementary medicine together with biomedicine and go from one medicine to another without perceiving contradictions in their approach (Schmitz 2006). There is indeed a certain permeability in the use of these different categories of medicines. Most of the parents I met preferred to treat themselves primarily with non-biomedical care approaches but still relied on biomedicine, including for their childbirth care and for monitoring their child's health. Furthermore, the holistic character of their midwife's follow-up allowed the parents to reconcile their different aspirations, being at a pivotal point between biomedicine and complementary medicine.

From the parents' perspective, *parole au bébé* consultations fit into the range of complementary medicine practices offered by their midwife, despite a lack of theoretical basis, certifying training, or acknowledgement by insurances. In addition to the *parole au bébé* consultations, some parents also turned to traditional "healers" who held a transmitted "gift", similar to Le Dû's touchers. In the French-speaking part of Switzerland, these healers are called "secret makers" and often address specific issues like burns or infant thrush. Léa and Guillaume called one of these practitioners after Simone's first and only vaccine, at two years old. "It completely changed Simone. It felt like she was not the same baby anymore. She was always opposing us", explained Léa. When Léa called the healer a fortnight after the vaccination, she confirmed the vaccine's detrimental impact: "She said that Simone was completely unbalanced. Simone was near the phone and asked to talk to the lady, and in the evening, it was over". Again, the act of a "gifted" or skilled person "speaking" to Simone solved the problem, similarly to the *parole au bébé* session described above. Léa had already contacted this secret maker earlier when she was facing issues with Simone and could not find satisfactory answers from other biomedical and non-medical practitioners. Consistent with Le Dû's (2017) research, parents used *parole au bébé* practitioners, or secret makers, as a complement to their midwife's and paediatrician's follow-ups, primarily to reassure themselves and to fill the gaps in a medical discourse that did not address their concerns. In the first months after birth, parents often consulted these therapists to ease their baby's transition to extra-uterine life, sometimes to solve issues that appeared at the moment of delivery, like Gaëlle, in the situation described above. Later, as in the case of Léa and Guillaume, the consultation with a practitioner was aimed at fixing a specific problem or to soothe transitions in the baby's life, like the baby's first vaccination.

Observation-driven communication

The midwives I followed during their postpartum consultations placed the child's observation at the centre of their practice, and they did their best to transmit this sensitivity to parents. In this way, the observation of the baby corresponded to the first stage of communication. For Alto mothers, observing babies helps to determine whether they are eager to communicate with their parents and other relatives (Scheper-Hughes 1992). These mothers look within their newborns for qualities showing that they are ready for "the struggle that was life" and prefer children demonstrating early physical, psychological, and social characteristics of "fighters" (1992: 316), manifested by a strong desire for interactions. If their observation was inconclusive, mothers postponed the baby's entry into communication. While the communication skills of newborns showing a desire to interact were stimulated, conversely, mothers did not encourage low-demand babies to be more active. In this value system, "active, quick, responsive and playful" children were preferred to "quiet, docile" children, with the latter nevertheless being closer to the "civilised" and self-sufficient neoliberal ideal child (ibid. 1992: 316).

Midwives have challenged this neoliberal model by suggesting that parents adjust to their baby's rhythm and not the opposite. In their recommendations for on-demand breastfeeding, they encouraged parents to anticipate their infant's wishes by being attentive to the warning signs of hunger that s/he was expressing. Before voicing an explicit request, babies would open their mouth, in front of which they would place their hands, or they would make small noises. Midwives translated this set of attitudes through the expression "S/he is seeking". The underlying reasoning was that a newborn whose desires are anticipated will be calmer and, therefore, will suckle more efficiently at the breast. Parents employed this argument. For example, Maud explained to me that she was offering her breast to her two-month-old daughter as soon as her daughter might be interested: "I never wait for Rose to cry to feed her. I know that they [babies] are a lot more Zen before that, and they drink better if they are not screaming before going to the breast". Tamara and Jérome also preferred to breastfeed Camille when she started making "little noises": "We give right away. We do not wait for you to groan!" said Tamara to Camille. Moreover, parents attributed influences on their child's behaviour to this principle, beyond the feeding moments. Following her midwife's recommendations, Patricia decided to feed Wilson, her son, as soon as he manifested an interest, advice she had not received at her daughter's birth, seven years earlier. She was pleased to observe a positive behaviour difference between her children: "I had never thought about the fact that a baby who is asked to wait is a much more nervous baby who also sleeps worse at night. [...] so Wilson is a very calm baby. I have also a lot more fun breastfeeding and living out my maternity". More broadly, parents and midwives sometimes also linked the childbirth's circumstances—in a peaceful place, without medical intervention—with the infant's character, consistent with Pruvost's (2016) findings. Sarah and Cédric proudly said to their midwife, Isabelle, and to me that their relatives were impressed by their daughter's behaviour: "Everyone thinks she's so cool!" "They are not used to babies born without trouble", answered Isabelle.

Midwives' observation of babies also served to enhance the newborns' skills, as a process of "anthropomorphizing" them (Scheper-Hughes 1992). During a visit to Olivia and Alain, after weighing Peregrine—their nine-day-old daughter—Pauline talked playfully to her, still naked and "smiling" on the changing table. Alain observed the "smile" and said, "We want to believe that it's a real smile, but it's not possible", implying that Peregrine was too young to perform a "real smile". Olivia evoked the notion of "reflex smiling" commonly attributed to these early "smiles". Pauline disagreed: "why wouldn't it be a real smile? Here, I think she really smiled to me". Pauline discredited standardising psycho-developmental theories by granting newborns the social ability to smile from birth. By recognising newborns as full-fledged individuals, midwives encouraged parents to rely on their newborn's signals and to learn to understand their means of communication and to "trust" them.

Skilled babies to be trusted

Beyond careful observation of babies' behaviour, midwives encouraged mothers to consider breastfeeding as a relationship process with their child. They urged mothers to "trust" their babies regarding the babies' feeding needs. This notion of trust breaks with the dominant biomedical approach of breastfeeding as a milk transfer and conflicts with ordinary Euro-American paediatric practices, in which weighing the child acts as the main—if not the only—measure of breastfeeding success (Sachs 2005, 2013).

As the baby regulates the course of feedings, the notion of trust also implies shared responsibilities between mother and child. By placing it at the centre of their rhetoric, midwives assign babies a role of social actors in their own right. As asserted by Anne to new parents, "Breastfeeding is already the beginning of communication".

Challenging a dominant representation of babies, characterised first and foremost by their vulnerability, midwives were committed to highlighting their skills: "The mom doesn't have full responsibility for breastfeeding. The baby has a very strong survival instinct!" and "She knows her needs. Trust her!" were midwives' recurring statements symptomatic of this intention.

The success of breastfeeding, perceived as "teamwork", was based on the commitment and collaboration of the two main protagonists involved in the physiological breastfeeding process. For example, Capucine encouraged a mother–baby pair: "You are both perfectly capable of achieving it!" This type of discourse was based on a representation of newborns as pre-programmed beings guided by their "survival instinct". This instinct would allow successful breastfeeding if adequately supported by mothers. The prescription "follow your baby" appeared multiple times in midwives' speeches.

Primarily identified as mothers' assistants, fathers were absent from such statements issued by midwives and were directly oriented on breastfeeding. In practice, they were fully invested in this teamwork and contributed in multiple ways to the achievement of breastfeeding.

Fathers compensating for a dry chest

Some fathers were frustrated about being excluded "by nature" from the exchanges between mothers and babies allowed by the feeding process. Two months after his daughter's birth, Alain expressed regrets: "I think the thing she prefers is to be at the breast. I think the father, in there, it's a little more work. You feel that there's still a delay". Alain's words showed his internalisation of an ideological hierarchisation of newborns' needs, placing nutritional needs—especially if met through breastfeeding—as a top priority. This hierarchy reflects the emphasis put on breastfeeding in contemporary Euro-American societies (Avishai 2004, 2007, 2011; Blum 1999; Faircloth 2013; Lee 2008).

To compensate for this perceived delay, Alain explained to me that he had developed a way of identifying whether his daughter's crying indicated that she was hungry or if she was expressing another need. By presenting his nose to her, the part of his body that he considered the most similar to the maternal nipple, he could deduce from her reaction whether she was hungry or not. In a similar way as his spouse through breastfeeding, Alain reinvented his body and adapted it to his new parental function. As observed by Miller (2011), "Emerging paternal identities are made visible and narrated through particular practices which are cited by men" (1102). Deprived of the possibility of feeding their babies, fathers sought to develop other means of communication.

> Jonathan was bathing Rose, his one-year-old daughter every night. Since she had learned sign language, and more specifically, the sign "to suckle", which she immoderately used to ask for a feed—Rose frequently addressed it to her father, which left him powerless. Maud, his spouse, told me that he sometimes got angry with her because of her biological advantage: "He reproaches me. 'You put your breasts under her nose, and you give her to me to go in the bath! I'd like to breastfeed her, but I can't!'"

In another family, Céline and Julien ended up supplementing their baby, Morgane, with formula, using a supplemental nursing system. As they were describing how they were adjusting to this new way of feeding their infant, Julien pointed out, "It's the first time that I can feed one of my babies". To feed Morgane, he would fix the supplemental nursing system spout on his finger, whereas Céline would fix it on her nipple. I asked Julien if he had considered fixing it on his chest and nipple. "No!" answered Julien, laughing, with the idea of offering Morgane his own nipple seeming totally incongruous to him. In this case, the desire to connect with his child physically as intimately as his spouse did with breastfeeding collided with a moral and social reluctance to transgress the gender order by performing "chestfeeding" (Walks 2018).[6]

Following babies' "natural" rhythm

Based on the WHO recommendations, on-demand feeding appeared as essential to successful breastfeeding in midwives' discourses. However, both parents and midwives constantly redefined the terms of the demand. Although midwives encouraged parents to allow infants unlimited access to their mother's breasts during the first days and weeks of life, it struck me that their recommendations changed significantly depending on the baby's age or weight.

Midwives unconditionally agreed on the principle of following the newborn's demand in the early postpartum period. For example, a few days after Milo's birth, Anne explained to Aurélie and Fabien, "Here, we are still in the phase where we must not try to understand. We must put him on the breast right away". This professional stance was also linked to risk management regarding newborns' growth: feeding them multiple times a day favours quick and steady weight gain and optimal stimulation with which to settle lactation.

Several weeks or months after birth, however, midwives strived to safeguard breastfeeding's continuity by widening both the notion of demand and the baby's adaptability. For example, Pauline reassured Maud and Jonathan when they asked for a breastfeeding consultation just before Maud resumed work, as Rose was six months old. Maud was worried about continuing to feed Rose two to three times per night once she returned to work. Pauline tempered, "Breastfeeding is a two-part story. There is no idea of sacrifice. She [Rose] can adapt".

A baby's rhythm therefore emerges, built through parents' and midwives' interpretations and evolving through the different moments of the day—daytime or night-time—and through various functions attached to feedings—nutritive or nurturing.

Building the natural

Mansfield (2008) showed that the "naturalness" of "natural" childbirth is accomplished through a range of social practices, including active birth preparation, gestures, and movements during childbirth and adequate social support. Similarly, respecting newborns' "natural" rhythm requires substantial investment from parents, in carefully observing babies, identifying their signals, and responding to them, agreeing to be unconditionally available. These precepts are related to babies' feeding needs but also to other physiological needs like sleeping or eliminating. In the longer term, this applies to diversification as well—when the baby is ready and shows an obvious interest—and to weaning.

From the midwives' invitation to "follow the baby's rhythm" comes a valuation of parents' "creativity": their ability to improvise and the adaptation they demonstrate in adjusting to this rhythm. Isabelle, a midwife, thus encouraged mothers "to put themselves in their baby's shoes".

> Marion was in her late twenties and was a self-employed worker in the health sector. She lived in a small town with her spouse, Laurent, an employee in an insurance company. When her water broke, after twenty-four hours without dilatation, Isabelle took Marion to the maternity ward because of infection risks. Although Marion's labour was induced, she was still satisfied with the care she received and the overall course of her delivery. She left the hospital the next day, against hospital staff's advice. Laurent had three days off and resumed work afterwards.

> During a postpartum visit two weeks after birth, Marion's daughter, Émilie, was agitated and cried. Isabelle invited Marion to try seeing things from Émilie's point of view: "It's interesting to just search for positions. Before, she could do it in the womb, but now, she cannot do it anymore; you have to try finding tricks". While continuing the discussion, she installed Émilie in different ways on the living room couch, surrounded by a nursing pillow raised by a sheepskin. Émilie momentarily stopped crying and started cooing. Isabelle commented, "She is chatting with you. These are other language codes, but you can't easily understand them, which causes frustration". Émilie started crying again. Isabelle asked Marion, "Do you think she'd like to eat a little more?" Marion responded, "She divides [feedings]. It's hard to know if it's a sucking reflex or hunger". Isabelle answered, "Tell yourself that African women do not ask themselves this question". Marion complied and installed Émilie at the breast. Isabelle commented joyfully, singing to Émilie, "Your mom agrees. She agrees!"

> After the feed, Isabelle offered to install Émilie back on the couch but insisted on preheating the place with a hot water bottle: "As long as you do not want to be in her place, she has the right to say it's not great". Émilie was no longer crying and resumed her cooing. Marion's interpretation was rather negative: "She's whining today". Isabelle corrected, "I'd rather say that she's chatting; she's experimenting. Sometimes, we have the impression that we have to distract them [babies] all the time,

but it's enough for them to connect some neurons. We must never forget the autonomy they had for nine months".

This excerpt reveals a tension between Marion's desire to "civilise" Émilie, as reflected in her reluctance to propose a new feed and her slight irritation with Émilie's "chatting", and Isabelle's perspective, who strived to value Émilie as an individual in her own right, with legitimate needs and desires to fulfil such as hunger, comfort, and security. Like Anne in a situation described earlier, Isabelle was taking on the role of the baby's spokesperson.

Since the beginnings of the "natural" childbirth movement in the 1930s, supporters of this approach have used representations referring to nature, from which modern industrialised societies would have distanced themselves and whose rediscovery would be beneficial (Moscucci 2002). Dick-Read's arguments were based on cultural stereotypes associated with so-called "primitive" societies, in which women would give birth easily and without feeling pain, while in contrast, women in industrialised societies—corrupted by the capitalist, urban, and consumerist way of life—could no longer give birth physiologically. Some midwives' references to "African women", like Isabelle in the excerpt above, allude to the Rousseauian representation of the noble savage. Midwifery discourses frequently reflected the idea of "natural" parenthood, which is critical of the neoliberal parenting model and its underlying ideology of separation between children and their parents.

In the sequence described above, Isabelle deployed different strategies with and around Émilie until Émilie stopped crying. The desire to "respect" the baby's rhythm is discordant with the gestures and interventions made to adjust to this rhythm. Parents and midwives are constantly acting on this supposedly natural rhythm by observing and interpreting the newborn's behaviour. During visits, there were times when it seemed appropriate to leave an observing posture and perform care, by waking up a sleeping baby when the visit ended if s/he had not been weighed for several days or showing how to give her or him a massage. These situations justified interventions to align the baby's rhythm with the temporalities of postpartum visits and parental organisation.

During another follow-up, I attended Mireille's first visit to Léa and Guillaume, Simone's new parents.

> Léa and Guillaume were both in their early thirties and lived in a small apartment in the city. Both were working as employees, Léa in the health sector and Guillaume in the tourism sector. While the couple's plan was to give birth in a birth centre, Léa ended up having a caesarean section at the hospital. The labour was lengthy. Simone, their daughter, was engaged in the birth canal but remained stuck in Léa's pelvis.
>
> I met them for Mireille's first postpartum consultation, nine days after birth. When I arrived, Léa was alone with Simone, sleeping in her

basket. Léa invited me to sit and chat in the living room while waiting for Mireille's and Guillaume's arrivals. Léa was disappointed by the course of her delivery but very pleased with her breastfeeding initiation: "Breastfeeding has been perfect since the first feed. During pregnancy, I already had a lot of colostrum", she commented, smiling.

Mireille arrived, and after half an hour of discussion on different topics, Simone woke up. Mireille spoke to her: "It's good that you are waking up. We'll be able to weigh you!" We moved to the parental bedroom, which was also Simone's. Her mother undressed her and placed her in the small hammock of her scale. Mireille lifted her and commented, "Well, it's good. Tomorrow, she'll be at her birth weight". Guillaume then arrived and joined us.

Mireille offered to take advantage of Simone's nudity to show her parents how to shower her in the bathroom sink—"That way, they will learn something on the level of motor development, and they love water flowing on their sacrum". She took Simone in her arms, put her on her stomach on one of her forearms, and vigorously swung her arm back and forth. This exercise allowed Mireille, according to her, to develop the baby's motor skills. She showed how Simone clung to her arm: "This way, your child will never fall from a tree. She has this skill now, and later, she'll lose it. You have to take advantage of it now", Mireille explained to the parents. We moved to the bathroom. Mireille was still holding Simone and placed her in the sink, making sure that her feet were placed flat against the bottom of the sink. According to Mireille, this allowed Simone to become aware of the boundaries of the space. Similarly, Mireille made Simone touch the edge of the sink with her hands. Mireille turned on the water faucet, adjusted the temperature and positioned Simone so that lukewarm water ran down her lower back and her buttocks. All this, according to Mireille, contributed to developing Simone's motor skills. She stopped the water and wrapped the baby in a towel. She went back to the room, dried her, and placed her on the changing table to massage her. Mireille put some baby oil in her hands and began the massage, explaining her gestures. She integrally oiled Simone, insisting on the necessity of not forgetting the folded areas of the body: behind the ears, under the arms. She then accentuated her gestures on the rest of the body, forming a roll of skin she slipped "to detach the skin from the muscles". Léa and Guillaume were attentive and sometimes amused.

Simone had remained relatively calm until the end of her shower in the sink, when she looked astonished by the treatment she was receiving. She began to cry louder and louder from the beginning of the massage. Mireille stopped massaging her and held the screaming baby above her: "Oh, that was really an event, wasn't it?" she said, amused. Mireille commented to Léa and Guillaume, emphasising the unprecedented nature of physical contact for newborns, "We never touched them. In the womb, they were weightless". She compared Simone's reaction with that of a "small animal unaccustomed to human contact", whose first reaction is fear but who then learns and lets itself be approached and manipulated. She concluded, "We are in full observation when we have a baby, to know who s/he is and how s/he reacts".

This sequence highlights how Mireille's speech wavered between a generic baby—"they love the water that flows on the sacrum"—and an individual one, with the enhancement of the observations of each baby's reactions. However, in this excerpt, it appears that Mireille judged it more important, at that moment, to complete her demonstration for educational purposes than to worry about Simone's reactions, who seemed reluctant to receive a massage. In this way, Mireille exempted herself from the injunction directed at the parents to follow their child's rhythm.

In the situation described above, Simone was compared to a "small animal" who, if properly trained during her first weeks of life, would never "fall from a tree". This animalisation of children, referring to their mammal status, evokes once again the imaginary of the "natural" birth (Odent 2011 [1990]). As a "product" of natural childbirth, children are defined by their "naturalness". This natural baby is shaped as opposed to a civilised baby, who is the fruit of the neoliberal education model.

Answering the demand, negotiating cadence

In midwives' discourse, on-demand breastfeeding is constructed as closest to nature while simultaneously being physiologically suitable for the lactation to settle. In this perspective, according to Marianne, "We are small mammals who must eat often. Breast milk is low in fat and high in carbohydrates that make the brain work. In the wild, the small mammals that we are, are not programmed [to respect a schedule]". Through the experiences of several families I observed in my fieldwork, I show in this section how a shift occurs, from an initial conception of on-demand breastfeeding to a readjustment over time, depending on parents' desires and obligations.

Odile and I had just arrived at Céline and Julien's apartment, the morning after Morgane's home birth. Odile laughed upon seeing Morgane at the breast: "I laugh because I tell myself that it will not be very complicated, this breastfeeding!" She elaborated, "Those babies who are at the breast all the time in the first days, it's just fine!" Céline and Julien agreed, and all three jokingly conjured up "the clichés still circulating of babies who are at the breast all the time" and would supposedly become capricious or too demanding in the future because of this permissiveness. Céline believed, on the contrary, that "plugged in at the breast, it's so easy!", compared to what parents willing to limit their newborn's access to the breast were experiencing.

The discussion continued a few days later during another visit, while we were enjoying a cup of coffee in Céline and Julien's living room. Their two-year-old daughter Yvonne was playing with a puzzle on the coffee table. Morgane was sleeping on her parents' bed. Odile said that she was clearly seeing a difference in the children's behaviour based on whether they breastfed on demand. She distinguished two categories of mothers: "those who do not wait and put the baby back at the breast even if he/she ate two hours earlier and those who fear that it will always be like that" and who therefore seek to regulate the frequency of feedings. According to her, babies who have unlimited access to maternal breasts will be calmer. She pointed out to Céline, "You are doing it like that, but you are not wondering how it will be in three months. It's a personal question: there are some women who immediately think about what will happen in the future, so it's useless because it will not work for them". Julien intervened and came back in the early days after Yvonne's birth. He observed, "I was still sensitive to all this at the beginning, saying to myself, 'She will not learn frustration!'" He continued about the notion of on-demand feeding and his initial reluctance: "It was a goal in itself, breastfeeding on demand. Whatever happens, if she wants to suckle, she suckles. I had to drop a lot of principles. You were alone against everyone at times" [speaking to Céline].

As Julien explained, he had to make an effort to distance himself from cultural expectations regarding children's behaviour. Since its emergence as a science in the early twentieth century in France, targeting mothers' education, childcare has been underpinned by the idea that children's education starts from birth (Neyrand 2000; Thébaud 1986). In this perspective, it is important not to allow behaviours perceived as undesirable in newborns to be established. The adequate way to feed infants does not proceed from their desire but from maintaining a strict, unchangeable feeding schedule (ibid. 1986). Midwives endeavour to deconstruct these ideas during breastfeeding initiation, relying on neuroscientific theories. For example, neuroscience and child psychology studies have identified letting babies cry as causing lasting brain damage (Gueguen 2014; Leach 2010). Therefore, midwives encouraged parents not to leave their child crying alone but to accompany their crying.

Midwives explained to parents the difference between "addressing a need" and "educating". For example, Pauline said to new parents worried about their newborn daughter's frequent feeding demands, "To reassure you, she is not throwing a tantrum here; she is just expressing her needs!" In another family, Jérôme asked Capucine about babies' cries: "And crying, is it happening anyway, or not necessarily?" "Crying is an alert, but if there is no stress, there is nothing to unload. Some emotional security factors are physical contact and the feeling of being heard. She has the opportunity to communicate emotion and to be reassured", Capucine answered. Jérome's relatives had told him that they maintained a two-hour interval between feedings with their own babies, while leaving them crying in between. Jérome did not want Camille to cry while waiting for her next feed but asked for Capucine's approval: "Is putting her at the breast when she cries not necessarily wrong?" "No, why would it be wrong?" she answered. Jérome explained that he and his spouse were pleased with their approach but wanted to make sure that they were not out of control, because they constantly improvised: "We would still like to stay on a path, even if it is a very wide one". Capucine finished reassuring him: "It's not about education but about trying to meet her needs. If you already feel that it is right ... My opinion is that there is no right and wrong way".

In another holistic care visit attended by Capucine, Patricia described how she adapted her breastfeeding and infant care practices.

> Patricia and Vincent were in their mid-thirties. They were both self-employed, part-time workers, Patricia in the entertainment sector and Vincent as an IT specialist. They lived in a caravan, in the garden of a squat. Even though they could easily access all of the commodities (kitchen and bathroom) in the main house twenty meters away from the caravan, they chose to give birth in a birth centre. However, the labour was so fast that their son, Wilson, was actually born in the caravan, under Capucine's guidance.
>
> One month after Wilson's birth, while he was sleeping in Patricia's arms, Patricia and I were talking over a cup of coffee in the squat kitchen about the different advice she had received during her first postpartum follow-up, seven years ago, versus this time. When Patricia gave birth to her first child—also a home birth attended by another independent midwife—she was very sceptical regarding on-demand breastfeeding: "I knew there were people who were breastfeeding on demand, but I didn't want to do it. It gave me a feeling of slavery". At the time, her first midwife had told her to respect a three-hour interval between feedings: "We clearly made her wait to keep this strict three-hour thing". As she had suffered a severe postpartum haemorrhage, requiring a hospital transfer for her immediately after birth, her midwife primarily focused on her health, and they had little discussion about breastfeeding or other baby care topics.
>
> For this second birth, she talked a lot with Capucine about breastfeeding, including during pregnancy. Capucine changed Patricia's mind regarding on-demand breastfeeding: "All these discussions we had, it changed a lot of things, on my way of thinking about my breastfeeding

... I decided at that time, can I not try to breastfeed on demand and see what it's like?" Patricia made a connection between her reluctance to breastfeed on demand and "a Protestant theory that one should not abuse what is good": "I feel like I grew up in it, I don't know how it's built ... and suddenly, at thirty-five, I deconstruct all that". "It's very important, what you are told right after birth. I have not really tried to do what suited me [after her first child's birth]. I tried to do well, but I did not listen to myself that much. I'm not the same age either; I've asserted myself a lot", observed Patricia.

Like Julien earlier, Patricia explained that she had to distance herself from cultural expectations regarding infants' self-sufficiency. More specifically, she told me about the highly controversial practice of breastfeeding children in order to help them fall asleep: "I had been told that you should not let a baby fall asleep at the breast. There is a cultural idea that a baby who falls asleep at the breast is a dependent baby". Even in the context of home birth parenting, parents may perceive producing a "dependent" baby as a failure. In this way, the holistic childcare approach differs from the dominant model but shares the same value of autonomy as an ultimate educational goal.

Feeding around the clock

One of the parents' main concerns was infants' sleep—and more particularly, the notion of "sleeping through the night" in relation to night-time feedings—as reflected by the tremendous amount of discussion on this topic on Internet parenting sites and groups, specialised media sources, and childcare books.

Mireille was used to asking mothers during her postpartum follow-up "how many times between midnight and 6 am" the baby was fed, assuming "that before midnight we do not really sleep yet and that from 6 am it is already the morning", in order to put the number of nocturnal feedings into perspective. Furthermore, frequent feedings are critical to stimulating lactation sufficiently during breastfeeding initiation, which also explains Mireille's concern with giving little importance to the frequency of parents' wakings.

When Mireille met again with some mothers whose deliveries she attended two months earlier, at the occasion of postnatal classes, her speech had slightly evolved: she pointed out to Léa that Simone, two months old at that time, was very chubby and had "enough reserves to hold up for a whole night". At that point, the stakes were not the same, lactation was well established and the elimination of a nocturnal feed would not endanger lactation. She encouraged mothers to probe their feelings and the message sent to their babies about night-time feedings: "It's always a question of how tired you are. S/he [the baby] feels whether you still agree. It's just important not to lie to yourself: you have the right to enjoy it [night-time feedings], but the day you get up clenching your teeth, you become toxic to your child". At that time, Léa did not want to encourage Simone to give up night feeding, which she did not consider a constraint. Simone was sleeping in a co-sleeper bed.[7] To breastfeed her, it was not necessary to get up or to turn on the light, and Léa's maternity leave would continue for a few more months. When I met again with Léa three months later, she explained that she had begun "wanting to skip a feed in order to really sleep seven or eight hours, really well" and reminded me that Mireille had already suggested that Simone had enough reserves when she was two months old to sleep through the night. Her five-month maternity leave would end a month later, and she was worried about her ability to cope with her unrelenting pace of work if her nights were still interrupted.

Some mothers indeed already had anticipated their return to work already in the first days after birth. The baby's behaviour therefore was interpreted mainly in light of this ultimatum.

It was Pauline's first consultation, on the day Olivia and her baby, Peregrine, had returned home from their hospital stay. Olivia described to Pauline her experience the night before at the maternity ward: "Last night, I was completely lost. She suckled a lot for a very long time at each breast. I heard she was struggling. I was afraid of giving her too much". Olivia called the nurse for advice, who told Olivia that she had to be careful not to give Peregrine her breast more than every two hours, or else there would otherwise be a risk of falling into a vicious circle (implying that if babies eat too often, they will not have time to digest between the two feeds and will suffer from colic). Pauline reminded Olivia and Alain that Peregrine's digestive system was setting itself up, according to the idea that Peregrine "knows her needs" and "does her baby's job well by stimulating lactation". Olivia was not convinced and expressed her worries: "You ask yourself, 'Will it be like this all the time? When will I sleep?'" She put her concerns regarding Peregrine's very close feedings into perspective: "It's about comfort, I think. On the one hand, we think, 'She's good; she had her sixth time [feeding]', and on the other hand, we want to do something else". Alain stepped in: "It may be about parental comfort, but can we encourage her to suckle less often but more milk at once?" Pauline gently dismissed this idea, drawing Alain's attention to the "gap between a baby's needs and the modern Western lifestyle".

The day after, Olivia was nursing Peregrine when Pauline and I arrived at their apartment. She commented, "It lasts an eternity. You see that the ratio time/efficiency … there is still something to improve!" Peregrine was taking a lot of breaks. Olivia tried to remove her each time, but Peregrine would start suckling again. Olivia explained to us that Alain was stunned to see Peregrine suckling that often: "Yesterday, he said three times, 'It's not possible!'" Alain reacted, upset, "I also think about our sleep. If she asks to suckle every hour, it's not bearable". Pauline asked them if they had tried anything to soothe Peregrine besides putting her at the breast. Alain answered, "It seems to me that certain positions are better than others. I can make her wait longer by taking her in a certain way". Pauline observed that seeking to "make her wait" maybe was not the most strategic choice. She explained that in the early times after birth, a baby woke up mostly to eat; therefore, it was better to put her at the breast as soon as she was awake, rather than waiting for tears. Alain was not pleased with this explanation: "Basically, she has the right not to have a rhythm, and we have the duty to endure it". Peregrine was four days old then, but Olivia already had concerns about her ability to maintain breastfeeding after resuming work, in five months, due to the chaotic, time-consuming rhythm of the feedings.

Two months later, I visited Olivia and Alain on my own to catch up on their breastfeeding situation. At the one-month check-up, their paediatrician advised them not to feed Peregrine more often than every two hours in order to rest her digestive system. While difficult to follow at first—"The first days, the last fifteen minutes were tough to go through", observed Olivia—this recommendation actually suited them. Peregrine seemed to suffer less from colic. "There were two transitional weeks between her evolution and our adjustment", said Alain. I reminded them that this was the advice a nurse gave them during their hospital postpartum stay. At that time, they did not follow it and chose to stick to Pauline's recommendation to feed Peregrine on demand. Olivia commented, "This did not convince me because I saw that she drank a lot, and often. She also stabilised her weight very quickly. It's the proof that it worked well". Alain added, "At that time, it was not appropriate, but two or three weeks later, it was appropriate". "The moment we started spacing [feedings], I think I was starting to feel like I was only doing that [feeding Peregrine]", observed Olivia.

Olivia and Alain were then very reluctant to put Peregrine at the breast to soothe her if they were not sure that she "really" was hungry because they were afraid that it might trigger colic. They were very concerned about Peregrine's "evening crying": "I find the evening crying the hardest to manage. Holding her or the rocking motions don't always soothe her", said Alain. He explained, "We try to make her understand that she can't continue to fall asleep only in our arms". Olivia conceded that she had "reused once or twice" the strategy of putting her at the breast to soothe her, pointing out that this was not the solution she wanted to use anymore. During our discussion, Peregrine fell asleep in Olivia's arms after feeding. Alain noticed it: "Oh no. Tonight won't be okay!"

Olivia and Alain finally managed to space their feedings while maintaining a consistent line of thought in their eyes: Peregrine had matured, and her needs had evolved. Her feeding and sleeping patterns, however, remained a major concern, as they kept in mind that the way they managed Peregrine's schedule during the day was determining the quality of their sleep at night. At the time of the discussion described above, Alain had already returned to work (he had two weeks off after his daughter's birth), while Olivia was halfway through her maternity leave.

Céline and Julien's situation described earlier was different: Céline was a stay-at-home mother, and Julien managed to take five weeks off after Morgane's birth. Despite working full-time, Julien's very irregular schedules allowed them flexibility. At the time of Odile's visits, they were easily accepting the "temporal chaos" brought by breastfeeding without projection into the future. For them, it was part of a certain continuity with their usual patterns: Julien's work schedules made them strangers to the idea of a routine, and they had no notion of maternity leave as a countdown that started ticking at birth, as experienced by other mothers.

As suggested in both situations above, the holistic care model is difficult to apply in the long term if both parents are employed full-time. Breastfeeding practices are caught up in the temporal organisation of neoliberal society, requiring regular schedules and the establishment of a "routine" and allowing parents to meet their own physiological needs while being able to fulfil the demands of their workday. It seems that only a looser work schedule, allowed by part-time working, teleworking, or self-employment, is compatible with the uncertainties of the baby's ever-changing feeding and sleep patterns.

Professionals and parents adjust to the baby's rhythm according to their expectations and interpretations of the baby's signals. Depending on practical circumstances—where the baby sleeps, the duration of the maternity leave, etc.—parents would seek to act around their baby's demands more or less actively. As Odile noted, the notion of projection is central to the experiences of new parents, who often express great concern about the high frequency of feedings during the first days of their child's life, and the representative character of this initial rhythm on their long-term breastfeeding journey.

Yet, more than the request frequency or the actual time spent on each feeding, the unpredictability of the process seemed to be the most disturbing aspect for parents, specifically not knowing when their baby would want to eat again and being unable to organise their schedule accordingly. The notion of rhythm is therefore crucial: the most important thing is the predictability of the baby's schedule, no matter how intense.

Chloé was a friend of one of the midwives I worked with. We first met at a fundraising event organised by independent midwives. At that time, she was only three months pregnant, and I was still in the exploratory phase of my research. Her midwife friend told her about my research after her son's birth, and Chloé was interested in participating. She had planned to give birth in a birth centre but was eventually transferred to a maternity ward due to her exhaustion and her desire to have an epidural. She came back home a few hours after her son Jules's birth. Chloé was in her early thirties. She had a degree in human sciences and was unemployed when Jules was born. She was the only mother to mention Bowlby's attachment theory specifically (about which she had learned during her studies) as inspiring the parenting practices she had implemented. I never had the opportunity to meet her spouse, Patrick, who was employed in a technology company. They lived in an apartment in the city.

Chloé and I met for our first interview when Jules was one month old. She told me about her choice to breastfeed on demand: "The rhythm has settled. Very quickly, he started to suckle every two hours. Breastfeeding on demand is a choice. You must expect to be called often". She continued, "It's not a big constraint after all, or it becomes less and less. At first, I told myself that every two hours would be too much, that I would be fed up with it". For Chloé, this adaptation to the breastfeeding rhythm was "rather complicated intellectually: you want to meet the needs of the baby, but there are surrounding pressures—the return to work, the longing for a full night of sleep". Chloé and Patrick had already planned to sleep with Jules before birth. They had invested in a co-sleeper bed. In practice, Jules came closer during the night and ended every night in his parents' bed. From the beginning, however, they had set the end of this arrangement: the project was to keep Jules sleeping next to them for another two months, assuming that he would have developed "more skills" at four months. "We know that at four months, the baby can understand when you differ from his needs because the brain structure is there", explained Chloé. Jules would then be able to wait a little longer for his night-time feeding than when he was within reach of his mother's breasts. The predictability of the baby's rhythm, as well as the idea of having a pre-established plan to determine the end of the bed-sharing period, seemed to reassure Chloé.

To rationalise her practices, Chloé relied on biomedical knowledge regarding children's psycho-emotional and brain development. Again, the educational model of holistic care is inscribed in the biomedical model and home birth parents are strongly inculcated with biomedical culture and knowledge, which also justify their childcare and educational choices. In this way, parents digress from the singularised care approach defended by holistic midwives, resting solely upon contextualised observation of each child.

It occurred to me that most mothers who breastfed on demand were nonetheless used to recording the timing and duration of their baby's feedings, in either a notebook or a smartphone application. The monitoring of quantitative data on smartphone applications inscribed these parents as being within dominant biomedical practices. However, other parents precisely resisted the spread of technological tools to all aspects of their daily life, including their parenting experience, by refusing to acquire adapted devices or by restraining the devices' use.

On the contrary, Olivia and Alain were keen users of perinatal smartphone applications. They told me about the "Baby Tracker", an application designed to record the baby's feeds and time per breast as well as to monitor sleep and diapers, which Olivia used every day since their baby's birth and which, according to her, enabled her "to have a bit of an idea of how the day is going". She clarified: "Sometimes, we think that she may be hungry, and we look at the application, and if it's been three hours and a half [since the last feed], we say, 'Ah, maybe'". Alain observed that he found it amusing to compare his baby's feeding rhythms from one day to the next, even if "it does not lead to anything". They took no effective measures in relation to this careful count. It seemed that the simple fact of documenting the feedings allowed Olivia and Alain to maintain a feeling of control over their schedule. This use of a quantification device is reminiscent of—and is perhaps encouraged by—midwives' inquiries on feeding rhythms during their postpartum consultations, such as when Mireille asked about the number of night-time feedings. After their midwife's follow-up, these parents kept the habit of tracking their child's schedule.

More generally, while spending time with new mothers, I was struck by a contradiction: despite a desire to breastfeed on demand, the clock often validated the baby's manifestation and the mother's interpretation: "Are you hungry? Ah, yes, it's time".

Nevertheless, as the breastfeeding relationship develops and matures, a mother and her baby establish a dialogue, so that they seem to reach a "compromise" about the feeding rhythm, which leads to breastfeeding being based not only on the baby's demand but with both protagonists involved. Laura, mother of four-month-old Maïlis, clearly differentiated the early stage of breastfeeding, which she defined as "on-demand", from the later breastfeeding pace. She explained that her daughter "doesn't really ask anymore" but that both "find themselves at the right moment": "A dialogue has been put in place, and now, we are adapted to each other". She developed this further: "Sometimes, I tell her, 'You're hungry, but I have to finish this, I'll feed you in fifteen minutes'. I ask her to adapt a lot, and she doesn't seem to suffer from it". The feeding rhythm had reciprocally adapted. Laura's expectations had evolved. She would not tolerate being interrupted in her activities, as was the case in the first weeks of Maïlis's life anymore, and Maïlis seemed well adjusted to this situation. An evolution had taken place between an initial desire to respect the baby's rhythm without interfering and the establishment of communication around breastfeeding. The baby was subsequently seen as a partner, with whom negotiation was possible.

Night-time routines

All of the parents I met chose to sleep with their baby for a more or less extended period, with variable settings and often with the intention of facilitating night-time breastfeeding, as encouraged by their midwives. Although bed-sharing was part of a premeditated plan, almost all of the parents had also set up a nursery for their baby. For example, during one of my visits to Jelena's apartment, she showed me the room she and her spouse had prepared for their daughter, commenting humorously, "All that, it's pretty, but it does not correspond to the real things we are practising at night. You see this bed? It's useless!"

While some parents chose to invest in a dedicated co-sleeper bed, others simply shared their bed with their infant, as was the case for Céline and Julien. Morgane slept on Céline's chest, who would cover herself with a quilt only up to her waist and, in addition, would put on a sweater so Morgane would not get cold since Morgane was born in winter. A nursing pillow was installed between the parents so that Julien would not disturb them with sudden movements. Céline alluded to online videos of mothers filming themselves at night, showing that they were always aware of the baby's position in their movements: "I was told that moms who are really breastfeeding [implied to be on demand] have a radar for the baby". Céline was referring to biological anthropology works about the physiological interrelationships between mothers and infants during sleep, according to which they would mutually regulate their sleep patterns, playing an important role in making night-time feedings easier. Mothers would respond to subtle signals from their babies and breastfeed them while neither they nor their babies are completely awake (McKenna & Gettler 2016). Without specifically quoting these works, the Facebook breastfeeding support group mentioned earlier, of which Céline was a member, frequently shared information about "breastsleeping" (McKenna & Gettler 2016).

As pointed out by Tomori (2015), in modern industrial societies, sleep is thought of as a time of withdrawal from social life, and lonely, uninterrupted sleep is erected as an ideal sleeping mode that would be the most beneficial, physiologically. In this respect, bed-sharing is a controversial practice, raising safety and moral concerns from laypersons and birth professionals. Moreover, in line with a conception of education as starting from birth, parents should not tolerate behaviour considered unsuitable in the long term (Delaisi de Parseval & Lallemand 1998; Neyrand 2000; Thébaud 1986).

Tomori (2015) showed that parents who sleep with their children view sleep as a time allowing close emotional ties to be knit, with sleeping thus becoming family time. I discussed this aspect with Fabienne, who was feeding her three-month-old daughter Malia on demand. When I met Fabienne at her apartment, she was about to return to work. She and her spouse,

Gaëtan, a stay-at-home father, supported bed-sharing. The floor of the parental bedroom was lined with mattresses, intended for their two elder daughters, if they wanted to join their parents at night. Malia slept on a dedicated mattress attached to her parents' mattress. Fabienne and Gaëtan had proceeded in the same way with both their elder daughters and were convinced that this arrangement was decisive in facilitating their breastfeeding experiences. Fabienne explained, "As we did the co-sleeping thing, I was nursing several times at night, and it was not a problem. I was told, 'You will be tired'. I said no. It's integrated. It's integrated into a movement. I do not wake up. I do not get up. I just breastfeed". For her, bed-sharing went hand-in-hand with breastfeeding, so that she had "trouble conceiving that it [breastfeeding] can be done with the baby in a separate room". She continued, referring to her upcoming return to work and the continuation of breastfeeding, "I am putting everything in place to make it possible". Fabienne saw bed-sharing as a way to make up emotionally for the time spent away from her baby during the day and to help maintain her lactation, despite a reduction of feedings. Bed-sharing would thus allow breastfeeding management that was both rational—maintaining lactation—and emotional—maintaining affective ties.

In this perspective, Tomori (2015) proposed an analysis of bed-sharing as a reproduction of capitalist ideology: breastfeeding and sleeping practices take place in a capitalist society that governs employment modalities. With co-sleeping, families adapt to—and thereby contribute to reproducing—capitalist practices striving to maximise employees' work potential and offering only minimal arrangements to articulate family and work lives adequately. Parents would only opt for specific sleeping setups like bed-sharing to reconcile the imperatives of their workday with those of breastfeeding: bed-sharing would optimise parents' rest by sparing them the effort of getting up to feed their babies while protecting lactation because they would remain in close contact with their children, allowing them to nurse on demand during night-time. However, in practice, some parents reported that sleeping with an agitated, noisy baby was not necessarily the best way to get the most of their night-time rest.

Before becoming parents, most people attribute daytime to work, while leisure and rest take place at night and on weekends. Thus, temporality is largely conceived of through work schedules. Yet, historians like Thoemmes (2009) theorised a paradigm shift in the conceptualisation of time and identified a major evolution of social temporalities since the 1980s. This development would manifest in a blurred separation between private life and work life, enabled by new information and communication technologies but also by lifestyle changes. In practice, this evolution would translate into flexible practices with regard to work schedules and place, particularly through teleworking. However, these new flexible arrangements are not accessible to all professional sectors. In my fieldwork, some of the parents had access to this type of arrangement, while others did not. Nevertheless, even for parents with a downshifting strategy, the requirement of productivity during the workday remained, so that Tomori's (2015) analyses are still relevant.

Parents adjust their own bodies to coordinate with their child's body: they become used to their baby's small sounds and establish measures regarding space distribution and sleep positions to prevent possible risks generated by bed-sharing. Alongside this work upon their own bodies, they also exercise authority over their baby's body to achieve preferred sleep patterns. These nocturnal negotiations highlight how capitalist work organisation shapes sleep experiences but also testify to the emergence of incorporated moralities, aimed at reconciling the maintenance of breastfeeding with the return to work. These sleep practices challenge and reproduce capitalist regimes of temporality and how they model kinship relations (Tomori 2015). Parents reinvent sleep as a shared family time to meet childcare and motherhood ideals, as embodied by breastfeeding, as well as optimise productivity through sufficient recovery time at night.

Based on her ethnography on the meaning of touch among Japanese families, Tahhan (2008, 2010) used the concept of skinship to describe the relational intimacy created by physical proximity, including by sharing a familial bed. On the premise that tactility inevitably leads to intimacy, she showed how sleeping together builds family ties. As highlighted by Fabienne's own analysis of her night-time arrangement, from this perspective, bed-sharing may be seen as a way to produce and maintain intimacy despite constraints such as time spent apart.

In Tomori's (2015) research, parents identified night-time infant feeding as "the most labor-intensive aspect of supporting breastfeeding", in which fathers were playing a key role (161). Based on my observations, fathers' night-time support varied. Some fathers left the parental bed to their spouse and baby and slept on a couch or in a guest room. Others preserved their lactating spouses' rest by taking their babies to sleep with them and bringing them to the mothers only for feeding sessions or caring for them once they were awake in the morning. At night, some fathers systematically changed their babies' diapers after they fed. More broadly, fathers' acceptance of bed-sharing was an essential prerequisite for the smooth operation of this practice.

Some parents talked about the pleasure of sleeping with their child and the skinship they created during night-time, especially if the father could not spend as much time with his child as his spouse could. As Chloé described, "At first, it was hard, with his little noises, but we got used to it". She continued, mentioning her spouse's feelings regarding sleeping with their son, Jules: "It makes him happy to see him [Jules] sleep and also to see him waking up. He [Jules] wakes up, and he is smiling; we can only be happy to wake up". Another mother, Marion, highlighted the positive influence of bed-sharing on the father–baby relationship in her family: "Falling asleep with his baby against him—he enjoys it. He can sleep close to him ... It also creates a bond for the dad". Tomori (2015) emphasised this emotional function of co-sleeping: "For fathers who slept next to their children and wives, incorporating the child into the parental bed also constituted a set of important embodied practices and produced powerful affective bonds that brought the three sleepers together into a family unit" (163). Sleep is reinvented during a period of skinship, from a solitary activity to a pleasurable group experience and a productive time, aimed at tightening family bonds. Through this sensual proximity, the baby's body becomes a medium of relationality, on the basis of which parents build their new parental identities (Brownlie & Sheach Leith 2011).

Beyond reinventing bedding equipment and sleeping positions, which sometimes required parents to sleep apart, the child's presence in the parental bed sometimes was also alluded to as impeding bodily contact between spouses and sexual intercourse. In this discourse, bed-sharing was identified as a "gift" from parents to the child, implicitly recognising some level of self-denial regarding conjugal, intimate life.

> A couple's life, if we stay long enough together, it's long. We have time, so … We slept together before, we'll sleep together after and now it's a moment that we are offering to this child. We also offered the same time to our two eldest children. It's a time we offer, and … Well, at some point, it will be part of our memories. And we'll be happy that we have been able to offer this to our children. It's really done naturally and simply. There are also times when my husband really has intense working days, a very big week, that we have the possibility, we have a guestroom above, so he will sleep through the night. He can at least recover well and not be woken up every hour by the baby, who may have a toothache or not be well. We also know that it's a moment that will pass. It's not a concern if we sleep apart for a while, in order to recover.
>
> (interview with Delphine, transcription)

At the time of my meeting with Delphine, her son was 11 months old. She had planned to sleep with him until he was at least one year old, like she had done with both her eldest children. In this excerpt, Delphine described a demanding routine, which also was reflected in her insistence on the temporary character of their night-time arrangement. Cécile also emphasised the boundaries of bed-sharing with Gaëlle: "Sometimes, we fancy more privacy in our bed with Jonas. We know it's a special time. When it's time, we'll feel it, and everyone will adapt. For now, it's nice to have her close and to be able to cuddle her".

These parents accepted putting their comfort and desires aside for a time because they believed it will make a difference in their child's affective development. The same reasoning led mothers to embrace the affective functions of feeding and to delay weaning if their child does not seem "ready" to stop breastfeeding, regardless of the parents' own feelings.

Suckling for comfort

Beyond the nutritive function of feedings, parents in my fieldwork acknowledged that their children had a "sucking need" to satiate, which they could answer by putting them at the breast or by proposing a substitute, like a parent's finger or a pacifier. Midwives also supported this idea during their postpartum follow-up. These "sucking needs" were identified as more or less intense depending on the baby. Midwives identified some newborns as "nipple nibblers": "Hey, you're a real nipple nibbler!" said Marianne to a baby, for example. For some parents, the idea of giving a pacifier to their baby was not appealing because they associated it with a restraining measure regarding their child's communication. Corinne, the mother of one-month-old Tom, explained at the postnatal classes led by Mireille, her midwife, that her son was suckling for a very long time every night and became upset at the breast. Mireille proposed giving him a pacifier, but Corinne was uncomfortable with this idea: "For me, a pacifier is like, 'Shut up, I don't want to hear you'". Corinne, like other mothers, preferred to offer her nipple to her child, even for non-nutritional purposes, rather than give him a pacifier.

For other women, putting their child at their breast as a first gesture of comfort was an easy solution, somehow making them lax mothers. Even for mothers who chose a care model underpinned by the values of attachment parenting, the use of breastfeeding as a source of comfort remains subversive in a cultural context dominated by values of autonomy (McBride-Henry & Shaw 2010). When breastfeeding is established over time, a clear division seems to appear between mothers reducing breastfeeding to a nutritional function and those who prefer to let their children access their breast each time they express the desire to.

Some, like Céline, fully recognised that feedings were "no longer nutritional at all". When I first met her, she was seven months pregnant and breastfed her two-year-old daughter Yvonne. Pregnancy inhibited her lactation, so that her breasts no longer ejected milk. She noticed that for several months, she had not heard Yvonne swallow during feedings: "She uses me as a comforter. You see, the other children, they have a comforter, a pacifier. Yvonne has her mom". As much as she enjoyed the breastfeeding experience, another mother, Olivia, evoked a mind shift in accepting the idea of a comforting feed: "I feel that a great complicity has developed in a really physical relationship, in saying to yourself, 'Here, you're not eating—you're sucking—but I agree to play along and accept it'".

However, mothers also perceived consenting to meet their babies' emotional needs using breastfeeding as a very efficient parenting tool to soothe a fussy child or console a physical or affective pain. Comforting feedings were underpinned by an idea of productivity and efficiency because parents saw them as the quickest and most radical way to calm down an upset child. For example, Lauriane greatly appreciated the convenience of using feeds to soothe her daughter: "Putting her at the breast is the first thing I do if she whines, if she's not okay. I'm not going to rack my brain. I don't care if she only nibbles; for me, it's always good for something". From this perspective, nutritional and emotional needs merge and are both satisfied by feedings. For mothers, there is therefore no point in identifying why their child wants to breastfeed.

Long-term breastfeeding: an investment in the future

Faircloth (2013) led research in the United Kingdom with a network of women who were breastfeeding their children "to full term"—until they outgrew the need or desire to breastfeed. In line with a "supposed hominid blueprint of care",[8] the end of full-term breastfeeding can be reached at any point between one and eight years, and would most often occur between two and five years (Faircloth 2010: 358). Faircloth's (2013) interlocutors based their commitment to long-term breastfeeding on health-related and emotional arguments of building "secure emotional foundations" for their infants (68). According to this perspective, breastfeeding practices could shape an individual's personality.

> Corinne was in her late thirties. She worked as an office employee at a private company and lived with her spouse in an apartment in a small town. She gave birth to her son, Tom, in a birth centre with her midwife, Mireille. Her spouse was an employee in the financial sector. He resumed working two days after Tom's birth, and shortly after, the three of them left for a month in the mountains, where a local midwife took over Mireille's follow-up. As a result, I never met Corinne's spouse and could only attend one postpartum consultation before their departure. I met Corinne again two months later at Mireille's postnatal classes. Corinne was already complaining about Tom becoming very fussy in the evening.
>
> Five months later, I met her at her apartment to discuss the evolution of her breastfeeding experience. She told me right away, "Breastfeeding is not easy, but it's due to Tom's character". She explained: "He's pretty complicated, Tom. He isn't very calm, and he isn't very patient, so breastfeeding is a little complicated". She explained that she and her spouse had decided "to follow him until at least six months". "We will try to follow his rhythm, to not impose a rhythm. It's part of the birth centre project", added Corinne. Tom was still very fussy each evening. Corinne and her spouse had a hard time getting him to sleep, and Tom would wake up multiple times during the night. In this demanding situation, Corinne identified breastfeeding as a major asset: "I don't know how you survive when you don't have the breast. At least he's relatively calm for a moment". For her, breastfeeding also has long-term

impacts on individuals and develops willpower: "The child engages in breastfeeding. I think for his development, it's good too". Corinne had resumed work one month before. She was facing a very hostile work environment and did not dare to claim her right to paid breastfeeding leave. She secretly pumped during her lunch breaks, while eating, in the bathroom or a "windowless meeting room", fearing interruption by a co-worker. As she had unsurprisingly encountered difficulties with pumping enough milk during her workday, she had introduced a daily bottle of formula into Tom's diet.

The next time I met with Corinne, Tom was one year old. She stopped pumping her milk at work two months before then, "to steer us towards weaning". She told me that this was a process requiring time and that she was not in a hurry: "I'd like him to stop by himself. As long as he wants to suckle, I want him to be able to suckle". Our discussion was interrupted frequently by Tom's yelling and overall extreme agitation. The living room was filled with toys, including an imposing children's slide, which Tom hit loudly against the tiled floor. Again, Corinne referred to Tom's "particular character" to explain that he might need to suckle more than another child would. Even though she still highly appreciated nursing him as a parenting tool—"It calms him, it refocuses him a lot, it allows him to stop being agitated"—she considered that "the time has come". She added, "He has acquired some level of independence. He must also fly from the nest in regard to that. [...] We try to teach him other ways to calm down. It's good for him too because he also enjoys self-sufficiency and independence". She breastfed him in the morning and at night, including night-time awakenings, and in special circumstances (while travelling or if Tom was sick). Despite Tom's agitation during my visit, she did not offer him her breast. Corinne spent time explaining to Tom that he was ready for weaning: "I tell him that he can stop if he wants, that he has suckled for a long time and that it was good".

One year later, Corinne told me how Tom's breastfeeding ended. She eventually had to initiate the weaning: "I had hoped he'd stop, but he didn't want to stop! It went well, he was ready, but it was not his decision". She took stock of their breastfeeding experience: "We built a very strong relationship. It's difficult to dissociate from his character, but I see that he is a very cuddly child who gives back the attention he receives. I see many aspects of him showing that he has not had emotional emptiness. He is fulfilled with his emotions. He is able to express his emotions, and he is independent too. I have the impression that children who are not breastfed are less independent. I think it's pretty conclusive".

Even though Corinne wanted to breastfeed Tom to full term, she eventually induced weaning because she no longer enjoyed breastfeeding: "I couldn't do it anymore, in terms of patience. The situation pushed me to my limits". However, she was pleased with her breastfeeding experience and relied on it to justify Tom's personal qualities. Interestingly, the notion of autonomy was central to her plea for breastfeeding: long-term breastfeeding provided solid emotional foundations for Tom, allowing him to reach self-sufficiency. Other parents shared this idea. For example, Fabien also associated long-term breastfeeding with increased self-reliance: "After the first few months, it's more like a habit, a bond. These children [who were breastfed long-term] are more confident, less afraid".

Despite their initial will to respect their child's natural rhythm, when it comes to weaning, parents often set up boundaries to restrict feedings to specific times of the day. Therefore, a long-term breastfed infant no longer would be breastfed on demand. On the contrary, feedings are subject to close negotiations between mother and child. For example, Céline's daughter Yvonne became very demanding after her sister's birth. Six months later, while Céline wanted to wean Yvonne, she was determined to "not impose it on her". During feedings, she asked Yvonne to count down from ten or twenty and then let the breast go: "At one point, she suckled so often that I told her, 'Okay, but you have to count'. At least she feels like she's managing something". She also explained to Yvonne that the situation was different between her and her sister since Morgane could only drink breast milk.

One year later, Yvonne, then three-and-a-half years old, was still not weaned, but her feedings were restricted to one in the morning: "She asks very rarely during the day, but I have to put a strict barrier in the evening", said Céline. Julien, her spouse, was no longer supportive of his eldest daughter's breastfeeding. He never attended the morning feeding scene and thought it would feel "really weird" for him to see that: "Breastfeeding belongs to the world of babies. I am beginning to feel the discrepancy".

Guillaume also considered that it would be desirable to wean their two-and-a-half-year-old daughter, Simone: "Léa [his spouse] always said that Simone will decide. It does not bother me that Léa has breastfed her for a long time. Well, I used to think this, but for some time now, I've wanted it to stop. I'm not categorical because I don't want to traumatise Simone and Léa. I do not want to break this link". Léa interrupted him: "It's not your role, either". Guillaume associated Simone's frequent wakings to breastfeeding: "When she wakes up, it's for a feed. She wakes up and says, 'Suckle'. We'd like to have uninterrupted nights". However, he still supported Léa's breastfeeding: "In the evening when I tell a story, when Simone says 'Suckle', I call Léa to come and give her a feed because it's an important moment for their relationship". He also attributed Simone's personality to breastfeeding: "Breastfeeding has contributed to her receiving a lot. She's never felt abandoned. At the emotional level, she's really cute—she's the best. I really feel like she's happy. As soon as she has a small scratch, with breastfeeding, she feels safe. She really feels that we love her".

Guillaume's words reflected his ambivalence. As a breastfeeding supporter, he recognised the benefits of continuing breastfeeding; simultaneously, he attributed Simone's sleeping issues to her desire for night-time feedings, and he took over a recurrent argument according to which a formula-fed child would more easily sleep through the night.

In order to embrace a long-term breastfeeding journey, parents must deal with their own prejudices and deconstruct cultural norms regarding breastfeeding. For example, most of the women I met initially had a negative view of long-term breastfeeding. They refused, for example, the idea of breastfeeding a child who could walk, speak, or spontaneously come to undress them to gain access to their breast. Cécile's perspective on long-term breastfeeding, for example, was influenced by a friend breastfeeding her three-year-old daughter. Cécile had the feeling that her friend's daughter was imposing it on her friend. Consequently, Cécile did not picture herself breastfeeding her daughter, Gaëlle, beyond two years: "If it works, if I want to … I don't set limits, but there is no pressure to breastfeed as long as possible. Maybe until she's two. We'll see. I wouldn't want it to become something completely directed by her and to become a power thing: that she demands her right to the breast. I know it's not necessarily easy to handle, this weaning. I think if it's not enjoyable for me anymore, I'll say to stop".

This attitude contrasts with the self-denial demonstrated by other women regarding weaning, like Céline, who continued to breastfeed Yvonne long after reaching her saturation point. She developed coping strategies, like reading content about weaning in line with the attachment parenting philosophy, which gave her "a second wind". These readings reminded her about the theoretical foundations of her commitment, inspired by Bowlby's attachment theory. In this way, she managed to hold on until Yvonne's self-guided weaning.

Some women experience awkwardness or even disgust when they face the evolution of their child's attitude at the breast. For example, Lauriane told me about her unease: "She was licking and looking at me with a big smile. I explained to her that Mom did not really feel comfortable". Chloé expressed the same awkwardness with Jules, at one year old: "We have trouble with the idea of a baby who walks and suckles. There is a representation according to which walking means that he is not really a baby anymore. His behaviour is different. He clearly grabs it [the breast] more by himself. It would bother me that he'd come and grab my breast. Already now, when he manipulates my breast, it annoys me, it bothers me. This is perhaps a sign that it is beginning to be a little too much for me. Now, he's pushing it, hitting it. It hurts me too". These thoughts reflect a cultural bias identifying breasts as primarily sexual in a Euro-American context (Mahon-Daly & Andrews 2002). In this perspective, a walking and talking infant who is consciously manipulating the maternal breast is perceived as transgressive. In addition, the heteronormative order intimates to women that breasts must remain their spouse's prerogative. As the sexual and maternal functions of women's bodies are thought of as being incompatible (Stearn 1999), long-term breastfeeding contradicts the social injunction to resume sexual intercourse quickly.

Several mothers also had concerns that their child's fondness for them would be solely based on their devotion to breastfeeding, like Maud with her one-year-old daughter: "Am I something else other than a milk provider? I'd like her to give me a hug without thinking about my milk, this fucking milk … I wonder if she'd love me without it". Remarkably, the argument that breastfeeding promotes attachment between mother and child is reversed here: in the long term, the appeal of feedings to children could indeed undermine their mothers' confidence regarding their bond.

In my fieldwork, I witnessed older children feedings multiple times, which did not fit within traditional breastfeeding imagery. Older children asked to breastfeed, sometimes loudly and insistently. They were not always calm at the breast but instead were excited. Some children liked to play with their mother during feedings, clapping her hand, or shaking their own legs, while others enjoyed manipulating the breast by stroking or squeezing it. They verbally asked for a feed, with a sign or a word that they often invented themselves—for example, "titi" for Yvonne—or with explicit gestures, while pulling their mother's clothes. Feedings sometimes occurred in the middle of a game and were very quick. At other times, toddlers did not want to end their feed and tirelessly moved from one breast to the other one, as was the case for Simone during one of my visits. Léa amusingly said to her, while unsuccessfully trying to lay her down and get up, "Come on, let's go and say goodbye to Caroline! Sweetie, we can't do that all day long!" These examples show a range of active attitudes among toddlers regarding breastfeeding, often perceived as disturbing through the prism of a neoliberal ideal of individuality and what is considered appropriate behaviour for infants. Breastfeeding still provides some nutrition to toddlers, but they mostly suckle for comfort and because they like the taste of maternal milk, as some of them told their mother.

A baby's tailor-made world: on other communication tools and practices

Besides on-demand breastfeeding, the parents I met set up a range of child-centred practices to favour communication with their children and, more broadly, their empowerment. In this perspective, the parents focused on how they could arrange their living environment to make it suitable for their child, and not the other way around. For example, they were critical of standard infant furniture, like cribs with bars, safety gates, or a playpen, referring to these items as "jails". For Tamara and Jérome, adjusting their house so that Camille "can frolic everywhere rather than putting her in a playpen" was part of their educational plan, as inspired by the Montessori method. "The way we educate her … we know that it has an influence on her development and her self-esteem: empowering her, meeting her needs, her autonomy, the way in which we installed her room" explained Tamara. Similarly, an enormous playpen (large enough to contain a children's slide) occupied half of Corinne's living room, allowing Tom to play safely while enjoying an extensive space. "Well, I don't want to put him in jail", she observed. These arrangements, sometimes detrimental to parental comfort, were in line with the idea of "putting oneself in the baby's shoes", as defended by midwives during their postpartum follow-ups.

In the following section, I first discuss elimination communication, another communication-oriented practice that parents favoured, which midwives supported and sometimes induced. In the second part, I analyse how the parents negotiated their initial parenting project while facing the obligation of entrusting their child with other caregivers, typically day care workers. More broadly, I discuss the reframing by parents when the ideal parenting model is not compatible with their daily life requirements and socio-economic contexts.

"On-demand" elimination

Delaisi de Parseval and Lallemand (1998) considered toilet training as "one of the longest learning experiences of early childhood and most loaded with ethical values" (177). Starting in the early twentieth century, in France, educators influenced by the hygienist movement advocated for early toilet training, starting from the first weeks after birth, by regularly placing infants on a container so that they could get into the habit of eliminating in it (ibid. 1998). After the 1960s, educators condemned these methods, insisting on the necessity of letting the child's physical and psycho-emotional system develop. The infant's consent and interest are now considered essential prerequisites for toilet training. For example, Swiss paediatrics guidelines indicate that the acquisition of toilet-training skills is relative to the child's development and cannot be accelerated by early training (Wilhelm-Bals, Birraux & Girardin 2010).

The toilet-training style I observed in my fieldwork was quite different from the model described by Delaisi de Parseval and Lallemand (1998), based on conditioning the child through a reward–punishment system. Ingrid Bauer (2001) coined the term "elimination communication" in her book *Diaper Free! The Gentle Wisdom of Natural Infant Hygiene*. Her method was inspired by Jean Liedloff's book, *The Continuum Concept: In Search of Happiness*, published in 1975 and based on her ethnography among the Yequana people in Venezuela. Liedloff (1975) argued that parents must keep their infants physically close to them to answer their needs quickly, including elimination, while babies are kept diaper-free to facilitate the process. In this way, infants would quickly learn to identify their elimination needs and become continent. As Walker (2014) highlighted, in one rare socio-anthropological publication on the topic, the reinvention of elimination communication relied heavily on a romanticisation of childrearing in so-called "traditional", non-industrialised societies. Through her study on elimination communication in the United States, she pointed out a mismatch between North American society and the application of this method, creating undue stress on mothers (Walker 2014: 233). Among other attachment-parenting practices like long-term breastfeeding or child carrying, she focused on elimination communication as the most paradigmatic example of a parenting model disconnected from the socio-economic contexts of neoliberal societies, as confirmed by some of the condescending reactions I noticed.

Indeed, this particular aspect of my fieldwork sparked some passionate feedback from my relatives when I mentioned it, including from advocates of home birth and attachment parenting practices like bed-sharing or long-term breastfeeding. Elimination communication, practised by more than one-third of the parents I met, interestingly appeared to be the most controversial aspect of my research. Non-initiated parents appeared to perceive it as a time-consuming form of enslavement or as cruel for children, on whom it would put "too much pressure", too early in their development. Parents who carried out elimination communication therefore often felt uncomfortable talking about it. For example, Léa told me that friends came to visit her and were astonished to see her offering Simone a container to eliminate after a feed: "It immediately seems very extreme". Another mother, Laura, commented, "I often see quite hallucinated gazes": when out, she would crouch her diaper-free baby, Maïlis, at the foot of a tree so that Maïlis could eliminate. Even her spouse, although supportive of the method, was embarrassed when Laura pulled a container out of her bag at their friends' house: "If we're inside, I put a little pot under her bottom, close it and put it back in my bag". In my fieldwork, non-user parents were often aware of this method. For some of them, it appeared to be an inaccessible ideal, which made them feel guilty, as in the case of Lauriane: "I feel bad about using diapers on them, but it seems too complicated for me at the moment". Although elimination communication was widely known in holistic care circles, it remained confined to these marginal social environments, unlike other practices like child wearing, which have become popular in dominant parenting practices. As an "underground" practice, elimination communication has little visibility outside of initiated circles and has been very seldom addressed in social science. It is, therefore, difficult to trace the history of its implementation in Switzerland or to evaluate its spread.

Elimination communication also leads to a specific market for parents willing to invest in dedicated items designed to support the child's learning process, specifically split trousers and overalls, potties, and underpants. Even though parents who use elimination communication obviously do not all invest in these tools, the abundance of consumer goods related to natural parenting raises the question of its democratisation and strengthens the prejudice of its restricted access to economically privileged parents.

The parents I met who practised elimination communication insisted that their purpose was not to toilet train their babies but rather to make them aware of their sensations and to accompany their children's bodily discovery. A precociously toilet-trained baby would only be a collateral advantage. Elimination communication was mainly described as a communication tool and was particularly connected to the notion of on-demand breastfeeding: "I don't want to bother him too much about it. I do not make it a doctrine. The idea is not to toilet train him but rather to make him conscious. It's a communication approach. You want to communicate with your baby. It goes in the same direction as on-demand breastfeeding", Corinne explained. The method consists of identifying clues of a need to urinate or defecate and offering the infant the opportunity to do so in a dedicated container or space (usually a sink or toilet) while emitting a motivational noise or word so that the infant can associate it with the elimination process.

> Chloé practised elimination communication, as part of her commitment to the attachment parenting approach, including on-demand breastfeeding and bed-sharing: "These are concepts that all come together around communication and building a special bond with the baby". To prepare for its implementation, Chloé had read a book on the method during pregnancy. She tried to apply it when Jules was three months old but felt it was too taxing and postponed doing so until Jules was four months old.

> At one of our meetings, Jules, who was five months old, slept throughout my visit and eventually woke up just before I left. Chloé offered him a chance to urinate in the toilet. I followed them into the bathroom. Chloé undressed Jules and held him by supporting him by the thighs above the toilet. Jules's back rested against Chloé's stomach. She whispered into Jules's ear, "Psss". Jules quickly urinated. Chloé congratulated him: "Yeah, well done!" Despite her reading, she explained that she did not follow any rules: "I do it my way, I think. There isn't one way to do it. It's intuitive". She perceived elimination time as a bonding time, like breastfeeding, to which she frequently referred to explain the understanding she had developed with Jules: "We look at each other, we smile at each other and we tell each other things".

> Six months later, Chloé and I were catching up on her breastfeeding and her overall parenting experience. She told me about the elimination communication's development. She had started a new part-time job a few months ago, and Jules spent a few days a week at day care. She and her spouse continued to practice elimination communication, when they were available and willing to do it. "We try to do it without stress, so that it's something natural and non-mandatory. It's more of a pleasure, too. Patrick is also happy to do it because he sees that it works", explained Chloé. They did not mind, for example, that the childcare workers did not apply the method when Jules was at day care.

The notion of pleasure, highlighted by Chloé, also contrasts with the hygienist model of infant toilet training described by Delaisi de Parseval and Lallemand (1998), which they referred to as an ascetic dressage of the child. In this perspective, the child is conceptualised as a machine that requires adequate tuning. As analysed by Delaisi de Parseval and Lallemand (1998), "Everything happens as if the ideal desired by the authors was to reign over a mechanised body; from early childhood, the child underwent a training to make her or him a machine and a clock, eating and excreting at fixed times" (192).

This is precisely what was contested by parents enthusiastic about elimination communication, who perceived diaper parenting as a denial of their child's individuality and resulting needs. As Laura said, "It's another communication, kind of magical, based on, I don't really know what, but it works. When you answer a need rather than a schedule, you treat the baby more as a person than as an object".

Some midwives also explicitly supported elimination communication, although this practice was not systematically talked about, unlike bed-sharing or babywearing. As one of these midwives supporting elimination communication, Mireille invited an elimination communication instructor to deliver a presentation during one of her postnatal classes.

Postnatal classes took place in the birth centre where Mireille was working. Three women and their babies participated in this class, including Léa and Corinne, who participated in my research. The four of us were sitting on large pillows on the floor while Mireille introduced the instructor, Florence, who had given birth under Mireille's surveillance a few years ago.

Florence began by telling us her own journey. She was very disappointed by the premature end of her first child's breastfeeding, and the discovery of elimination communication had allowed her to heal her frustration by getting back to a privileged way of communicating with him. She explained that babies are continent from birth but are conditioned by adults to become incontinent. Mireille intervened to specify that during her training at midwifery school, she learned that children cannot control their sphincters before two years old and that it was, therefore, traumatising to ask them to do so. Florence evoked an imprisonment of the child in diapers and insisted on the dialogue allowed by elimination communication between parents and babies: "You don't only learn to communicate around the pee and poo. These children [trained with elimination communication] know how to communicate their needs in general". Mireille referred to African women: "Over there, you will never see a woman with a wet back. It creates Pavlov reflexes, and the child holds back".

Florence immediately presented elimination communication as linked to breastfeeding—in her case, to cope with a disappointing breastfeeding experience. As with crying, the idea was to "accompany" babies' elimination needs, whereas letting them urinate or defecate in a diaper would mean ignoring those needs. Again, Mireille referred to "African women" as a model of mothering uncorrupted by the socio-economic requirements of neoliberal societies, corroborating Walker's (2014) analysis of elimination communication as a racialised, imaginary idealisation of childrearing in non-industrialised societies.

In addition, elimination communication goes hand-in-hand with cloth diapers, another staple of the holistic care model. Their lower absorbency—compared to disposable diapers—would enable children to be "more uncomfortable" when they urinate. According to elimination communication reasoning, this would, therefore, stimulate infants' will to signal their need in order to avoid discomfort. Even though the method uses a discourse that revolves around communication, thus refuting the idea of training or efficiency, this argument refers to the hygienist model and the idea that constraints imposed on the child today will ensure a brighter, diaper-free future.

Outside the bubble of home birth parenting: negotiations and renunciations

For many parents, the end of maternity leave marks the end of the period when they could fully supervise their children's care. When they start day care, they must accept that a part of their infant's diet, sleep, elimination habits, and schedules will be out of their control. At the same time, parents perceived maintaining breastfeeding despite being apart during the day as protective against health and emotional risks, as noted by Faircloth (2013): "The drive to protect their children's purity from infection by the outside world was manifested at all ages" (122).

For example, Maud regretted that her and her spouse's parenting choices and practices were determined by day care requirements: "What really broke me in all this stuff was to put her in day care. It broke a lot of things. For example, they do not know the 'baby-led weaning' method. It's a shame not having done that. For the second [child], I'd dream of staying at home. But financially, it's not going to work". Maud and Jonathan stopped breastfeeding exclusively and accelerated the transition to solid food earlier than they would have liked in order to prepare Rose for day care. In their perspective, continuing to breastfeed her, including during the night, was a strategy to counterbalance the perceived negative effects induced by day care: "I insist on my milk, so she drinks it well. At night, I breastfeed on demand, as she wants" explained Maud. Another mother, Léa, contested that day care standardised rules, including mealtimes, which are the same for all babies, regardless of their hunger. Her daughter Simone did not have fixed schedules, and Léa was concerned that Simone would not eat properly if her mealtimes were imposed. In general, most of the parents complained about the meals provided at day care, which did not suit their children's usual diet (often organic, plant-based, or low in sugar and in processed foods), and about the impossibility of using cloth diapers or practising elimination communication at day care. More broadly, parents regretted that day care did not provide personalised care in tune with each child's individual rhythm and specific needs.

Beyond the necessary adjustments required by a day care centre or other arrangements, parents' own physical or emotional limits would sometimes interfere with their parenting project.

> Lauriane was in her early thirties. She had stopped working as a secretary after giving birth to her first child and started teaching private language lessons. Her thirty-year-old spouse, Mathieu, was completing his apprenticeship in the building sector, a professional reconversion after long-term unemployment despite his engineering degree. When I first met them, they were living with Mathieu's parents and siblings in an apartment in the city. At that time, they had just given birth to their second child, Nadine, in a birth centre. I met with Lauriane numerous times over the years since she had never stopped breastfeeding during the entire period of my fieldwork.

> She gave birth to her third child, Mathilde, at home. The delivery went smoothly, but Lauriane had a severe postpartum haemorrhage and had to be transferred to the hospital. When she wrote to me the next day to announce Mathilde's birth, she was exhausted and in shock. I was very upset to hear this news, and I went to visit her at the maternity ward with a friendly, non-ethnographic purpose.

> Three months after Mathilde's birth, we met at Lauriane's apartment to debrief on her experience and catch up on her breastfeeding situation. She and her family had just left Mathieu's parents' apartment and moved to a new place of their own. Lauriane was pleased with this change. However, she seemed very tired because her in-laws were no longer around to help with her eldest children while Mathieu was away during the day. He was taking his final exams and had to spend a lot of time studying. She returned to the circumstances of her last delivery and their impacts on her breastfeeding initiation. She was exposed to radioactivity as part of the procedure to stop the haemorrhage, so she could not give colostrum to Mathilde in the first twenty-four hours after the treatment. Her midwife managed to provide her with some breast milk, donated by a new mother among her midwife's colleagues. As hospital staff also provided a syringe of formula for Lauriane's disposal, she accidentally confused it with the syringe of maternal milk and gave it to Mathilde. This was the first time that one of her children had ingested formula, and she was very upset about it. Lauriane also had to let go of some of her parenting principles during her one-week hospital stay due to her exhaustion. For example, she consented

to entrusting hospital staff with Mathilde's care in order to get some rest during the night, while Mathilde was sleeping in the nursery. The seriousness of her health situation led her to take a step back regarding these deviations from her parenting ideal: "Surprisingly, I did not experience it badly".

She also told me that she had decided to leave parenting groups on Facebook, in which she had been very active in the last few years. "It's tiring ... having a third child, and the beautiful ideas of people without children ... I don't like to go on these groups anymore because there are such irrevocable opinions. It lacks nuance. For example, with baby-led weaning, it's all or nothing. If you're talking about mashed vegetables, it's like dropping an atomic bomb", she explained. Being exposed to these groups gave her a feeling of failure, as she compared her parenting practices with those of other parents. Similarly, she told me how disappointed she was that she could not carry out babywearing: "I love the idea, but despite what is said, that it is physiological and everything, it ruins my back. It's just not something practical for me in the long run".

This extract highlights the normativity of the parenting approach favoured by home birth parents, which calls to mind the biomedical model's formality. Parents do not feel comfortable recounting their non-compliant experiences, constrained by the social expectations of fellow home birth parents. In order to reconcile her parenting model with the requirements of her daily life and her well-being, Lauriane had to deconstruct this model to which she once adhered unreservedly and renounced some aspects of her parenting project. Similarly, other parents confided some concessions regarding their parenting style. For example, even though they had planned to share their bed with Simone and carry her, Léa and Guillaume eventually had to purchase a pushchair and a crib—"with bars and everything" specified Léa—because Simone did not sleep very well with them, and Léa suffered from a backache. Céline, for her part, was enthusiastic about tandem nursing in the early days after Morgane's birth: "I'm having a ball—it's pure happiness! I didn't know I would like it so much; I was afraid of feeling overwhelmed. I like when they exchange looks". At the same time, Julien, her spouse, was taking a picture of the tandem feed. A few months later, Céline commented that she did not at all enjoy the tandem feeds anymore: "The two of them simultaneously, it tends to annoy me and get on my nerves. Their two suctions are not the same, and it's unpleasant".

If parents theoretically adhere to a parenting practice and are forced to give it up when confronted with the realities of its implementation, their convictions are shaken. As highlighted by Faircloth (2013), parenting practices structure parents' "identity work", defined as "The active processes by which identity is constructed, as well as the inherent social nature of this enterprise (as opposed to it being simply a means of self-expression)"

(31–32). Therefore, as in the case of mothers who interrupt breastfeeding sooner than planned, renouncing some practices supported by the holistic care model—and by their midwife, as a spokesperson of this model—can foster a feeling of transgression or failure in parents' experiences. This deviation from the initial holistic care script requires a readjustment in parents' narratives to preserve the coherence of their reflexive project (Giddens 1991).

Conclusion

The temporal modalities of holistic care, such as the period when the relationship between parents and midwife is built or the duration of postpartum visits, break with the institutional logic and the technocratic hierarchy implying the individual's subordination to the institution (Davis-Floyd & St. John 1998). Thus, midwives distance themselves from institutional schedules and advocate for a relational assessment of breastfeeding. By presenting the baby as a full-fledged breastfeeding partner, they invite a shared responsibility for successful breastfeeding and dismiss a reductive conception of the newborn as primarily helpless. Focused on observing babies, highlighting their skills, on the one hand, and stimulating mothers' "creativity", on the other hand, midwives' discourses support an "ethic of maternal availability" that contributes to the (re)production of an unequal distribution of responsibilities between mothers and fathers (Garcia 2011: 12). In this perspective, the holistic model of care—like the technocratic model, to which it developed as a response—is loaded with injunctions, mainly addressed to mothers. Scheper-Hughes (1992) noticed that, in line with the biomedical script of mother and child "bonding", mothers are buried under information on appropriate behaviours and feelings. As a result, women experiencing alternative feelings regarding their child are stigmatised. Scheper-Hughes (1992) highlighted the links between the bonding theory and mothers' isolation in the context of the neoliberal nuclear family model, which requires a heavy maternal commitment to infant care. The bonding theory would naturalise this socio-economic context.

Although my interlocutors joined a neoliberal vision of individuality as an extension of biological data—the "natural" body (Conklin & Morgan 1996)—they also adhered to a conception based on social relations. They took a critical stance towards the dominant autonomist ideology, in favour of a more progressive formation of individuality over time. In this regard, the baby's dependence on her or his parents and their duty to constant availability are seen as a necessary and even desirable transition step with which to access self-sufficiency. This reasoning is consistent with the arguments underlying the attachment theories. Autonomy thus remains the ultimate goal, although the path taken to civilise the baby varies.

Beyond the material and economic circumstances specific to each family, the experience of on-demand breastfeeding and its continuation past several weeks or months depend on the parents' ability to rethink their temporal organisation. When facing their babies' frequent solicitations, mothers rely on various interpretive registers, corresponding to different strategies of adaptation to on-demand breastfeeding's requirements. In order for breastfeeding to evolve from a limited and extraordinary parenthesis to a sustainable, lasting practice in mothers' ordinary life, it is also necessary not to consider it as time-consuming. In this perspective, mothers experiencing a prolonged liminality rely on adjustment strategies and constructions of meaning so that the temporal chaos can meet the expectations and requirements of normal life (Sachs 2005). Although breastfeeding is first perceived as a moment of emotional sharing between mother and child, it is not relevant to count the time spent doing so or worry about feedings taking up too much time in a day. In their discourses, midwives present breastfeeding as a key part of mothers' relationship with their baby and, therefore, engage parents in a co-construction of meaning around the rhythm of feedings. Interestingly, my analysis is consistent with the recent shift in breastfeeding initiation and support, resulting in the notion of responsive feeding, as a relational process relying on mutual responsiveness among mothers to their infants' cues as well as infants' responses to their mothers' proposal diminishing pressure on parents (Aryeetey & Dykes 2018; Dykes & Flacking 2010).

In practice, this conception of breastfeeding requires flexibility and self-reliance regarding work planning and, therefore, excludes parents who work full-time in a dedicated workplace, away from their child. In my fieldwork, families nevertheless developed coping strategies to achieve their breastfeeding goals and downshifted their lifestyle to free up time. For example, in one case, both parents were able to work part-time—the father worked in the morning, and the mother in the afternoon—so that one of them could always be with their children. Two other mothers renounced working outside their home. Some parents also drastically revised their consumption habits. However, being able to set up a downshifting strategy also demands specific organisational resources, meaning that this model cannot fit the most financially and educationally disadvantaged families.

When breastfeeding settles over time, the understanding of on-demand breastfeeding widens. Nevertheless, how feedings—and their attributed nutritive or emotional functions—are mobilised still refers to the chosen care model and the degree of acceptance of an "ethic of maternal availability" (Garcia 2011: 12). In line with the notion of "parental determinism", mothers agree to maintain breastfeeding, sometimes against their own needs and desires, because they believe in a long-term positive impact on their child's psycho-emotional development. Parents rely on "science"—namely, evidence derived from psycho-developmental studies—to legitimate their breastfeeding practices. According to Faircloth (2013), "women's use of the discourses of science is a critical element of their identity work, serving as an accountability strategy par excellence, which—like recourse to nature—serves to edify their marginal position and foreclose further debate about their non-conventional breastfeeding" (144). This accountability strategy also applies to other attachment parenting practices or principles such as not leaving babies to cry alone.

The child-centred care and practices elected by parents are underpinned by a specific representation of the child, whose singularity must be enhanced and strengthened from birth, or even before birth.[9] This conceptualisation of the infant's personhood fits into a broader picture of contemporary individuality in neoliberal societies, raising the self as a fundamental and unquestionable value and driving each of our choices, interests, and actions (Rose 1998). Rose (1998) anchored the construction of our contemporary regime of the self in the emergence and development of "psychosciences and disciplines" since the second half of the nineteenth century in Europe and North America, which has determined the modalities of our current understanding of the self and the emphasis of this notion (2). As a way to produce contemporary individualities, parenting practices implemented by home birth parents are aimed at singling the baby out by enhancing the specific features of her or his physiological needs and addressing them in a personalised way. These practices challenge a standardised and standardising childcare approach, according to which each infant should conform to a schedule regarding her or his feeds or meals, sleep, and elimination needs.

Simultaneously, these practices produce a set of normative rules, forming a quite rigid parenting model that appears to some parents as an out-of-reach ideal that is difficult to maintain in the long term. This normativity, precisely denying the singularity of each family's life situation, echoes the biomedical model, which establishes normal child development based on average data.

Anchored in the baby's and the mother's bodies but also, to a lesser extent, in the father's body, the parenting practices I observed in my fieldwork were aligned with an understanding of the body as a necessary foundation for the expression of personhood (Memmi 2014). However, bodily substances or physical attributes are not sufficient by themselves; rather, parental identities are produced through the uses that parents make of their bodily attributes. Breasts and breast milk do not "make" mothers, but on-demand breastfeeding or long-term breastfeeding make the home birth mother. Through these practices, home birth infants are also produced with specific features—at least, in the minds of their caregivers. They are calm, communicating, affectionate, emotionally secure, independent, and self-confident.

Notes

1 This surveillance specifically targets the prevention of shaken baby syndrome (SBS), a phenomenon largely covered by Swiss media in recent years after the

death of a Swiss celebrity's child in 2001. This case raised medical awareness, leading to an inventory of SBS cases in Switzerland (Lips 2002).

2 This original French concept lacks an official English translation to this day. Therefore, I refer to it using the French expression.

3 The related information in this chapter is based on a discussion with a *parole au bébé* practitioner, whom I contacted separately from my fieldwork and on conversations with parents.

4 A respiratory support system designed for neonates.

5 Foetal macrosomia is identified as one of the most important foetal/maternal complications resulting from gestational diabetes (Tran, Boulvain & Philippe 2011).

6 "Chestfeeding" has emerged as a gender-inclusive term to design male, trans, and gender-fluid individuals who breastfeed (Walks 2018). Initially intended for lactating individuals, I suggest that this term could also fit for a non-lactating man feeding his child with the help of a supplemental nursing system fixed on his chest.

7 An infant bed open on one side and designed to be attached to the side of the parents' bed.

8 On this topic, see Dettwyler (1995a).

9 As argued by some psycho-developmental specialists, foetuses would also develop singular sensory skills in utero, which parents-to-be must strengthen with appropriate techniques and behaviours (see, for example, Herbinet & Busnel 2009 [1981]).

Conclusion

My ethnography focused on a birth model that concerns a small proportion of parents, out-of-hospital births with an independent midwife accounting for 3 per cent of births in Switzerland. This research thereby questions the dominant biomedical model, highlighting differences, as well as similarities, in discourses and practices, and it shows how an ethnographic attention "to the margins" can reveal much about the dynamics of power and culture "at the centre". Through the lens of my fieldwork analyses, I discuss in this conclusion the symmetry at play between the holistic and technocratic models of care, readdressing the transversal themes of risk, its anticipation and management, bodies and technologies, and temporalities. I conclude with considerations on gender regimes in holistic care and raise questions of a broader scope on this modality of care.

In my fieldwork, I witnessed a specific expression of the holistic care model, led by independent midwives and shaped by the local cultural context and healthcare system. In Switzerland, this model, while providing a critical alternative, also fits within the dominant biomedical model. The holistic care I observed is characterised by its continuity, a non-interventionist approach to birth, conceived as a "normal", physiological process, and the resulting choice of home as the place of delivery and postpartum care. The holistic model includes a particular vision of infants' care, partially referring to the attachment parenting philosophy, based on Bowlby's attachment theory, but also influenced by the "natural motherhood" movement (Bobel 2002). I suggest that the holistic care model presumes an ideal type script regarding postpartum and parenting practices, in which breastfeeding appears as a central element, leading to and justifying other body-centred parenting practices, such as babywearing or bed-sharing. However, the application of the holistic care script raises some difficulties and confronts parents about challenges and contradictions when facing the specificities of their life circumstances and requirements. More broadly, these tensions reflect inconsistencies and breaches in the model with respect to modern neoliberal policies, sustaining an ideology of individual parenting choices and responsibilities. Switzerland, in particular, stands out with minimal and sparse family policy, in comparison with other European countries. The

DOI: 10.4324/9781003124108-102

2021 introduction of paternity leave is an emblematic example because, before that, its inexistence deeply impacted the parents' organisation and made it more challenging to adopt equalitarian parenting practices.

In general, I observed that achieving their breastfeeding project requires dedication from parents and body work from mothers—the workload varying greatly from one situation to another. As a result, women's bodies are subject to a heavy management to sustain the lactation process. This makes me wonder, if the most committed parents, granted with one-on-one care, are facing various kinds of breastfeeding difficulties, leaving them sometimes overwhelmed, how could the majority of parents follow the WHO recommendations?

Overall, my research contributes to the existing debate by offering new perspectives on the conceptualisation of breastfeeding as a collective process, co-produced by parents liaising with their midwife. It shows that the individual-based approach of public health promotion fails to address the complexity of breastfeeding as a childcare practice resting not only on the mother but also on her child, partner, family and relatives, and health professionals. It is shaped by the social contexts in which breastfeeding is performed. Not only is this individual-based paradigm ineffective, but it also has the effect of heightening women's feeling of guilt and failure as well as gendered parental responsibilities.

Parents, alongside their midwife and their baby, are collectively building a "negotiated breastfeeding". This co-production of meanings evolves as the child is growing, confronting parents with different challenges and raising questions along the way, regarding the management of health risks, construction of the lactating body, or communication with the child. Tensions and conflicts may appear between the different protagonists—parents and midwife, parents and baby, or between parents—producing diverging meanings around breastfeeding practices. My research analyses the ways in which meanings are produced through interactions, highlighting tensions and negotiations. Moreover, negotiations also take place between parents and the holistic care script, including their breastfeeding project, because their expectations do not always comply with their everyday life requirements.

To support my analyses, I based my ethnographic material on a close follow-up of each family. I had the opportunity to observe routine, ordinary practices and discussions during the postpartum consultations, as well as the handling of specific problems and the underlying negotiations between midwives and parents. The design of my study allowed me to revisit these events with parents and, to a lesser extent, with midwives. I spent time with some of the midwives for the entire duration of my fieldwork, and I continued meeting some of them after I stopped attending their consultations. Similarly, I followed families for up to two years. It enabled me to confront discourses and practices as well as produce in-depth, contextualised material for a long-term understanding of breastfeeding experiences. This favoured the development of reflexivity for parents, who would take a step back from the immediate postpartum period and their initial breastfeeding project.

Following individual breastfeeding journeys, my research highlights the continuity—and in some cases the ruptures—of holistic care, from an out-of-hospital birth project to postpartum follow-ups, and the way it is experienced by parents, including breastfeeding initiation as well as breast-feeding practices in the long term. If most parents I met had established a breastfeeding project, they were unequally equipped to achieve it with regard to their parental leave, work organisation, the presence or absence of other children, or support received from relatives. The "fetishization of the will" tends to overshadow these structural socio-economic constraints (Ruhl 2002: 651). The informed choice ideal reduces to the individual-level decisions regarding childcare and parenting practices. However, I did not notice a significant social homogeneity among my interlocutors, who do not reflect the home birth parents' ideal type as described by other researchers: white, middle-class, urban, and with a higher education (Gouilhers-Hertig 2017; Hildingsson et al. 2006; Jacques 2007; Perrenoud 2016; Pruvost 2016; Quagliariello 2017b; Viisainen 2001).

Interestingly, fellow social science researchers have often questioned the socio-economic background of the home birth parents I met, expecting priv-ileged socio-economic categories. My research population was significantly heterogeneous regarding their socio-economic status and cultural affilia-tions. All of them were nevertheless well integrated into the local popula-tion, and in each family, at least one parent had mastered French, enabling easy access to information regarding the model of care they chose and, more broadly, to local health systems. My discussions with midwives on this topic confirmed that they regularly attend births with families who contrast with the usual portrait of home birth parents. In comparison with other studies in Switzerland and in Europe on out-of-hospital birth, my fieldwork in the canton of Vaud presented a great diversity between city and countryside res-idents, possibly explaining this heterogeneous population, which seems to be a special feature of my research. I also believe that information regarding holistic care tends to become more widely accessible, leading to a democra-tisation of this modality of care. However, the condition that at least one of the parents has to master French excludes some of the most disadvantaged populations—for example, immigrant allophone people. More than a third of the parents I met were foreigners but mainly from European countries. They were already living and working in Switzerland for at least a few years and were familiar with the local health system.

In addition, all the couples I met were heterosexual. Based on my obser-vations, if the holistic care model is heteronormative, it is merely a reflection of the Swiss perinatal landscape and, more broadly, of the Swiss political cli-mate. I rather believe that the holistic care model, due to the continuity and individualisation of care, is potentially more inclusive than the dominant technocratic one. In Switzerland, in 2020, most biomedical informative material is still markedly heterocentric. In contrast, in holistic care, no graphic-containing leaflets or other paper information are distributed, which might also feel more inclusive. Overall, the access and experience of holistic care and of out-of-hospital birth in general by lesbian couples remain to be addressed in Switzerland and in other countries.

Breastfeeding and risk management

My fieldwork unfolded in a context where breastfeeding was identified as the most appropriate infant-feeding mode by public health agencies as well as nutrition and child health experts. Its promotion has increasingly become an important public health concern, arousing feelings of failure and guilt for some women who do not meet the officially recommended terms and durations. Breastfeeding promotion discourses base their argumentation on risk, presenting in a mirror effect the health benefits attributed to breastfeeding and the threats constituted by formula feeding. The underlying project aims at the emergence of a "healthy body and mind" society—since breastfeeding is also supposed to prevent social issues by favouring an optimal psycho-emotional development of children. Based on a biopolitics logic, the goal of public health campaigns is to produce qualitatively optimised citizens. Breastfeeding practices are part of a "delegated biopolitics" (Memmi 2004): women are thought to be responsible for the achievement of breastfeeding objectives, in compliance with public health agencies' guidelines. Independent midwives bridge the "intermediate space of social and political regulation between the state and social practices" and take on the role of transmitting public health messages to families (Fassin & Memmi 2004: 24). As part of a holistic care philosophy, the moral injunction to breastfeed is even more heavily felt by mothers. As a result, some of them experienced "early" weaning as a transgression of the model of care they favoured. Jeopardising their "reflexive project", this deviation from the planned script required some adjustment to create a new, coherent sense of self (Giddens 1991).

Paradoxically, the biomedical authoritative knowledge underlying breastfeeding promotion is challenged by the institutional standards of infants' weight gain measurement. The holistic care model constitutes a privileged observatory of the negotiations between these competitive knowledge standards, alternatively embodied by midwives and parents. These antagonistic postures also coexist in the decisions and practices of each individual midwife, imbued with risk culture, as well as with past hospital experiences and knowledge.

The midwifery training takes place within the biomedical model. Holistic care falls within the biomedical system, and even the most critical independent midwives master biomedical protocols and rely upon them to a greater or lesser extent, depending on the requirements of each follow-up. Tensions between their holistic care ideals and their biomedical background and reference framework are omnipresent in midwives' follow-up. They incorporate these tensions into their practice, which eventually integrate the holistic care model. For example, in the case of a baby's failure to thrive, midwives rely on daily weighing, overcoming their reluctance to introduce a hospital protocol at home. In this way, midwives become experts at juggling principles of holistic care and requirements of the biomedical model. This interpenetration of the two models is also precisely what ensures the durability of the holistic care model: while midwives are taking liberties with hospital protocols, they also master how to conform to a biomedical approach of risk management when necessary.

Similarly, while parents primarily turn to complementary medicine and "natural" remedies, they also rely on biomedicine for their child's care or health monitoring. In the context of medical pluralism, characteristic of the Swiss healthcare and perinatal landscape, parents do not perceive contradictions in combining the biomedicine and holistic care approaches. This weaving of both care approaches is a key reason for choosing their midwife, situated at a pivotal point between them.

My research shows the dominance of the notion of risk in the holistic care practice, structuring the experience of breastfeeding initiation. It appears to me that, in circles that are most critical regarding a risk-based management of birth and childcare, risk remains an important criterion in decision-making processes and practices: an "inversed" relation to risk takes shape, as the hospital is perceived by home birth parents as a source of iatrogenic risk, potentially hindering breastfeeding initiation. My observations, like those of Gouilhers-Hertig (2017), highlight that the risk as an interpretative framework of birth spreads from hospital to home and from delivery to postpartum. This spread is two-dimensional. First, biomedical norms and recommendations, including the imperative to breastfeed, are internalised by midwives and parents. Second, by anticipative measures, giving birth out of the hospital is perceived by parents and midwives as a way to bypass the risks, which are perceived as institution related.

In parallel, holistic care redistributes knowledge hierarchy by valuing experiential knowledge and recognising the validity of emotion-based management of risks. Midwives endeavour to support parenting practices defined as "risky" from a biomedical perspective, such as bed-sharing or non-vaccination, and challenge institutional protocols like daily weighing in order to preserve breastfeeding. In this configuration, paediatricians occupy a secondary position, although their intervention in the children's health follow-up is not questioned: they act as children's protectors against rare and severe risks that could jeopardise their health. Unlike risks induced by weight loss or premature weaning, these types of risks remain abstract and invisible, and parents think of them as undetectable by laypeople and irreversible. These risks are in this way perceived similarly to risks occurring during childbirth, constructed as a "fateful moment" (Scamell & Alaszewski 2012).

In the long term, the prolongation of breastfeeding beyond the maternity leave is thought by parents as a means to maintain a protective hold on their children, breastfeeding acting as a "natural vaccine", in line with a central focus on the immune system in the conception of children (Brownlie & Sheach Leith 2011; Lupton 2013a). Moreover, the continuation of breast-feeding, despite physical separation between mothers and infants during the day, is perceived as protection against emotional risks, creating a reassuring bubble around children. Breastfeeding therefore acts as an extension of family bonds, which alleviates the hazards of the outside world (Faircloth 2013).

While breastfeeding is readily perceived as a "natural vaccine", parents together with midwives are very critical in regard to vaccination. Based on my observations, it is also a topic about which parents are very actively seeking information in an attempt to build their own opinion and make an "informed" choice. In the past ten years, non-vaccination has become a hot topic, raising major controversies and alarming public health agencies in most Euro-American countries, including Switzerland (see for example Boseley 2019). As non-vaccination was not my principal focus, I mainly approached it in relation to breastfeeding and as a background feature of the holistic care model. Although this topic remained peripheral from my perspective, it constantly came back in parents' and midwives' discourses and definitely deserves further investigation from social scientists.

Lactating bodies and interembodiment

Memmi (2014) suggests that when facing birth medicalisation and tech-nologisation, women and parents refocus on their corporal experience and sensations: their "mindful body", as described by Scheper-Hughes and Lock (1987). Holistic care and home birth are characteristic expressions of this "revenge of the flesh" (Memmi 2014). After birth, breastfeeding, combined with other body-based parenting practices, is believed to foster attachment between babies and parents. Attachment bonds are forged through the body, which constitutes the support of parental identity. By breastfeeding, mothers share their bodies with their baby. Reciprocally, the baby's body is perceived by parents as "a site of relationality" (Brownlie & Sheach Leith 2011: 202), where identities merge and are reinvented. "Skinship" is created by way of body-based parenting practices (Tahhan 2008, 2010), to which breastfeeding is central. In midwives' discourses, newborns would acquire self-consciousness by means of their bodies and, in particular, through their physiological needs and the way parents address them. In parallel, parents would also develop a new perception of themselves, reshaped by these bod-ily interactions. There is no determinist relation between body and identity, but the body becomes a "necessary support" for the expression of identity (Memmi 2014: 227). According to this perspective, as part of the holistic care "lifestyle" (Giddens 1991), body practices "make" parents, whereas breastfeeding, through the body work deployed to achieve it, "makes" mothers.

As a locus of biopower, women's lactating bodies are submitted to medical surveillance, pushing them to use specific techniques and tools to execute their breastfeeding project. This biopower extends to infants, whose bodies are also measured and regulated through different interventions (weighing, positioning, cutting a tongue-tie). Sachs (2005) noticed on her hospital fieldwork a lack of body techniques to improve the milk transfer between mothers and babies, with hospital staff mainly proposing to express breast milk in order to give it to infants with a bottle or supplementing them with formula milk, in an attempt to objectify the milk quantity absorbed. On the contrary, I observed a multitude of body techniques to optimise the breastfeeding process: repositioning the child or the mother, applying pressure on the breast, increasing lactation with galactogenic foods and drinks, incorporating additional feeds, or using a supplemental nursing system. The emphasis put on these body techniques, instead of resorting to tools, such as a breast pump, or to industrial products, such as formula, is in line with the midwives' moderate use of technologies during pregnancy and at the time of delivery. Nevertheless, the underlying project of production of the lactating body refers to the technocratic model, as women's bodies are the subject of a heavy management and the lactation process is not left to chance. The midwives' discourse, relating to an industrial rhetoric to talk about breastfeeding (for example, the milk "production"), reflects this productivist perspective.

To sustain their lactating body and nurture their breastfeeding relationship with their child, mothers engage in significant body and emotional work, sometimes regardless of their feelings (pain, soreness) or affects (disgust, tiredness, rejection). While this testimony of self-denial and self-discipline is part of a "delegated biopolitics" (Memmi 2004: 137), it also reflects an ideological vision of motherhood. In the era of "intensive motherhood", women are expected to comply with strong expectations regarding their parenting practices, requiring adjustments to ensure their child an optimal physical and psycho-emotional development. As part of a "parental determinism", parenting choices must be evaluated in the light of child health experts' recommendations.

By adopting "child-centred" practices, parents aim to enhance their child's singular personhood from birth, in line with a neoliberal conception of the self as a fundamental value. Our contemporary regime of the autonomous self is based on a psychological definition of the individual as a territory of self-realisation and self-development (Rose 1998). Psychosciences and disciplines have thus importantly reshaped professional practices of "those who exercise authority over others: social workers, managers, teachers, nurses—such that they nurture and direct these individual strivings in the most appropriate and productive fashions" (ibid. 1998: 17). As part of the professional categories defined by Rose, independent midwives practising holistic care contribute to the production of new regimes of the self, based on attachment parenting practices. These body-based practices both challenge and reproduce the model of the autonomous self. As they require constant physical closeness between babies and parents, practices such as on-demand breastfeeding, bed-sharing, child wearing, or elimination communication often surprise and upset supporters of the dominant autonomist childcare practices among the home birth parents' relatives. As a result, subscribers to holistic practices frequently feel stigmatised by their parenting style and are reluctant to share their experiences.

Moreover, inscribed in the legacy of the hygienist model, dominant educational practices condemn attachment parenting practices, out of fear of producing an overly dependent child. At the same time, parents practising elimination communication are perceived as enslaved both to their child and to the parenting style they have chosen. Yet, in the long term, they share the same value of self-sufficiency as the final education goal: the specificity of the parenting model I observed lies in the path taken to reach autonomy but does not fundamentally question the legitimacy of this value.

In holistic care, midwives, as part of a child-centred approach, inscribe babies as full-fledged social actors in their postpartum follow-up, working towards "anthropomorphizing" them (Scheper-Hughes 1992). In an effort to enhance their individualities, midwives act as babies' spokeswomen, translating their gestures positively into communication attempts or skills. Through their lens, newborns would "show" that they enjoy being at the breast or would address a "real" smile to their caregivers. However, this child-centred approach reaches its limit when the baby's behaviour does not comply with the midwife's agenda. For example, babies are woken up if they are asleep when the midwife wants to weigh them, or they will bear a massage at a time when they are obviously not enjoying it.

At the beginning of my fieldwork, in order to embrace an emic perspective on the babies I met and to respond to Gottlieb's (2000) invitation to an "anthropology of infants", I had the intention to integrate babies as full-fledged actors of my ethnography. However, I quickly realised that it was an ambitious goal. Babies, especially newborns, were most often asleep, suckling at their mother's breast or enduring an action conducted on them by their midwife or parents: diaper changing, bathing, or medical interventions such as a Guthrie test. The range of their actions was restrained, and for a layperson like me—neither a parent nor a birth professional—it was challenging to notice and interpret the subtleties of each child's behaviour and gestures. If I made an effort to integrate newborns in my ethnographic descriptions (the space they occupy, their activity, or their attitude), I did not directly address how they were acting but rather by whom, in which manner, and with what intention they were acted on. As a result, my research does not directly contribute to an "anthropology of infants" but rather to an anthropology of their caretakers (Gottlieb 2000).

Time to breastfeed

As an "intensified" approach to parenthood, the parenting style I observed involves time-consuming parenting practices, of which on-demand breast-feeding and long-term breastfeeding are a significant part. In order to achieve their breastfeeding project, parents have to reframe their relationship to time, reduce time spent apart from their child to a greater or lesser extent, and optimise family time, for example, by extending it through co-sleeping. In comparison with the dominant Euro-American educational model, home birth parents stand out by the time allotted in the first months and years after birth to transitionally lead their child to autonomy. This time is therefore conceptualised as an investment in the future: by building "secure emotional foundations" for their infants through on-demand, long-term breastfeeding and other child-centred practices, they ensure long-lasting benefits (Faircloth 2013: 68). Their altered relationship to time is justified by a higher interest than the contingencies of daily life. Therefore, parents agree to surrender their time and efforts to a demanding childcare approach. Coupled with this self-denial, they proceed to structural and work arrangements to devote as much of themselves as possible to their parenting role, their child becoming a life project in her- or himself.

More specifically, on-demand breastfeeding requires a shift in the parents' relationship to time, towards a more flexible and expansive time conception. This reconceptualisation of time and daily routines corresponds to a state of liminality, experienced by all parents during the postnatal period, and strongly accentuated by breastfeeding, as a prolongation of body sharing between mothers and babies (Sachs 2005). The liminality maintained throughout the breastfeeding period as a transitory stage also concerns children. They are "moving from two-in-one to a highly dependent existence" as breastfed babies, before eventually becoming autonomous selves (ibid. 2005b: 178).

Greenhouse (1995) proposed a definition of time as a cultural formulation of agency—the ability of individuals to act—and the compatibility or incompatibility of that agency with specific institutional forms (in Bartlett 2010b). According to Bartlett (2010b), in this perspective, breastfeeding and maternity generally become "a radical alternative to standard life trajectories which revolve around transitions from school to work to retirement" (126). The very concept of "maternity leave" would circumscribe maternity as a "liminal, temporary and transitory" period (ibid. 2010b: 127). Motherhood concentrates tensions between women and work, and breastfeeding seems to exacerbate these tensions: breastfeeding time does not match institutional and economic time, and it radically subverts these dominant models based on the notion of temporal linearity.

Dykes' ethnographic work showed that women's breastfeeding initiation in a hospital setting is deeply shaped by linear time (2006):

Breastfeeding was then experienced as time-consuming, and impeding, or potentially impeding, more pressing calls upon their time. The sense of urgency in relation to time was powerfully reinforced by the ways in which midwives communicated their own time pressures to women. This required women to compete for time in order to protect themselves from time "going" elsewhere. (Dykes 2006: 170)

In this context, women's time conception is framed, on the one hand, by pressures associated with linear time: fears and projection in the future, requiring a rational and efficient management of present time. On the other hand, the institutional organisation of midwives' work fosters a feeling of competition among mothers to capture midwives' time and attention.

Embracing the "maialogical time" of breastfeeding, the parents I met had reconceptualised their relationship to time, as well as their everyday organisation (Kahn 1989). Nevertheless, parents' understanding of on-demand breastfeeding widened as it extended over time, so negotiations would take place between mothers and children, leading to compromises regarding the rhythm of feedings. As communication became more elaborate, the child was perceived as a partner, with whom the schedule of feedings had to be bargained. These observations are also in line with the shift in health policies to the notion of "responsive feeding", emphasising a conception of breastfeeding as a relational process based on mutual responsiveness between the mother and child (Aryeetey & Dykes 2018; Dykes & Flacking 2010).

Reciprocally, the temporalities of the holistic care offered by independent midwives also contrast with the institutional time. As midwives adopt an "expansive" understanding of time (Simonds 2002), time devoted to each family mainly depends on the demands of their specific situation and not on a strict, pre-established schedule. Parents do not have to compete for their midwife's time, as she is uniquely focusing on one family at a time. These circumstances favour the development of an "authentic presence" by midwives, described by Schmied, Beake, Sheehan et al. (2011) as an empathetic, person-centred approach, enabling feelings of connectedness between midwives and parents. The exclusive attention of their midwife promote parents' satisfaction and allows them and their midwife freedom to digress and chat, increasing the pleasure of meeting on both sides.

More broadly and in the long term, breastfeeding temporalities concentrate on women's struggles with contradictory injunctions. On the one side, women feel morally obliged to breastfeed, which is in line with public health policies. On the other side, they feel social disapproval if they breastfeed "too often" or "too long", disrupting the ordinary time allowed to dive into the blur of "babydaze" (Bartlett 2010b: 121).

Gender regimes and breastfeeding

The ability to breastfeed is inscribed in women's bodies, and mothers often take full responsibility for achieving it. However, in the marginal model of care I observed in my fieldwork, most fathers fully embraced the breastfeeding project, and a large majority of them engaged in all aspects of childcare to sustain it, thereby redistributing and "undoing" traditional gendered patterns (Deutsch 2007). My observations thus differ from those of Bobel (2002), who highlighted, based on her study on "natural" mothers, the reproduction mechanisms of the gender system and inequalities, manifested in a biologically determined division of labour between parents. However, unequal fathers' participation might have filtered out those most attached to traditional gender roles. The fathers most committed to breastfeeding were perhaps also the most interested in my research and more likely to meet with me. On the contrary, I could only appreciate the involvement of the fathers I did not have the chance to meet on the basis of their spouse's discourse.

An ethnography among lesbian parental couples where both parents would endeavour to breastfeed would be illuminating to explore the influence of breastfeeding practices on gender parental roles and on the sharing of parental tasks and responsibilities.[1] Another interesting perspective on these issues could be gained among men "chestfeeding" by means of hormonal supplementation and mechanical stimulation. Marie-Claire Springham, then an English student in design, developed a "chestfeeding kit", intended to ease lactation induction by expecting fathers (Pochin 2018). The creation of this kit has been reported by local tabloids and social media, raising passionate debates. As I occasionally observed in my fieldwork, when the topic of fathers' chestfeeding was mentioned, the idea often aroused hilarity, or even disgust, evoking a gender transgression. During conversations with midwives, I also incidentally had the opportunity to ask some of them about their opinions on men chestfeeding. I was surprised by the vigorous indignation of one of them, Mireille, who argued that it would be dispossession of women and that men's lifestyle (poor diet choices, alcohol consumption, and smoking habits) would be prejudicial for babies. These strong prejudices reflect her difficulties in challenging traditional roles, symptomatic of an acceptance of social and parental roles as a direct result of body design (Bobel 2002).

Based on my observations, most of the time, fathers' high degree of involvement in childcare was not reflected in midwives' discourses. Midwives primarily focused on the mother and child duo, especially regarding breastfeeding and the underlying injunction of maternal "availability" to honour the baby's demand. Midwives' difficulty in detaching themselves from a matricentric approach clashes with the natural childbirth ideal, which emphasises the importance of spouses' support and involvement in the birth project. It also opposes the well-defined role of partners during delivery outside the hospital, usually revolving around specific massages and technical gestures taught by the midwife. On this occasion, fathers are acting as midwives' partners, unlike in the situation of a hospital delivery, in which fathers report feelings of helplessness and oddness (Reed 2005, Truc 2006).

The fathers' role during the postpartum period, especially regarding breastfeeding, was not the subject of a similar elaboration by midwives. Because of a then inexistent paternity leave in Switzerland, midwives were perhaps not used to relying on the fathers' presence during their follow-up. More broadly, midwives' matricentric approach reflects the gender system in Switzerland, which favours women's part-time employment and primary responsibility for infants' care. Therefore, I believe that midwives' heterocentric or sexist discourses are produced by the Swiss cultural context. Despite a commitment to provide an individualised and contextualised care, midwives' discourses often express gender stereotypes, as they are influenced by Swiss family policies favouring a traditionalist vision of gendered parental roles, in line with the male breadwinner/female carer schema.

In addition, midwives rely on biological determinism and hormone-based discourses to bolster mothers' confidence in their breastfeeding skills and, in general, reinforce their sense of competence during the postpartum period. The notion of "breastfeeding hormones" was frequently used to reassure mothers regarding their ability to breastfeed or, more broadly, provide adequately to their child. For example, "breastfeeding hormones" would ensure an efficient let-down reflex but also a state of alertness to prevent harming the baby while bed-sharing. In this way, midwives favoured a vision of parenting based on body design.

In their discourses, parents seemed to accept midwives' explanations and were not questioning their hormone-based approach. However, fathers' implication regarding breastfeeding challenged this conception, to varying degrees from a traditional role of protector of the family's interests and well-being, including breastfeeding, to forming a "breastfeeding team" with their spouse. The first posture of breastfeeding protector fits into traditional gender expectations, except when it comes to emotional and structural support—that is, taking charge of all the domestic chores or other aspects of infants' care. The second posture, implying hands-on lactation care and breastfeeding support, suggests a process of "undoing" gender (Deutsch 2007), as parents were working towards sharing even the most biological functions of parenting. Defying the hormone-based discourse, these fathers were not "helping" their spouse but were equally involved in each aspect of their child's care. Addressing all requirements to sustain breastfeeding, some fathers I met suggested that motherhood "intensification" extends to men, subverting traditional gendered norms.

Breastfeeding can be interpreted both as a gender performance, in line with moral expectations regarding maternal commitment to conform with public health recommendations, and as a gender transgression, as breastfeeding women are performing gender in a way that also subverts the gendered norm of women's body as available for sexuality. The relationship of gender and sexuality with breastfeeding, especially night-time breastfeeding and bed-sharing or long-term breastfeeding, remains little addressed. In the course of my research, it was mostly raised implicitly and in a peripheral way by my interlocutors. I was probably too concerned about respecting their intimacy to openly approach these topics with each of them, so only a few of my interlocutors spontaneously confided about it. There is a strong cultural ambivalence regarding breastfeeding promotion in a Euro-American cultural context, identifying breasts as primarily sexual. As women's sexual and maternal "functions" are thought of as incompatible (Stearns 1999), the injunction to breastfeed diverges from directives addressed to women on "getting their bodies back" after giving birth. Having internalised the ideal of female bodies virtually unchanged by the birth process, women often feel uncomfortable with their postpartum bodies (Fox & Neiterman 2015). Interestingly, the argument that breastfeeding would favour weight loss is precisely used by breastfeeding promotors (Avishai 2004, Blum 1999, Breastfeeding Promotion Switzerland 2017b). Moreover, the body is the means of motherhood, and mothers who no longer provide their child with their body after delivery—for example, by bottle-feeding—are deemed morally inferior.

At the same time, because women's lack of sexual desire during the postpartum period is thought of as a social problem requiring medical care, women feel the urge to quickly resume sexual intercourse after giving birth (Hirt 2005). However, most of my interlocutors reported a feeling of dispossession of their own body while breastfeeding because their bodies worked hard to provide for their babies' needs. Breastfeeding affects both the appearance and the physiology of the breast, and sexual arousal can trigger the let-down reflex. In this perspective, breastfeeding is often considered as an impediment to sexuality. These considerations reflect the heteronormative order, exhorting women that breasts must remain their male partner's prerogative.

Holistically caring

While Dykes's (2006) study challenged the suitability of the hospital institution to initiate breastfeeding, my fieldwork showed that breastfeeding initiation at home, with independent midwives providing one-on-one care, is reported as an efficient form of postpartum follow-up by its protagonists. Parents globally express a strong satisfaction regarding the care they received, and most of them highlight the crucial contribution of their midwife in their breastfeeding project. In the long term, and based on my observations and discussions with midwives, home birth children are breastfed for a much longer time than the Swiss average breastfeeding duration. In 2014, the Swiss average duration of exclusive breastfeeding was 12 weeks, whereas the total median duration of breastfeeding was 31 weeks (Dratva et al. 2014). More than a third of the babies in my fieldwork were exclusively breastfed for six months, while another third were breastfed exclusively for five months. The total duration of breastfeeding (with the addition of other food and liquid intake) was a year or more for half of the infants.

Parents' commitment to their breastfeeding project, combined with the holistic care provided by midwives, appeared to facilitate their observance of the WHO recommendations. Some of them actually reached the gold standard of six months of exclusive breastfeeding and the continuation of breastfeeding until two years of age or beyond but often with a high emotional and physical cost. The prolongation of breastfeeding to achieve child-led weaning, regardless of their own feelings and affects, even seemed traumatic for some women.

Interestingly, breastfeeding was mostly approached in a dogmatic way in my fieldwork. No midwife ever advised resorting to formula feeding in combination with breastfeeding to sustain it in the long term—and not as a temporary crutch in the case of a baby's failure to thrive. Some mothers explained that they had to supplement their breast milk supply with formula, sometimes for months or even years before weaning. In these cases, this topic remained unaddressed in the presence of their midwife. This can, however, be explained in part by the fact that the formula introduction usually occurred after the mother had resumed work and the midwife's follow-up had ended.

The specificities of the holistic care model—the continuity of care, associated with an expansive conception of time—promote a contextualised knowledge of each family by midwives, which favours the development of a trust relationship between parents and midwives and the exercise of an informed choice. This trust relationship also allows parents to question their midwife's recommendations. Highly committed from birth, parents are usually well versed in breastfeeding and do not always consider their midwife as the most reliable resource, especially if her advice feels inconsistent with their knowledge. As a result, all decisions taken during the postpartum period, including risk management, are constantly discussed and negotiated between midwives and parents.

Moreover, the space in which midwives' postpartum consultations takes place—the parents' home—participates in balancing power relations between parents and midwives. In the maternity ward, midwives are on their territory and parents are "guests", obliged to follow institutional rules. Quite the contrary, at the parents' home, midwives are "guests", respecting the household rules. They have to adjust to the parents' environment and not the other way around. For example, if during a visit a midwife needs equipment that she does not carry with her, she must ask her clients for it. Similarly, she has to reinvent how to perform a newborn clinical examination, depending on the house setting: searching for the best natural light to observe a baby's colouring or achieving a Guthrie test on a couch using a diaper filled with hot water to warm the baby's foot in order to improve blood flow. This constant adjustment required by the independent practice fosters a feeling of deference, as midwives are operating in an ever-changing work environment, positioning themselves as continuously learning, echoing the position of parents with their newborn. Nevertheless, power relationships, if not as manifest as in the dominant institutional model, are not absent from the holistic model of care, as midwives sooner or later impose limits to parents regarding risk management (see also Gouilhers-Hertig 2017).

Furthermore, midwives sometimes shift from an informative to a prescriptive attitude, at least from the parents' perspective, who, in turn, attribute expectations to their midwife regarding their parenting practices. The holistic model of care is underpinned by the ideal values of self-determination and informed choice. As pointed out by Malacrida and Boulton (2014), these well-intentioned values can translate into normative injunctions for parents embracing this model of care. Furthermore, values and expectations showing through midwives' discourses are at odds with the centrality of informed choice in the holistic care model. Acting as "experts of conduct", midwives favour a "counter-expertise", positioning themselves in critical opposition to the dominant highly medicalised birthing culture, while also accentuating women's accountability over their birth and postpartum choices (McCabe 2016). In this perspective, McCabe regretted that "neoliberal consumer logics that center choice, autonomy and empowerment become the means by which midwives and birth workers distinguish themselves from more medicalized obstetrical practices" (2016: 182). Furthermore, due to their close relationship, parents, particularly mothers, sometimes feel responsible for not disappointing their midwife, fostering a feeling of transgression in cases wherein they do not comply with the parenting model she represents.

Unlike childbirth, the postpartum period stretches over several weeks and is not perceived as a "fateful moment" (Scamell & Alaszewski 2012). This extended time allows decision processes to mature in a participative way. In addition, midwives' support does not end once the postpartum follow-up is over, and most of them remain available for parents should they encounter difficulties or questions—for example, their child's first disease or her or his adjustment to day care. While supporting them during decision-making processes, midwives make an effort to respect parents' rhythm of thinking—that is, they "walk with them as long as it takes", as described by Odile. The holistic care practices I observed were part of a "logic of care" where tasks are shared between midwives and parents, anchored in day-to-day life (Mol 2009).

In this way, midwives and parents collectively reinvent postpartum care based on an in-depth, contextualised knowledge of each other and shared healthcare and parenting values. However, tensions and conflicts emerge along the way, as power relationships inevitably infuse the holistic care model, while midwives engage with parents in a co-construction of meaning regarding risk, management of the lactating body, or interpretation of the child's behaviour. Through this production of meanings, which are not always shared, they are building together, at each step of the process, a negotiated breastfeeding.

Note

1 Mechanical stimulation is in principle sufficient to induce lactation in a woman who has not given birth, without hormonal support. For a description of this process, see, for example, the documentary *Breastmilk*, directed by Dana Ben-Ari, which followed the co-nursing experience of a lesbian parental couple (2014).

Bibliography

Adam Barbara. 1992. "Time and Health Implicated: A Conceptual Critique". In Frankenberg Ronald (ed.), *Time, Health and Medicine*. London: Sage, 153–164

Akrich Madeleine & Pasveer Bernike. 1996. *Comment la naissance vient aux femmes? Les techniques d'accouchement en France et aux Pays-Bas*. Paris: Les empêcheurs de tourner en rond.

Apple Rima D. 1987. *Mothers and Medicine. A Social History of Infant Feeding 1890–1950*. London: The University of Wisconsin Press.

Apple Rima D. 2014. "Medicalization of Motherhood. Modernization and Resistance in an International Context". *Journal of the Motherhood Initiative for Research and Community Involvement* 5 (1), 115–126.

Armstrong David. 1995. "The Rise of Medicine Surveillance". *Sociology of Health and Illness* 17 (3), 393–405.

Aryeetey Richmond & Dykes Fiona. 2018. "Global Implications of the New WHO and UNICEF Implementation Guidance on the Revised Baby-Friendly Hospital Initiative". *Maternal & Child Nutrition* 14 (3), e12637.

Avanza Martina. 2008. "Comment faire de l'ethnographie quand on n'aime pas «ses indigènes»? Une enquête au sein d'un mouvement xénophobe". In Fassin Didier & Bensa Alban (eds.), *Les politiques de l'enquête. Épreuves ethnographiques*. Paris: La Découverte, 41–58.

Avishai Orit. 2004. "At the Pump". *Journal of the Association for Research on Mothering* 6 (2), 138–149.

Avishai Orit. 2007. "Managing the Lactating Body: The Breast-Feeding Project and Privileged Motherhood". *Qualitative Sociology* 30 (2), 135–152.

Avishai Orit. 2011. "Managing the Lactating Body: The Breastfeeding Project in the Age of Anxiety". In Liamputtong Pranee (ed.), *Infant Feeding Practices. A Cross-Cultural Perspective*. New York: Springer, 23–38.

Badinter Elisabeth. 1980. *L'amour en plus. Histoire de l'instinct maternel XVIIe – XXe siècle*. Paris: Flammarion.

Badinter Elisabeth. 2010. *Le conflit. La femme et la mère*. Paris: Flammarion.

Ballif Edmée. 2017. *Du temps pour parler. Le gouvernement des grossesses dans le canton de Vaud (Suisse)*. Thèse de doctorat en sciences sociales, Université de Lausanne.

Ballif Edmée. 2020. "Policing the maternal mind: Maternal health, psychological government and Swiss pregnancy politics". *Social Politics* 27(1), 74–96.

Balsamo Franca, De Mari Gisella, Maher Vanessa & Serini Rosalba. 1992. "Production and Pleasure: Research on Breast-Feeding in Turin". In Maher Vanessa (ed.), *The Anthropology of Breast-Feeding: Natural Law or Social Construct*. New York: Berg, 59–90.

Bartlett Alison. 2005. *Breastwork*. Sydney: UNSW Press.

Bartlett Alison. 2010a. "Breastfeeding and Time. In Search of a Language of Pleasure and Agency". In Shaw Rhonda & Bartlett Alison (eds.), *Giving Breastmilk. Body Ethics and Contemporary Breastfeeding Practices*. Toronto: Demeter Press, 222–235.

Bartlett Alison. 2010b. "Babydaze: Maternal Time". *Time & Society* 19, 120–132.

Bauer Ingrid. 2001. *Diaper Free ! The Gentle Wisdom of Natural Infant Hygiene*. Salt Spring Island: Natural Wisdom Press.

Beaud Stéphane & Weber Florence. 1997. Guide de l'enquête de terrain. Paris: La découverte.

Beck Ulrich. 1992. *Risk Society*. Thousand Oaks: Sage.

Becker Howard S. 1963. *Outsiders. Étude de sociologie de la déviance*. Paris: Métailié.

Ben-Ari Dana (Director). 2014. *Breastmilk* [film]. Cavu Pictures.

Bensa Alban. 2006. *La fin de l'exotisme: Essais d'anthropologie critique*. Paris: Anacharsis.

Bensa Alban. 2008. "Conclusion. Remarques sur les politiques de l'intersubjectivité". In Fassin Didier & Memmi Dominique (eds.), *Le gouvernement des corps*. Paris: Éditions de l'École des hautes études en sciences sociales, 323–328.

Blaffer Hrdy Sarah. 2000. *Mother Nature. Maternal Instinct and the Shaping of the Species*. London: Vintage.

Bläuer Herrmann Anouk & Murier Thierry. 2016. *Les mères sur le marché du travail*. Neuchâtel: Office Fédéral de la Statistique. Available at: https://www.bfs .admin.ch/bfsstatic/dam/assets/1061096/master. Accessed: 14.03.2019.

Bloch Maurice & Bloch Jean H. 1980. "Women and the Dialectics of Nature in Eighteen-Century French Thought". In Maccormack Carol & Strathern Marilyn (eds.), *Nature, Culture and Gender*. Cambridge: Cambridge University Press, 25–41.

Blum Linda M. 1999. *At the Breast. Ideologies of Breastfeeding and Motherhood in the Contemporary United States*. Boston: Beacon Press.

Bobel Chris. 2002. *The Paradox of Natural Mothering*. Philadelphia: Temple University Press.

Boltanski Luc. 1977. *Prime éducation et morale de classe*. Paris: Mouton.

Boltanski Luc. 2004. *La condition fœtale. Une sociologie de l'engendrement et de l'avortement*. Paris: Gallimard.

Bolzman Claudio. 2002. "La politique migratoire en Suisse. Entre contrôle et intégration". *Écarts d'identité* 99, 65–71.

Bonapace Julie. 2016. *Trusting Birth with the Bonapace Method: Keys to Loving Your Birth Experience*. Montreal: Juniper Publishing.

Bonnet Doris & Pourchez Laurence. 2007. *Du soin au rite dans l'enfance*. Toulouse: Erès.

Borel Bernard, Burkhalter Anne, Fioretta Gérald, Midwives "Aquila" & Fasnart Bernard. 2010. "L'accouchement en maison de naissance plus physiologique: 4 fois moins de risques d'y accoucher par césarienne". Available at: http://www .nascerebene.ch/files/1513/4866/5900/Laccouchement_en_maison_de_naissance _plus_physiologique.pdf. Accessed 21.11.2017.

Boseley Sarah. 2019. "Half of New Parents Shown Anti-Vaccine Misinformation on Social Media – Report". *The Guardian*, 24.01.2019. Available at: https://www .theguardian.com/society/2019/jan/24/anti-vaxxers-spread-misinformation-on-s ocial-media-report. Accessed 17.04.2019.

Bosson Alain. 2002. "La lutte contre la mortalité des nourrissons en Suisse: enjeux et mesures de prévention (1876–1930)". *Cahiers d'histoire* 471/2, 93–126.

Boucher Debora, Bennett Catherine, Mcfarlin Barbara & Freeze Rixa. 2009. "Staying Home to Give Birth: Why Women in the United States Choose Home Birth". *Journal of Midwifery & Women's Health* 54 (2), 119–126.

Bourdieu Pierre. 1972. *Esquisse d'une théorie de la pratique.* Genève: Librairie Droz.

Bowlby John. 1969. *Attachment.* New York: Basic Books.

Bozon Michel. 2009. *Sociologie de la sexualité* (2nd ed.). Paris: Armand Colin.

Bradley R. M. & Mistretta C. 1975. "Fetal Sensory Receptors". *Physiological Reviews* 55 (3), 352–382.

Bramwell Ros. 2001. "Blood and Milk: Constructions of Female Bodily Fluids in Western Society". *Women & Health* 34 (4), 85–96.

Breastfeeding Promotion Switzerland. 2015. "Information aux médias, 1er juillet 2015". Available at: http://www.stillfoerderung.ch/logicio/client/stillen/archive/ document/aktuell/MM_Neuer Name_Stillforderungfr.pdf. Accessed 20.11.2017.

Breastfeeding Promotion Switzerland. 2017. *Breastfeeding: A Healthy Start to Life.* Bern: Breastfeeding Promotion Switzerland.

Breastfeeding Promotion Switzerland. 2020. "Films sur l'allaitement". Available at: https://www.stillfoerderung.ch/logicio/pmws/stillen__root_3_4__fr.html. Accessed 14.08.2020.

Bretherton Inge. 1992. "The Origins of Attachment Theory: John Bowlby and Mary Ainsworth". *Developmental Psychology* 28, 759–775.

Broderick Michael L. 2016. "Home Birth: The Wholeness of Absence". *Health Communication* 31 (3), 379–381.

Brosco Jeffrey P. 2001. "Weight Charts and Well-Child Care. How the Paediatrician Became the Expert in Child Health". *Archives of Pediatrics and Adolescent Medicine* 155 (12), 1385–1389.

Brownlie Julie & Sheach Leith Valerie M. 2011. "Social Bundles: Thinking Through the Infant Body". *Childhood* 18 (2), 196–210.

Bühlmann Félix, Elcheroth Guy & Tettamanti Manuel. 2010. "The Division of Labour among European Couples: The Effects of Life Course and Welfare Policy on Value-Practice Configurations". European Sociological Review 26 (1), 49–66.

Burton-Jeangros Claudine, Hammer Raphaël, Manaï Dominique, Issenhuth-Scharly Ghislaine. 2010. "Introduction générale. Droit, médecine et société", in Manaï Dominique, Burton-Jeangros Claudine, Elger Bernice (eds.), *Risques et informations dans le suivi de la grossesse : droit, éthique et pratiques sociales.* Bern: Stämplfi, 9–38.

Buskens Petra. 2010. "The Impossibility of 'Natural Parenting' for Modern Mothers. On Social Structure and the Formation of Habit". *Journal of the Association for Research on Mothering* 3 (1), 75–86.

Butler Judith. 1990. *Gender Trouble. Feminism and the Subversion of Identity.* New York: Routledge.

Butler Judith. 1993. *Bodies that Matter. On the Discursive Limits of "Sex".* New York and London: Routledge.

Butler Judith. 2004. *Undoing Gender.* New York: Routledge.

Campo Monica. 2010. "The Lactating Body and Conflicting Ideals of Sexuality, Motherhood and Self". In Shaw Rhonda & Bartlett Alison (eds.), *Giving Breastmilk. Body Ethics and Contemporary Breastfeeding Practices*. Toronto: Demeter Press, 51–63.

Carpenter Faedra C. 2006. "'(L)activists and Lattes': Breastfeeding Advocacy as Domestic Performance". *Women and Performance: A Journal of Feminist Theory* 16 (3), 347–367.

Carricaburu Danièle. 2007. "De l'incertitude de la naissance au risque obstétrical: l'accouchement en hôpital public". *Sociologie du travail* 47 (2), 123–144.

Carter Pam. 1995. *Feminism, Breasts and Breastfeeding*. London: Macmillan.

Castañeda Angela N. & Searcy Julie, Johnson. 2015. *Doulas and Intimate Labour. Boundaries, Bodies, and Birth*. Bradford: Demeter Press.

Cavalli Samuele & Gouilhers-Hertig Solène. 2014. "Gynécologues-obstétriciens et sages-femmes dans le suivi de la grossesse, une complémentarité sous contrôle médical?". In Burton-Jeangros Claudine, Hammer Raphaël & Maffi Irene (eds.), *Accompagner la naissance. Terrains socio-anthropologiques en Suisse romande*. Lausanne: Giuseppe Merrone Editeur, 85–106.

Charrier Philippe. 2004. "Comment envisage-t-on d'être sage-femme quand on est un homme ? L'intégration professionnelle des étudiants hommes sages-femmes". *Travail, Genre et Sociétés* 12, 105–124.

Charrier Philippe & Clavandier Joëlle. 2013. *Sociologie de la naissance*. Paris: Armand Colin.

Chautems Caroline. 2011. *Accoucher à l'hôpital ou hors de l'hôpital. Regard anthropologique sur les choix de naissance de femmes enceintes en Suisse romande*. Mémoire de Master, Université de Lausanne.

Chautems Caroline. 2019. "'À la demande', mais pas trop souvent. Enjeux temporels et contradictions autour de la notion d'allaitement en Suisse romande". In Herrscher Estelle, & Séguy Isabelle (eds.), *Premiers Cris, Premières Nourritures*. Marseille: Éditions PUP, Collection "Corps et Ames", 41–58.

Chautems Caroline & Guerra Sophie.2021a. "Des outils 'naturels' pour soutenir un processus 'inné': sélection d'aides à l'allaitement de sages-femmes indépendantes vaudoises" In Foehr-Janssens Yasmina, Dasen Véronique, Solfaroli Camillocci Daniela, & Maffi Irene (eds.), *Allaiter. Histoire(s) et cultures d'une pratique*. Bruxelles: Brepols.

Chautems Caroline & Guerra Sophie. 2021b. "Le tire-lait: entre responsabilisation et autonomisation des mères "In Foehr-Janssens Yasmina, Dasen Véronique, Solfaroli Camillocci Daniela, & Maffi Irene (eds.) *Allaiter. Histoire(s) et cultures d'une pratique*. Bruxelles: Brepols.

Cheyney Melissa J. 2008. "Homebirth as Systems-Challenging Praxis: Knowledge, Power, and Intimacy in the Birthplace". *Qualitative Health Research* 18 (2), 254–267.

Cixous Hélène. 1975. "Le rire de la méduse". *L'Arc* 61, 39–54.

Clifford James. 1983. "On Ethnographic Authority". *Representations* 2, 118–146.

Colson Suzanne. 2010. *An Introduction to Biological Nurturing. New Angles on Breastfeeding*. Amarillo: Hale Publishing.

Conklin Beth A. & Morgan Lynn M. 1996. "Babies, Bodies and the Production of Personhood in North America and a Native Amazonian Society". *Ethos* 24 (4), 657–694.

Crouch Mira & Manderson Lenore. 1993. "Parturition as Social Metaphor". *The Australia and New Zealand Journal of Sociology* 29 (1), 55–72.

Crouch Mira & Manderson Lenore. 1995. "The Social Life of Bonding Theory". *Social Science & Medicine* 41 (6), 837–844.

Csordas Thomas J. 1990. "Embodiment as a Paradigm for Anthropology". *Ethos* 18 (1), 5–47.

Csordas Thomas J. 1994. "Introduction: The Body as Representation and Being-in-the-World". In Csordas Thomas J. (ed.), *Embodiment and Experience. The Existential Ground of Culture and Self*. Cambridge: Cambridge University Press, 1–24.

Darmon Muriel. 2003. *Devenir anorexique. Une approche sociologique*. Paris: La Découverte.

Darmon Muriel. 2005. "Le psychiatre, la sociologue et la boulangère: analyse d'un refus de terrain". *Genèses* 1 (58), 98–112.

Davis Kathy. 2007. "Reclaiming Women's Bodies: Colonialist Trope or Critical Epistemology?" *Sociological Review* 55, 50–64.

Davis-Floyd Robbie E. 1992. *Birth as an American Rite of Passage*. Berkeley: University of California Press.

Davis-Floyd Robbie E. & Davis Elizabeth. 1996. "Intuition as Authoritative Knowledge in Midwifery and Homebirth". *Medical Anthropology Quarterly* 10 (2), 237–269.

Davis-Floyd Robbie E. & Sargent Carolyn F. (eds.). 1997. *Childbirth and Authoritative Knowledge: Cross-Cultural Perspectives*. Berkeley: University of California Press.

Davis-Floyd Robbie E. & St. John Gloria. 1998. *From Doctor to Healer. The Transformative Journey*. New Jersey: Rutgers University Press.

Davis-Floyd Robbie E. & Johnson Christine Barbara. 2006. *Mainstreaming Midwives. The Politics of Change*: New York: Routledge.

Davis-Floyd Robbie E., Barclay Lesley, Daviss Betty-Jane & Tritten Jan (eds.). 2009. *Birth Models that Work*. Berkeley and Los Angeles: University of California Press.

Delaisi De Parseval Geneviève & Lallemand Suzanne. 1998. *L'art d'accommoder les bébés*. Paris: Odile Jacob.

De La Soudiere Martin. 1988. "L'inconfort du terrain". *Terrain* 11, 94–105.

De Vries Raymond. 1996. *Making Midwives Legal. Childbirth, Medicine and the Law*. Colombus: Ohio State University Press.

De Vries Raymond, Wiegers Thérèse A., Smulders Beatrijs & Van Teijlingen Edwin. 2009. "The Dutch Obstetrical System: Vanguard of the Future in Maternity Care". In Davis-Floyd Robbie E., Barclay Lesley, Daviss Betty-Jane & Tritten Jan (eds.), *Birth Models that Work*. Berkeley and Los Angeles: University of California Press, 31–54.

Denis Brigitte. 2009. *La Parole au bébé*. Québec: Éditions Le Dauphin Blanc.

Dettwyler Katherine A. 1995a. "A Time to Wean: The Hominid Blueprint for the Natural Age of Weaning in Modern Human Populations". In Stuart-Macadam Patricia & Dettwyler Katherine A (eds.), *Breastfeeding: Biocultural Perspectives*. New York: Aldine de Gruyter, 39–74.

Dettwyler Katherine A. 1995b. "Beauty and the Breast: The Cultural Context of Breastfeeding in the United States". In Stuart-Macadam Patricia & Dettwyler Katherine A. (eds.), *Breastfeeding: Biocultural Perspectives*. New York: Aldine de Gruyter, 167–216.

230 *Bibliography*

Deutsch Francine M. 2007. "Undoing Gender". *Gender & Society* 21 (1), 106–127.
Dick-Read Grantly. 1933. *Natural Childbirth*. London: Heinemann Medical Books.
Dick-Read Grantly. 1944. *Childbirth without Fear*. New York: Harper & Bros.
Diserens Marc, Lavanchy Philippe, Holzer Valérie & Alvarez Caroline. 2006. *Programme cantonal de promotion de la santé et de prévention primaire enfants (0–6 ans) – parents*. Département de la santé et de l'action sociale, Service de la santé publique (SSP), Département de la formation et de la jeunesse, Service de protection de la jeunesse (SPJ). Suisse: Canton de Vaud.
Dolto Françoise. 1985. *La cause des enfants*. Paris: Robert Laffont.
Douglas Susan J. & Michaels Meredith W. 2005. *The Mommy Myth. The Idealization of Motherhood and How It Has Undermined All Women*. New York: Free Press.
Downe Soo & Mccourt Christine. 2008. "From Being to Becoming: Reconstructing Childbirth Knowledge". In Downe Soo (ed.), *Normal Childbirth: Evidence and Debate* (2nd ed.). London: Elsevier, 3–27.
Dratva Julia, Gross Karin, Spath Anna & Zemp Stutz Elisabeth. 2014. *Étude nationale sur l'alimentation des nourrissons et la santé infantile durant la première année de vie*. Bâle: Swiss TPH.
Droux Joëlle. 2005. "Pour le bonheur des dames ? Le rôle des écoles d'infirmières dans la diffusion de nouvelles normes d'hygiène maternelle et infantile en Suisse (1890–1940)". In Bourdelais Patrice & Faure Olivier (eds.), *Les nouvelles pratiques de santé. XVIIIe–XXe siècles*. Paris: Éditions Belin, 285–308.
Droux Joëlle. 2007a. "1936–1946: une ère de transitions". In Rieder Philip (ed.), *À l'orée de la vie. Cent ans de gynécologie et obstétrique à la maternité de Genève*. Genève: Médecine & Hygiène, 97–115.
Droux Joëlle. 2007b. "1946–1976: les Trentes glorieuses?". In Rieder Philip (ed.), *À l'orée de la vie. Cent ans de gynécologie et obstétrique à la maternité de Genève*. Genève: Médecine & Hygiène, 135–149.
Duffy Linda C., Faden Howard, Wasielewsji Raymond, Wolf Judy & Kryftosik Debra. 1997. "Exclusive Breastfeedings Protects against Bacterial Colonisation and Day Care Exposure of Otitis Media". *Pediatrics* 100, e7.
Dykes Fiona & Williams Catherine. 1999. "Falling by the Wayside: A Phenomenological Exploration of Perceived Breast Milk Inadequacy in Lactating Women". *Midwifery* 15 (4), 232–246.
Dykes Fiona. 2002. "Western Marketing and Medicine. Construction of an Insufficient Milk Syndrome in Lactating Women". *Health Care for Women International* 23 (5), 492–502.
Dykes Fiona. 2005. "'Supply' and 'Demand': Breastfeeding as Labour". *Social Science and Medicine* 60, 2283–2293.
Dykes Fiona. 2006. *Breastfeeding in Hospital. Mothers, Midwives and the Production Line*. London: Routledge.
Dykes Fiona & Flacking Renée. 2010. "Encouraging Breastfeeding: A Relational Perspective". *Early Human Development* 86, 733–736.
Elgin Duane. 1993. *Voluntary Simplicity: Toward a Way of Life that Is Outwardly Simple, Inwardly Rich*. New York: William Morrow.
Elias Norbert. 1973 [1969]. *La civilisation des mœurs*. Paris: Calmann Lévy.
Eyer Diane E. 1993. *Mother–Infant Bonding: A Scientific Fiction*. New Haven: Yale University Press.

Fage-Butler Antoinette Mary. 2017. "Risk Resistance: Constructing Home Birth as Morally Responsible on an Online Discussion Forum". *Health, Risk & Society* 19 (3–4), 130–144.

Fainzang Sylvie. 2006. *La relation médecin–malades: information et mensonge.* Paris: Presses Universitaires de France.

Faircloth Charlotte. 2010. "'if They Want to Risk the Health and Well-Being of Their Child, that's Up to Them'; Long-Term Breastfeeding, Risk and Maternal Identity". *Health, Risk and Society* 12 (4), 257–367.

Faircloth Charlotte. 2013. *Militant Lactivism? Attachment Parenting and Intensive Motherhood in the UK and France.* Oxford: Berghahn Books.

Faircloth Charlotte. 2014a. "The Problem of 'Attachment': The 'Detached' Parent". In Lee Ellie, Bristov Jennie, Faircloth Charlotte & Macvarish Jan (eds.), *Parenting Culture Studies*. Basingstoke: Palgrave Macmillan, 147–164.

Faircloth Charlotte. 2014b. "Intensive Fatherhood? The (Un)involved Father". In Lee Ellie, Bristov Jennie, Faircloth Charlotte & Macvarish Jan (eds.), *Parenting Culture Studies*. Basingstoke: Palgrave Macmillan, 184–199.

Fassin Didier & Memmi Dominique. 2004. "Le gouvernement de la vie: mode d'emploi". In Fassin Didier & Memmi Dominique (eds.), *Le gouvernement des corps*. Paris: Éditions de l'École des hautes études en sciences sociales, 9–33.

Fassin Didier. 2008. "L'éthique, au-delà de la règle. Réflexions autour d'une enquête ethnographique sur les pratiques de soins en Afrique du Sud". *Sociétés contemporaines* 3 (71), 117–135.

Faucon Céline & Brillac Thierry. 2013. "Accouchement à domicile ou à l'hôpital: comparaison des risques à travers une revue de la littérature internationale". *Gynécologie obstétrique et fertilité* 41(6), 388–393.

Favre Adeline. 2009. *Moi, Adeline, accoucheuse.* Lausanne: Éditions d'En Bas.

Favret-Saada Jeanne. 2009. "Être affecté". In Favret-Saada Jeanne (ed.), *Désorceler*. Paris: Éditions de l'Olivier, 145–161.

Federal Statistical Office. 2019a. "Full-/Part-Time Employed". Available at: https://www.bfs.admin.ch/bfs/fr/home/statistiques/situation-economique-sociale-population.assetdetail.7626102.html. Accessed: 14.03.2019.

Federal Statistical Office. 2019b. "Statistique médicale des hôpitaux. Accouchements et santé maternelle en 2017". Available at: https://www.bfs.admin.ch/bfsstatic/dam/assets/8369419/master Accessed 4.09.2020.

Foucault Michel. 1975. *Surveiller et punir: naissance de la prison.* Paris: Gallimard.

Foucault Michel. 1976. *Histoire de la sexualité 1. La volonté de savoir.* Paris: Gallimard.

Foucault Michel. 1977. *Disciplin and Punish: The Birth of the Prison.* Harmondsworth: Penguin.

Fox Bonnie & Neiterman Elena. 2015. "Embodied Motherhood. Women's Feelings about Their Postpartum Bodies". *Gender & Society* 29 (5), 670–693.

Froidevaux-Metterie Camille. 2018. *Le corps des femmes. La bataille de l'intime.* Paris: Philosophie Magazine Éditeur.

Furedi Franck. 2002. *Paranoid Parenting: Why Ignoring the Experts May Be Best for Your Child.* Chicago: Chicago Review Press.

Fuschetto Roxane. 2017. *La maternité de Lausanne. Un patrimoine pour la vie.* Lausanne: Éditions BHMS.

Gagnon John. 2008. *Les scripts de la sexualité. Essais sur les origines culturelles du désir.* Paris: Payot.

Gallenga Ghislaine. 2008. "L'empathie inverse au cœur de la relation ethnographique". *Journal des anthropologues* 114–115, 145–161.

Galton Bachrach Virginia R., Schwartz Eleanor & Bachrach Lela Rose. 2003. "Breastfeeding and the Risk of Hospitalization for Respiratory Disease in Infancy. A Meta-Analysis". *Archive of Pediatrics and Adolescent Medicine* 157, 237–243.

Galtry Judith. 1997. "Suckling and Silence in the USA: The Costs and Benefits of Breastfeeding". *Feminist Economics* 3 (3), 1–24.

Garcia Sandrine. 2011. *Mères sous influence. De la cause des femmes à la cause des enfants*. Paris: La Découverte.

Gardey Delphine & Löwy Ilana. 2000. *L'invention du naturel. Les sciences et la fabrication du féminin et du masculin*. Paris: Éditions des archives contemporaines.

Gaskin Ina May. 1975. *Spiritual Midwifery*. Summertown: Book Publishing Company.

Gatrell Caroline Jane. 2011. "Breastfeeding under the Blanket: Exploring the Tensions between Health and Social Attitudes to Breastfeeding in the United States, Ireland and the United Kingdom". In Liamputtong Pranee (ed.), *Infant Feeding Practices. A Cross-Cultural Perspective*. New York: Springer, 109–123.

Geertz Clifford. 1973. *The Interpretation of Cultures*. New York: Basic Books.

Gélis Jacques. 1988. *La sage-femme ou le médecin*. Paris: Fayard.

Gettler Lee T. & Mckenna James J. 2010. "Never Sleep with Baby? Or keep Me Close but Keep Me Safe: Eliminating Inappropriate Safe Infant Sleep Rhetoric in the United States". *Current Pediatrics Reviews* 6 (1), 71–77.

Giami Alain & De Colomby Pierre. 2002. "La médicalisation de la sexologie en France". *L'Évolution Psychiatrique* 67 (3), 558–570.

Giddens Anthony. 1990. *The Consequences of Modernity*. Cambridge: Polity Press.

Giddens Anthony. 1991. *Modernity and Self-Identity. Self and Society in the Late Modern Age*. Cambridge: Polity Press.

Gimlin Debra. 2007. "What is 'Body Work'? A Review of the Literature". *Sociology Compass* 1 (1), 353–370.

Giraud Olivier & Lucas Barbara. 2009. "Le renouveau des régimes de genre en Allemagne et en Suisse : bonjour 'néo maternalisme' ?" *Cahiers du Genre* 46, 17–46.

Goffman Erving. 1968. *Asiles. Études sur la condition sociale des malades mentaux*. Paris: Minuit.

Gojard Séverine. 2010. *Le métier de mère*. Paris: La Dispute.

Gottlieb Alma. 2000. "Where Have All the Babies Gone?: Toward an Anthropology of Infants (and Their Caretakers)". *Anthropological Quaterly* 73 (3), 121–132.

Gottlieb Alma. 2004. The Afterlife is Where We Come From: The Culture of Infancy in West Africa. Chicago: University of Chicago Press.

Goody Jack. 2001. *La famille en Europe*. Paris: Seuil.

Gouilhers Solène. 2010. "Le suivi de grossesse par les sages-femmes: vers une 'autonomie raisonnée' des femmes enceintes". In Manai Dominique, Burton-Jeangros Claudine & Elger Bernice (eds.), *Risques et informations dans le suivi de la grossesse: droit, éthique et pratiques sociales*. Berne: Stämpfli, 213–142.

Gouilhers-Hertig Solène. 2014. "Vers une culture du risque personnalisée. Choisir d'accoucher à domicile ou en maison de naissance en Suisse". *Socio-anthropologie* 29, 101–119.

Gouilhers-Hertig Solène. 2017. Gouverner par le risque: une ethnologie des lieux d'accouchement en Suisse romande. Thèse de doctorat en sociologie, Genève: UNIGE.

Greenhouse Carol J. 1995. *A Moment's Notice: Time Politics Across Culture*. Ithaca, NY: Cornell University Press.

Gribble Karleen. 2008. "'As Good as Chocolate' and 'Better than Ice Cream': What Breastfeeding Means to Children". *Early Child Development and Care* 179 (8), 1067–1082.

Gribble Karleen. 2010. "Receiving and Enjoying Milk. What Breastfeeding Means to Children". In Shaw Rhonda & Bartlett Alison (eds.), *Giving Breastmilk. Body, Ethics and Contemporary Breastfeeding Practices*. Toronto: Demeter Press, 64–82.

Grummer-Strawn Laurence M. & Mei Zuguo. 2004. "Does Breastfeeding Protect against Pediatric Overweight ? Analysis of Longitudinal Data from the Centers for Disease Control and Prevention Pediatric Nutrition Surveillance System". *Pediatrics* 113, e81–e86.

Grylka Susanne & Pehlke-Milde Jessica. 2019. *Rapport statistique des sages-femmes indépendantes en Suisse*. Berne: Fédération suisse des sages-femmes.

Gueguen Catherine. 2014. *Pour une enfance heureuse. Repenser l'éducation à la lumière des dernières découvertes sur le cerveau*. Paris: Robert Laffont.

Hall-Smith Paige, Hausman Bernice L. & Labbok Miriam (eds.). 2012. *Beyond Health, beyond Choice. Breastfeeding Constraints and Realities*. New Brunswick: Rutgers University Press.

Harder Thomas, Bergmann Renate, Kallischnigg Gerd & Plagemann Andreas. 2005. "Duration of Breastfeeding and Risk of Overweight: A Meta-Analysis". *American Journal of Epidemiology* 162 (5), 397–403.

Hardyment Christina. 2007. *Dream Babies: Childcare Advice from John Locke to Gina Ford*. London: Francis Lincoln.

Hausman Bernice L. 2004. "The Feminist Politics of Breastfeeding". *Australian Feminist Studies* 19 (45), 273–285.

Hausman Bernice L. 2012 "Feminism and Breastfeeding: Rhetoric, Ideology and the Material Realities of Women's Lives". In Hall-Smith Paige, Hausman Bernice L. & Labbok Miriam (eds.), *Beyond Health, Beyond Choice. Breastfeeding Constraints and Realities*. New Brunswick: Rutgers University Press, 15–24.

Hays Sharon. 1996. *The Cultural Contradictions of Motherhood*. New Haven: Yale University Press.

Herbinet Etienne & Busnel Marie-Claire (eds.). 2009 [1981]. "L'aube des sens. Ouvrage collectif sur les perceptions sensorielles fœtales et néonatales". *Les Cahiers du Nouveau-Né* 5, 1–56.

Hildingsson Ingegerd M., Lindgren Helena E., Haglund Bengt & Radestad Ingela J. 2006. "Characteristics of Women Giving Birth at Home in Sweden: A National Register Study". *American Journal of Obstetrics and Gynaecology* 195 (5), 1366–1372.

Hirt Caroline. 2005. *La baisse ou absence de désir sexuel après l'accouchement: analyse de la construction d'un problème social*. Mémoire de Licence en Ethnologie, Neuchâtel: Université de Neuchâtel.

Hughes Everett C. 1958. *Men and Their Work*. Westport: Greenwood Press.

Irigaray Luce. 1981. *Le corps à corps avec la mère*. Montréal: La pleine lune.

Jackson Wendy. 2004. "Breastfeeding and Type 1 Diabetes Mellitus". *British Journal of Midwifery* 12 (3), 158–165.

Jacques Béatrice. 2007. *Sociologie de l'accouchement*. Paris: Presses Universitaires de France.

Jenni Oskar, Bucher Hans Ulrich, Gosztonyi Laura, Hosli Irene, Honigmann Silvia, Sutter Martin & Aeschlimann Christine. 2013. "Bedsharing et mort subite du nourrisson: recommandations actuelles". *Paediatrica* 24 (5), 9–11.

Jordan Brigitte. 1978. *Birth in Four Cultures: A Crosscultural Investigation of Childbirth in Yucatan, Holland, Sweden and the United States*. Montreal: Eden Press.

Jordan Brigitte. 1997. "Authoritative Knowledge and Its Construction". In Davis-Floyd Robbie E. & Sargent Carolyn F. (eds.), *Childbirth and Authoritative Knowledge: Cross-Cultural Perspectives*. Berkeley: University of California Press.

Jordan Brigitte. 2014. "Technology and Social Interaction: Notes on the Achievement of Authoritative Knowledge". *Talent Development and Excellence* 6 (1), 95–132.

Kahn Robbie Pfeufer. 1989. "Women and Time in Childbirth and during Lactation". In Forman Frieda Johles & Sowton Caoran (eds.), *Taking our Time. Feminist Perspectives on Temporality*. Oxford and New York: Pergamon Press, 20–36.

Katz Rothman Barbara. 1991 [1982]. *In Labor. Women and Power in the Birthplace*. New York: W. W. Norton and Company.

Katz Rothman Barbara. 2007a. "Laboring Then. The Political History of Maternity Care in the United States". In Simonds Wendy, Katz Rothman Barbara & Norman Bari Meltzer (eds.), *Labouring On. Birth in Transition in the United States*. New York: Routledge, 2–28.

Katz Rothman Barbara. 2007b. "Laboring Now. Current Cultural Constructions of Pregnancy, Birth and Mothering". In Simonds Wendy, Katz Rothman Barbara & Norman Bari Meltzer (eds.), *Labouring On. Birth in Transition in the United States*. New York: Routledge, 29–93.

Kaufman Sharon R. & Morgan Lynn M. 2005. "The Anthropology of the Beginning and Ends of Life". *Annual Review of Anthropology* 34, 317–341.

Kaufmann Jean-Claude. 2004. *L'entretien compréhensif*. Paris: Armand Colin.

Kenney Martha & Muller Ruth. 2017. "Of Rats and Women: Narratives of Motherhood in Environmental Epigenetics". *BioSocieties* 12, 23–46.

Knaak Stephanie J. 2010. "Contextualising Risk, Constructing Choice: Breastfeeding and Good Mothering in Risk Society". *Health, Risk and Society* 12 (4), 345–355.

Knibiehler Yvonne. 2012. *Histoire des mères et de la maternité en Occident*. Paris: Presses universitaires de France.

Kristeva Julia. 1982. *Powers of Horros: An Essay on Abjection*. New York: Columbia University Press.

Kukla Rebecca. 2005. *Mass Hysteria. Medicine, Culture and Mothers' Bodies*. Lanham: Rowman & Littlefield Publishers.

Kukla Rebecca. 2006. "Ethics and Ideology in Breastfeding Advocacy Campaigns". *Hypatia* 21 (1), 157–180.

LA Leche League International. 1958. *The Womanly Art of Breastfeeding*. New York: Penguin Books.

Laqueur Thomas. 1990. *Making Sex: Body and Gender from the Greeks to Freud*. Cambridge, MA and London: Harvard University Press.

Lawrence Ruth. 1995. "The Clinician's Role in Teaching Proper Infant Feeding Techniques". *The Journal of Pediatrics* 126 (6), S112–7.

Le Du Maï. 2017. *Toucher pour soigner. Le toucheur traditionnel, le médecin et l'ostéopathe: un nourrisson entre de bonnes mains.* Thèse de doctorat en sociologie, Paris.

Le Goff Jean-Marie & Levy René. 2016. *Devenir parents, devenir inégaux. Transition à la parentalité et inégalités de genre.* Zürich: Seismo.

Leach Penelope. 2010. *The Essential First Year.* London: DK Publishing.

Leboyer Frédérick. 1974. *Pour une naissance sans violence.* Paris: Seuil.

Lee Ellie. 2008. "Living with Risk in the Age of 'Intensive Motherhood': Maternal Identity and Infant Feeding". *Health, Risk and Society* 10 (5), 467–477.

Lee Ellie. 2011. "Infant Feeding and the Problem of Policy". In Liamputtong Pranee (ed.), *Infant Feeding Practices. A Cross-Cultural Perspective.* New York: Springer, 79–91.

Lett Didier & Morel Marie-France. 2016. *Une histoire de l'allaitement.* Paris: Éditions de la Martignière.

Liamputtong Pranee (ed.). 2011. *Infant Feeding Practices. A Cross-Cultural Perspective.* New York: Springer.

Liedloff Jean. 1975. *The Continuum Concept. In Search of Lost Happiness.* Cambridge, MA: Perseus Books.

Lips Ulrich. 2002. "Recensement du 'syndrome de l'enfant secoué' par le Swiss Pediatric Surveillance Unit (SPSU)". *Paediatrica* 13 (4), 37.

Lock Margaret. 1993. "Cultivating the Body: Anthropology and Epistemologies of Bodily Practice and Knowledge". *Annual Review of Anthropology* 22, 133–55.

Lorenz Konrad. 1937. "The Nature of Instinct". In Schiller Claire H. (ed.), *Instinctive Behavior: The Development of a Modern Concept.* London: Methuen, 129–175.

Lupton Deborah. 1993. "Risk as Moral Danger: The Social and Political Functions of Risk Discourse in Public Health" *International Journal of Health Services* 23 (3), 425–435.

Lupton Deborah. 2013a. "Infant Embodiment and Interembodiment: A Review of Sociocultural Perspectives" *Childhood* 20, 37–50.

Lupton Deborah. 2013b. "Risk and Emotion: Towards an Alternative Theoretical Perspective". *Health, Risk and Society* 15 (8), 634–647.

Lupton Deborah & Barclay Lesley. 1997. *Constructing Fatherhood: Discourses and Experiences.* London: Sage Publications.

Mabilia Mara. 2005. *Breastfeeding and Sexuality. Behaviours, Beliefs and Taboos among the Gogo Mothers in Tanzania.* New York: Berghahn Books.

Maccormack Carol. 1980. "Nature, Culture and Gender: A Critique". In Maccormack Carol & Strathern Marilyn (eds.), *Nature, Culture and Gender.* Cambridge: Cambridge University Press, 1–24.

Macdonald Margaret. 2006. "Gender Expectations: Natural Bodies and Natural Births in the New Midwifery in Canada". *Medical Anthropology Quaterly* 20 (2), 235–256.

Macdonald Margaret. 2007. *At Work in the Field of Birth.* Nashville: Vanderbilt University Press.

Maffi Irene. 2012. "L'accouchement est-il un événement ? Regards croisés sur les définitions médicales et les expériences intimes des femmes en Jordanie et en Suisse". *Mondes contemporains* 2, 53–80.

Maffi Irene. 2013. "Can Caesarean Section Be 'Natural'? The Hybrid Nature of the Nature–Culture Dichotomy in Mainstream Obstetric Culture". *Journal for Research in Sickness and Society* 10 (19), 5–26.

Maffi Irene. 2014. "Les cours de préparation à la naissance dans une maternité suisse. Entre logiques institutionnelles, postures des sages-femmes et autonomie des couples". In Burton-Jeangros Claudine, Hammer Raphaël, & Maffi Irene (eds.), *Accompagner la naissance. Terrains socioanthropologiques en Suisse romande*. Lausanne: Giuseppe Merrone Editeur, 175–197.

Maffi Irene. 2016. "The Detour of an Obstetric Technology: Active Management of Labor across Cultures". *Medical Anthropology* 35 (1), 17–30.

Maher Vanessa (ed.). 1992. *The Anthropology of Breast-Feeding: Natural Law or Social Construct*. New York: Berg.

Mahon-Daly Patricia & Andrews Gavin J. 2002. "Liminality and Breastfeeding: Women Negotiating Space and Two Bodies". *Health & Place* 8, 61–76.

Malacrida Claudia & Boulton Tiffany. 2014. "The Best Laid Plans? Women's Choices, Expectations and Experiences in Childbirth". Health 18 (1), 41–59.

Marcus George E. & Saka Erkan. 2006. "Assemblage". *Theory, Culture and Society* 23(2–3), 101–106.

Mansfield Becky. 2008. "The Social Nature of Natural Childbirth". *Social Science and Medicine* 66, 1084–1094.

Marshall Joyce L., Godfrey Mary & Renfrew Mary J. 2007. "Being a 'Good Mother': Managing Breastfeeding and Merging Identities". *Social Science & Medicine* 65, 2147–2159.

Marshall Joyce L. & Godfrey Mary. 2011. "Shifting Identities: Social and Cultural Factors that Shape Decision-Making around Sustaining Breastfeeding". In Liamputtong Pranee (ed.), *Infant Feeding Practices. A Cross-Cultural Perspective*. New York: Springer, 95–108.

Marland Hilary & Rafferty Anne Marie. 1997. *Midwives, Society and Childbirth. Debates and Controversies in the Modern Period*. New York: Routledge.

Martin Emily. 1987. *The Woman in the Body: A Cultural Analysis of Reproduction*. Boston: Beacon Press.

Matsuoka Etsuko & Hinokuma Fumiko. 2009. "Maternity Homes in Japan: Reservoirs of Normal Childbirth". In Davis-Floyd Robbie E., Barclay Lesley, Daviss Betty-Jane & Tritten Jan (eds.), *Birth Models that Work*. Berkeley: University of California Press, 213–237.

Mauss Marcel. 1936. "Les techniques du corps". *Journal de psychologie*, XXXII, ne, 3–4.

Mcbride-Henry Karen & Shaw Rhonda. 2010. "Giving Breastmilk as Being-With". In Shaw Rhonda & Bartlett Alison (eds.), *Giving Breastmilk. Body, Ethics and Contemporary Breastfeeding Practices*. Toronto: Demeter Press, 191–204.

Mccabe Katharine. 2016. "Mothercraft. Birth Work and the Making of Neoliberal Mothers". *Social Science & Medicine* 162, 177–184.

Mccourt Christine & Dykes Fiona. 2009. "From Tradition to Modernity: Time and Childbirth in Historical Perspective". In Mccourt Christine (ed.), *Childbirth, Midwifery and Concepts of Time*. New York: Berghahn Books, 17–36.

Mckenna James J. & Gettler Lee T. 2016. "There is No Such Thing as Infant Sleep, There is no Such Thing as Breastfeeding, There is Only Breastsleeping". *Acta Paediatrica* 105 (1), 17–21.

Memmi Dominique. 2004. "Administrer une matière sensible. Conduites raisonnables et pédagogie par corps autour de la naissance et de la mort". In Fassin Didier & Memmi Dominique (eds.), *Le gouvernement des corps*. Paris: Éditions de l'École des hautes études en sciences sociales, 135–154.

Memmi Dominique. 2014. *La revanche de la chair. Essai sur les nouveaux supports de l'identité*. Paris: Éditions du Seuil.

Michaels Paula A. 2014. *Lamaze. An International History*. New York: Oxford University Press.

Millard Ann V. 1990. "The Place of the Clock in Pediatric Advice: Rationales, Cultural Themes and Impediments to Breastfeeding". *Social Science & Medicine* 31 (2), 211–221.

Miller Tina. 2011. "Falling Back into Gender? Men's Narratives and Practices around First-Time Fatherhood". *Sociology* 45 (6), 1094–1109.

Mol Annemarie. 2009. *Ce que soigner veut dire. Repenser le libre choix du patient*. Paris: Presses des Mines.

Morel Marie-France (ed.). 2016. "Introduction". In *Naître à la maison. D'hier à aujourd'hui*. Villematier: Éres, 9–20.

Moscucci Ornella. 1990. *The Science of Woman. Gynaecology and Gender in England 1800–1929*. Cambridge: Cambridge University Press.

Moscucci Ornella. 2002. "Holistic Obstetrics: The Origins of 'Natural Childbirth' in Britain". *Post-Graduate Medical Journal* 79, 168–173.

Mottier Véronique. 2000. "Narratives of National Identity: Sexuality, Race, and the Swiss 'Dream of Order'. *Revue Suisse de Sociologie* 26(3), 533–558.

Müller Marianne, Lanfranconi Lucia M., Fuchs Gesine & Rabhi-Sidler Sarah. 2017. "L'égalité dans le domaine de la parenté en Suisse". Lucerne University of Applied Sciences and Arts. E-Learning Box. Available at: http://gleichstellen .ch/src/media/gleichstellen-ch-Hintergrundinfos-Elternschaft_Franzoesisch.pdf. Accessed: 14.03.2019.

Muller Mike. 1974. *The Baby Killer*. London: War on Want.

Murphy Elizabeth. 1999. "'Breast is Best': Infant Feeding Decisions and Maternal Deviance". *Sociology of Health and Illness* 21 (2), 182–208.

Murphy Elizabeth. 2000. "Risk, Responsibility and Rhetoric in Infant Feeding". *Journal of Contemporary Ethnography* 29 (3), 291–325.

Murphy Elizabeth. 2003. "Expertise and Forms of Knowledge in the Government of Families". *Sociological Review* 51 (4), 433–462.

Naepels Michel. 1998. "Une étrange étrangeté. Remarques sur la situation ethnographique". *L'Homme* 38 (148), 185–199.

Négrié Laetitia & Cascales Béatrice. 2016. *L'accouchement est politique. Fécondité, femmes en travail et institutions*. Breuillet: Éditions l'instant présent.

Neyrand Gérard. 2000. *L'enfant, la mère et la question du père. Un bilan critique de l'évolution des savoirs sur la petite enfance*. Paris: Presses Universitaires de France.

Nice. 2014. "Intrapartum Care for Healthy Women and Babies". Guideline cg190. Available at: https://www.nice.org.uk/guidance/cg190/resources/intrap artum-care-for-healthy-women-and-babies-pdf-35109866447557. Accessed: 21.11.2017.

Oakley Ann. 1984. *The Captured Womb: A History of the Medical Care of Pregnant Women*. Oxford: Blackwell.

Obermeyer Carla Makhlouf & Castle Sarah. 1996. "Back to Nature? Historical and Cross-Cultural Perspectives on Barriers to Optimal Breastfeeding". *Medical Anthropology* 17, 39–63.

Oddy Wendy H. 2001. "Breastfeeding Protects against Illness and Infection in Infants and Children: A Review of the Literature". *Breastfeeding Review* 9(2), 11–18.

Odent Michel. 1976. *Bien naître*. Paris: Seuil.

Odent Michel. 2005. *Césariennes, questions, effets, enjeux. Alerte face à la banalisation*. Paris: Le Souffle d'Or.

Odent Michel. 2011 [1990]. *Le bébé est un mammifère*. Paris: Éditions l'Instant Présent.

O'driscoll Kieran, Meagher Declan & Boylan Peter. 1980. *Active Management of Labour*. London: Mosby.

Ólafsdóttir Ólöf Ásta & Kirkham Mavis. 2009. "Narrative Time: Stories, Childbirth and Midwifery". In Mccourt Christine (ed.), *Childbirth, Midwifery and Concept of Time*. New York: Berghahn Books, 167–183.

Olivier De Sardan Jean-Pierre. 1995. "La politique du terrain. Sur la production des données en anthropologie". *Enquête* 1, 71–96.

Olivier De Sardan Jean-Pierre. 2000. "Le 'je' méthodologique. Implication et explicitation dans l'enquête de terrain". *Revue française de sociologie* 41 (3), 417–445.

Olivier De Sardan Jean-Pierre. 2008. *La rigueur du qualitatif, les contraintes empiriques de l'interprétation socio-anthropologique*. Louvain-la-Neuve: Academia-Bruylant.

Olsen Ole & Clausen Jette A. 2012. "Planned Hospital Birth *Versus* Planned Home Birth". *Cochrane Database Systematic Review* 9, 1–39.

Oudshoorn Nelly. 1994. *Beyond the Natural Body. An Archeology of Sex Hormones*. Oxon and New York: Routledge.

Owen Christopher G., Martin Richard M., Whincup Peter H., Davey Smith George & Cook Derek G. 2006. "Does Breastfeeding Influence Risk of Type 2 Diabetes in Later Life? A Quantitative Analysis of Published Evidences 1'2'3". *The American Journal of Clinical Nutrition* 84 (5), 1043–1054.

Palmer Gabrielle. 2009 [1988]. *The Politics of Breastfeeding. When Breasts Are Bad for Business*. London: Pinter & Martin.

Pasveer Bernike & Akrich Madeleine. 2001. "Obstetrical Trajectories. On Training Women/Bodies for (Home)Birth". In De Vries Raymond, Benoit Cecilia, Van Teijlingen Edwin R. & Wrede Sirpa (eds.), *Birth by Design. Pregnancy, Maternity Care and Midwifery in North America and Europe*. New York: Routledge, 229–242.

Paumier Marie & Richardson Mary. 2003. "Le mouvement pour la reconnaissance des sages-femmes en France et au Québec". In Saillant Francine & Boulianne Manon (eds.), *Transformations sociales, genre et santé*. Paris: Éditions L'Harmattan, 247–262.

Paumier Marie. 2006. "Le corps enceint et la connaissance intuitive: la nature incorporée?". In Schmitz Olivier (ed.), *Les médecines en parallèle. Multiplicité des recours au soin en Occident*. Paris: Karthala, 77–90.

Perez-Rios Naydi, Ramos-Valencia Gilberto & Ortiz Ana Patricia. 2008. "Cesarean Delivery as a Barrier for Breastfeeding Initiation: The Puerto Rican Experience". *Journal of Human Lactation* 24 (3), 293–302.

Perrenoud Patricia. 2014. "Naissance et évolution des pratiques: entre Evidence-Based Medicine, expérience et intuition". In Burton-Jeangros Claudine, Hammer Raphaël & Maffi Irene (eds.), *Accompagner la naissance. Terrains socioanthropologiques en Suisse romande*. Lausanne: Giuseppe Merrone Editeur, 133–153.

Perrenoud Patricia. 2016. *Construire des savoirs issus de l'expérience à l'ère de l'Evidence-Based Medicine: une enquête anthropologique auprès de sages-femmes indépendantes en Suisse romande*. Thèse de doctorat en anthropologie, Lausanne.

Pochin Courtney. 2018. "Dads May Soon Be Able to Breastfeed Their Newborns Babies With First Ever 'Chestfeeding Kit'". *The Daily Mirror*, 25.10.2018. Available at: https://www.mirror.co.uk/news/weird-news/dads-soon-able-brea stfeed-newborn-13478225. Accessed 14.11.2018.

Praz Anne-Françoise. 2005. *De l'enfant utile à l'enfant précieux*. Lausanne: Éditions Antipodes.

Pruvost Geneviève. 2016. "Qui accouche qui? Étude de 134 récits d'accouchement à domicile". *Genre, Sexualité et Société* 16, 1–28.

Quagliariello Chiara. 2017a. "'Ces hommes qui accouchent avec nous'. La pratique de l'accouchement naturel à l'aune du genre". *Nouvelles Questions Féministes* 1 (36), 82–97.

Quagliariello Chiara. 2017b. "L'accouchement naturel contre l'hôpital moderne? Une étude de cas en Italie". *Anthropologie & Santé* 15, 1–21.

Quandt Sara A. 1995. "Sociocultural Aspects of the Lactation Process". In Stuart-Macadam Patricia & Dettwyler Katherine A. (eds.), *Breastfeeding: Biocultural Perspectives*. New York: Aldine de Gruyter, 127–144.

Quigley Maria, Kelly Yvonne J. & Sacker Amanda. 2007. "Breastfeeding and Hospitalization for Diarrheal and Respiratory Infection in the United Kingdom Millennium Cohort Study". *Pediatrics* 110(4), e837–e842.

Rao Shobha & Kanade Asawari N. 1992. "Prolonged Breast-Feeding and Malnutrition among Rural Indian Children below 3 Years of Age". *European Journal of Clinical Nutrition* 46, 187–195.

Reed Richard K. 2005. *Birthing Fathers: The Transformation of Men in American Rites of Birth*. New Brunswick: Rutgers University Press.

Rempel Lynn A. & Rempel John K. 2011. "The Breastfeeding Team: The Role of Involved Fathers in the Breastfeeding Family". *Journal of Human Lactation* 27 (2), 115–121.

Rich Adrienne. 1976. *Of a Woman Born: Motherhood as Experience and Institution*. New York: Bantam.

Richardson Sarah S. 2015. "Maternal Bodies in the Postgenomic Order. Gender and the Explanatory Landscape of Epigenetics". In Richardson Sarah S. & Stevens Hallam (eds.), *Postgenomics: Perspectives on Biology after the Genome*. London: Duke University Press, 210–231.

Rieder Philip. 2007a. "Accoucher avant la maternité". In Rieder Philip (ed.), *À l'orée de la vie. Cent ans de gynécologie et obstétrique à la maternité de Genève (1907–2007)*. Genève: Médecine & Hygiène, 17–23.

Rieder Philip. 2007b. "Former et assister: la première Maternité genevoise". In Rieder Philip (ed.), *À l'orée de la vie. Cent ans de gynécologie et obstétrique à la maternité de Genève (1907–2007)*. Genève: Médecine & Hygiène, 24–40.

Rochat Line. 2014. "Pratiques sensorielles, pratiques professionnelles: interactions quotidiennes entre infirmières et bébés au sein d'un service de néonatologie romand". In Burton-Jeangros Claudine, Hammer Raphaël & Maffi Irene (eds.), *Accompagner la naissance. Terrains socio-anthropologiques en Suisse romande*. Lausanne: Giuseppe Merrone Editeur, 155–174.

Rollet Catherine & morel Marie-France. 2000. *Des bébés et des hommes. Traditions et modernité des soins aux tout-petits*. Paris: Albin Michel.

Rose Nikolas. 1989. *Governing the Soul. The Shaping of the Private Self*. London and New York: Routledge.

Rose Nikolas. 1998. *Inventing Our Selves. Psychology, Power and Personhood.* Cambridge: Cambridge University Press.

Rose Nikolas. 2006. "Governing 'Advanced' Liberal Democracies". In Aradhana Sharna & Anil Gupta (eds.), *The Anthropology of the State: A Reader.* Oxford: Blackwell, 144–162.

Rowe-Murray Heather J. & Fisher Jane R. W. 2002. "Baby-Friendly Hospital Practices: Cesarean Section is a Persistent Barrier to Early Initiation of Breastfeeding". *Birth* 29 (2), 124–131.

Ruhl Lealle. 2002. "Dilemmas of the Will: Uncertainty, Reproduction, and the Rhetoric of Control". *Journal of Women in Culture and Society* 27 (3), 641–663.

Ruz Anne-Julie. 2018. "L'allaitement au travail, un droit encore méconnu". *24 heures* 31.01.2018, 3.

Sachs Magda, Dykes Fiona & Carter Bernie. 2005. "Weight Monitoring of Breastfed Babies in the UK – Centile Charts, Scales and Weighing Frequency". *Maternal and Child Nutrition* 1, 63–76.

Sachs Magda. 2005. *'Following the Line': An Ethnograhic Study of the Influence of Routine Baby Weighing on Breastfeeding Women in a Town in the Northwest of England.* Department of Midwifery Studies, University of Central Lancashire.

Sachs Magda. 2013. "Weighing it Up: The Reasons Breastfeeding Women Weight Their Babies". In Hall Moran Victoria (ed.), *Maternal and Infant Nutrition and Nurture: Controversies and Challenges.* London: Quay Books, 157–176.

Sadauskaite-Kuehne Vaiva, Ludvigsson Johny, Padaiga Zilvinas, Jasinskiene Edita & Samuelsson Ulf. 2004. "Longer Breastfeeding is an Independent Protective Factor against Development of Type 1 Diabetes Mellitus in Childhood". *Diabetes/ Metabolism Research and Reviews* 20(2), 150–157.

Sandre-Pereira Gilza. 2005. "La Leche League: des femmes pour l'allaitement maternel (1956–2004)". *CLIO.* Histoire, femmes et sociétés [online] 21. Available at: https://clio.revues.org/1462. Accessed 16.10.2017.

Scamell Mandie. 2011. "The Swan Effect in Midwifery Talk and Practice: A Tension between Normality and the Language of Risk". *Sociology of Health and Illness* 33 (7), 987–1001.

Scamell Mandie & Alaszewski Andy. 2012. "Fateful Moments and the Categorisation of Risk: Midwifery Practice and the Ever-Narrowing Window of Normality during Childbirth". *Health, Risk and Society* 14 (2), 207–221.

Scariati Paul D, Grummer-Strawn Laurence M & Fein Sara Beck. 1997. "A Longitudinal Analysis of Infant Morbidity and the Extent of Breastfeeding in the United States". *Pediatrics* 99, e5.

Scheper-Hughes Nancy & Lock Margaret M. 1987. "The Mindful Body: A Prolegomenon to Future Work in Medical Anthropology". *Medical Anthropology Quaterly* 1 (1), 6–41.

Scheper-Hughes Nancy. 1992. *Death without Weeping. The Violence of Everyday Life in Brazil.* Berkeley and Los Angeles: University of California Press.

Schmied Virginia & Lupton Deborah. 2001. "Blurring the Boundaries: Breasfeeding and Maternal Subjectivity". *Sociology of Health and Illness* 23 (2), 234–250.

Schmied Virginia, Beake Sarah, Sheehan Athena, Mccourt Christine & Dykes Fiona. 2011. "Women's Perceptions and Experiences of Breastfeeding Support: A Metasynthesis". *Birth* 38 (1), 49–60.

Schmitz Olivier. 2006. *Les médecines en parallèle: multiplicités des recours au soin en Occident.* Paris: Karthala.

Scholl Sarah. 2017. "Nourrir au lait de vache. L'alimentation des bébés entre nature et technique (1870–1910)". *Anthropozoologica* 52 (1), 113–119.

Schwartz Olivier. 1993. "L'empirisme irréductible". In Anderson Nél (ed.), *Le Hobo: sociologie des sans-abris*. Paris: Nathan, 265–307.

Scott Jane Anne, Binns Colin W. & Arnold Ruth V. 1997. "Attitudes toward Breastfeeding in Perth, Australia: Qualitative Analysis". *Journal of Nutrition Education* 29 (5), 244–249.

Scott Jane Anne. 2011. "Attitudes to Breastfeeding". In Liamputtong Pranee (ed.), *Infant Feeding Practices. A Cross-Cultural Perspective*. New York: Springer, 39–54.

Sears William & Sears Martha. 2001. *The Attachment Parenting Book : A Commonsense Guide to Understanding and Nurturing Your Baby*. London: Little, Brown and Company.

Sestito Rosanna. 2017. "Faire naître à la maison en France. L'invisibilité des radiations ordinaires de sages-femmes à domicile". *Anthropologie & Santé* 15, 1–21.

Shaw Rhonda. 2004. "Performing Breastfeeding: Embodiment, Ethics and the Maternal Subject". *Feminist Review* 78, 99–116.

Sheehan Athena & Schmied Virginia. 2011. "The Imperative to Breastfeed: An Australian Perspective". In Liamputtong Pranee (ed.), *Infant Feeding Practices. A Cross-Cultural Perspective*. New York: Springer, 55–76.

Shirani Fiona, Henwood Karen & Coltart Carrie. 2012. "Meeting the Challenges of Intensive Parenting Culture: Gender, Risk Management and the Moral Parent". *Sociology* 46 (1), 1–16.

Shorter Edward. 1984. *Le corps des femmes*. Paris: Éditions du Seuil.

Simonds Wendy. 2002. "Watching the Clock: Keeping Time during Pregnancy, Birth and Postpartum Experiences". *Social Science and Medicine* 55 (4), 559–570.

Sjoblom Ingela, Nordstrom Berit & Edberg Anna-Karin. 2006. "A Qualitative Study of Women's Experiences of Home Birth in Sweden". *Midwifery* 22 (4), 348–355.

Sjoblom Ingela, Idvall Ewa, Radested Ingela, Lindgren Helena. 2012. "A Provoking Choice—Swedish Women's Experiences of Reactions to Their Plans to Give Birth at Home". *Women and Birth* 25 (3), e11–e18.

Société Suisse de Néonatologie. 2002. "Prophylaxie à la vitamine K chez le nouveau-né: nouvelles recommandations". *Paediatrica* 13 (6), 56–57.

Société Suisse de Néonatologie. 2007. "Prise en charge des nouveau-nés ≥ 34 semaines avec risque élevé d'hypoglycémie ou hypoglycémie en salle d'accouchement et à la maternité". *Paediatrica* 18 (6), 11–13.

Stearns Cindy A. 1999. "Breastfeeding and the Good Maternal Body". *Gender & Society* 13, 308–325.

Stearns Cindy A. 2009. "The Work of Breastfeeding". *Women's Studies Quaterly* 37 (3–4), 63–80.

Stearns Cindy A. 2010. "The Breast Pump". In Shaw Rhonda & Bartlett Alison (eds.), *Giving Breastmilk. Body Ethics and Contemporary Breastfeeding Practice*. Bradford: Demeter Press, 11–23.

Stearns Cindy A. 2013. "The Embodied Practices of Breastfeeding: Implications for Research and Policy". *Journal of Women, Politics and Policy* 34, 4, 359–370.

Strub Silvia & Bannwart Livia. 2017. "Analyse der Löhne von Frauen und Männern anhand der Lohnstrukturerpolitische 2014". *Schlussbericht*. Bern: Büro für arbeits und sozialpolitische Studien BASS.

Stuart-Macadam Patricia & Dettwyler Katherine A. (eds.). 1995. *Breastfeeding: Biocultural Perspectives*. New York: Aldine de Gruyter, 217–142.

Swiss Anthropological Association. 2010. "Une charte éthique pour les ethnologues?". *Tsantsa* 15, 148–165.

Swiss Society of Paediatrics. 2011. "Checklist pour les examens de prévention". Available at: http://www.swiss-paediatrics.org/sites/default/files/membres/chec klists/pdf/checklisten_201204_f_office.pdf. Accessed 25.04.2018.

Swiss Society of Paediatrics. 2017. "Recommandations pour l'alimentation des nourrissons". Available at: http://www.swiss-paediatrics.org/sites/default/files/20 17.07.21_empfehlung_sauglingsernahrung_f_korr.pdf. Accessed 02.05.2018.

Tahhan Diana Adis. 2008. "Depth and Space in Sleep: Intimacy, Touch and the Body in Japanese Co-Sleeping Rituals". *Body & Society* 14 (4), 37–56.

Tahhan Diana Adis. 2010. "Blurring the Boundaries between Bodies: Skinship and Bodily Intimacy in Japan". *Japanese Studies* 30 (2), 215–230.

Taylor Janelle S., Layne Linda L. & Wozniak Danielle F. 2004. *Consuming Motherhood*. New Brunswick, New Jersey and London: Rutgers University Press.

Thebaud Françoise. 1986. *Quand nos grands-mères donnaient la vie. La maternité en France dans l'entre-deux-guerres*. Lyon: Presses Universitaires de Lyon.

Thirion Marie. 1994. *L'allaitement. De la naissance au sevrage*. Paris: Éditions Albin Michel.

Thoemmes Jean. 2009. "Les temporalités sociales: mise en marché et conflits". *Temporalités* 10, 2–7.

Thompson Anne. 1997. "Establishing the Scope of Practice: Organizing European Midwifery in the Inter-War Years 1919–1938". In Marland Hilary & Rafferty Marie (eds.), *Midwives, Society and Childbirth. Debates and Controversies in the Modern Period*. New York: Routledge.

Tomori Cecilia. 2015. *Nighttime Breastfeeding. An American Cultural Dilemma*. New York: Berghahn Books.

Tomori Cecilia, Palmquist Aunchalee E. L. & Dowling Sally. 2016. "Contested Moral Landscapes: Negotiating Breastfeeding Stigma in Breastmilk Sharing, Nighttime Breastfeeding, and Long-Term Breastfeeding in the U.S. and in the U.K.". *Social Science & Medicine* 168, 178–185.

Tomori Cecilia. 2018. "Breastfeeding in Four Cultures. Comparative Analysis of a Biocultural Body Technique". In Tomori Cecilia, Palmquist Aunchalee E. L. & Quinn E. A. (eds.), *Breastfeeding. New Anthropological Approaches*. Oxon: Routledge, 55–68.

Tran Christel, Boulvain Michel & Philippe Jacques. 2011. "Prise en charge du diabète gestationnel: nouvelles connaissances et perspectives futures". *Revue Médicale Suisse* 7, 1250–1254.

Truc Gérôme. 2006. "La paternité en maternité. Une étude par observation". *Ethnologie française* 36, 341–349.

UNICEF. 2017. "Hôpitaux et maisons de naissance Amis des Bébés". Available at: https://www.unicef.ch/sites/default/files/documents/170424_bfhi_spitalliste_fr.p df. Accessed 10.10.2017.

United Nations. 2017. "International Migration Report 2017. Highlights". New York. Available at: http://www.un.org/en/development/desa/population/migrat ion/publications/migrationreport/docs/MigrationReport2017_Highlights.pdf. Accessed: 15.03.19.

Van Esterik Penny. 1988. "The Insufficient Milk Syndrome: Biological Epidemic or Cultural Construction?". In Whelehan Patricia (ed.), *Women and Health Cross-Cultural Perspectives*. Boston: Bergin and Garvey, 97–108.

Van Esterik Penny. 1989. *Motherpower and Infant feeding*. London: Zed Books.

Van Esterik Penny. 1995. "The Politics of Breastfeeding: An Advocacy Perspective". In Stuart-Macadam Patricia & Dettwyler Katherine A. (eds.), *Breastfeeding: Biocultural Perspectives*. New York: Aldine de Gruyter, 145–166.

Van Gennep Arnold. 1909. *Les rites de passage: étude systématique des rites*. Paris: E. Nourry.

Vervatidis Aurélie. 2016. *Quand l'allaitement maternel prend corps. Ethnographie et autoethnographie dans le contexte vaudois de rencontres et consultations petite enfance*. Mémoire de Master, Université de Lausanne.

Victora Cesar G., Bahl Rajiv, Barros Aluisio J. D., França Giovanny V. A., Horton Susan, Krasevec Julia, Murch Simon, Sankar Mari Jeeva, Walker Neff, & Rollins Nigel C. 2016. "Breastfeeding in the 21st Century: Epidemiology, Mechanisms, and Lifelong Effect". *The Lancet* 387, 475–490.

Viisainen Kirsi. 2000. "The Moral Dangers of Home Birth: Parents' Perceptions of Risks in Home Birth in Finland". *Sociology of Health and Illness* 22 (6), 792–814.

Viisainen Kirsi. 2001. "Negotiating Control and Meaning: Home Birth as a Self-Constructed Choice in Finland". *Social Science & Medicine* 52, 1109–1121.

Vuille Marilène. 2000. "Les sages-femmes face à 'l'accompagnement global'". *Perspective soignante* 7, 125–143.

Vuille Marilène. 2004. "L'expérience des femmes dans l''Accouchement Sans Douleur' (ASD): une expérience collective?". In Bos Marguerite, Vincenz Bettina & Wirz Tanja (eds.), *Erfahrung: Alles nur Diskurs? Zur Verwendung des Erfahrungsbegriffs in der Geschlechtergeschichte*, Zürich: Chronos Verlag, 357–365.

Vuille Marilène. 2005. "Le militantisme en faveur de l'Accouchement sans douleur". *Nouvelles Questions Féministes* 24 (3), 50–67.

Vuille Marilène, Malbois Fabienne, Roux Patricia, Messant Françoise & Pannatier Gaël. 2009. "Comprendre le genre pour mieux le défaire". *Nouvelles Questions Féministes* 28 (3), 4–15.

Wacquant Loïc J. D. 1995. "Pugs at Work: Bodily Capital and Bodily Labour among Professional Boxers". *Body & Society* 1 (1), 65–93.

Walentowitz Saskia. 2013. "Importance et signification des rituels d'intégration en pays touareg". In Morel Marie-France (ed.), *Accueillir le nouveau-né, d'hier à aujourd'hui*. Toulouse: Erès.

Walker Madeline. 2014. "Intensive Mothering, Elimination Communication and the Call to Eden". In Ennis Linda Rose (ed.), *Intensive Mothering. The Cultural Contradictions of Modern Motherhood*. Bradford: Demeter Press, 233–246.

Walks Michelle. 2018. "Chestfeeding as Gender Fluid Practice". In Tomori Cecilia, Palmquist Aunchalee E. L. & Quinn E. A. (eds.), *Breastfeeding. New Anthropological Approaches*. Oxon: Routledge, 127–139.

Wall Glenda. 2001. "Moral Construction of Motherhood in Breastfeeding Discourse". *Gender & Society*, 15 (4), 592–610.

Walsh Denis, El-Nemer Amina M. R. & Downe Soo. 2008. "Rethinking Risk and Safety in Maternity Care". In Downe Soo (ed.), *Normal Childbirth: Evidence and Debate* (2nd ed.). Edinburg: Elsevier, 117–127.

Weber Florence. 1989. *Le travail à côté. Étude d'ethnographie ouvrière*. Paris: INRA, EHESS.

Wertz Richard W. & Wertz Dorothy C. 1989 [1977]. *Lying-In. A History of Childbirth in America*. New Haven: Yale University Press.

West Candace & Zimmerman Don H. 1987. "Doing Gender". *Gender & Society* 1, 125–151.

World Health Organization. 1981. *International Code of Marketing of Breast Milk Substitutes*. Geneva: Word Health Organization.

World Health Organization. 2001. *The Optimal Duration of Exclusive Breastfeeding. A Systematical Review*. Geneva: Word Health Organization.

World Health Organization. 2003. *Global Strategy for Infant and Young Child Feeding*. Geneva: World Health Organization.

World Health Organization. 2006. *WHO Child Growth Standard*. Geneva: World Health Organization.

World Health Organization. 2015. *WHO Statement on Caesarean Section Rates*. WHO/RHR/15.02. Geneva: World Health Organization, Department of Reproductive Health and Research. Available at: http://apps.who.int/iris/bitst ream/10665/161442/1/WHO_RHR_15.02_eng.pdf. Accessed 06.10.2017.

World Health Organization. 2018. *Implementation Guidance. Protecting, Promoting and Supporting Breastfeeding in Facilities Providing Maternity and Newborns Services: The Revised Baby-Friendly Hospital Initiative*. Geneva: World Health Organization.

Wilhelm-Bals Alexandra, Birraux Jacques & Girardin Eric. 2010. "Troubles mictionnels de l'enfant. Groupes suisses de travail de néphrologie pédiatrique". *Paediatrica* 21 (5), 25–30.

Williams Stephen. 2008. "What is Fatherhood? Searching for the Reflexive Father". *Sociology* 42 (3), 487–502.

Wolf Joan B. 2006. "What Feminists can Do for Breastfeeding and What Breastfeeding can Do for Feminists". *Signs* 31 (2), 397–424.

Wolf Joan B. 2007. "Is Breast Really Best? Risk and Total Motherhood in the National Breastfeeding Awareness Campaign". *Journal of Health Politics, Policy and Law* 32 (4), 595–636.

Wolf Joan B. 2011. *Is Breast Best? Taking on the Breastfeeding Experts and the New High Stakes of Motherhood*. New York: New York University Press.

Woolridge Michael W. 1995. "Baby-Controlled Breastfeeding: Biocultural Implications". In Stuart-Macadam Patricia & Dettwyler Katherine A. (eds.), *Breastfeeding: Biocultural Perspectives*. New York: Aldine de Gruyter, 217–142.

Young Iris. 2005. *On Female Body Experience. 'Throwing Like a Girl' and Other Essays*. New York: Oxford University Press.

Zanardo Vincenzo, Svegliado Giorgia, Cavallin Francesco, Giustardi Arturo, Cosmi Erich, Litta Pietro, & Trevisanuto Daniele. 2010. "Elective Caesarean Delivery: Does it Have a Negative Effect on Breastfeeding?". *Birth* 37 (4), 275–279.

Index

animalisation (of babies) *see* babies, as
    mammals
Apple Rima 54, 66–68, 163
attachment parenting 6, 75–77
attachment theory 6, 76, 163; and
    breastfeeding 76, 192
authoritative knowledge (*vs.*
    experiential knowledge) 45–46, 85,
    114–120, 212
Avishai Orit 80, 124, 151–152

babies: as breastfeeding partners
    172–174, 186, 204; and child
    psychiatry 73–74, 179; conceptions
    of 72–75, 162, 164–166, 206; as
    mammals 10, 135, 159, 178
Bartlett Allison 66, 159–216
bed-sharing 187–190; and autonomy
    214–215; and breastfeeding 164, 187,
    189; and intimacy 190, 219–220;
    and safety 85–86, 117–118, 129; and
    "skinship" 189–190
birth *see* childbirth
birth centre *see* home birth
Blum Linda 54, 58, 64, 70
Bobel Chris 6, 34, 35, 75, 80–81, 114,
    217–218
body: biopower 10, 50, 52, 214;
    boundaries 74, 79, 155–156, 159,
    216; lactating bodies 127–128,
    150–158, 213–215; as machine
    9, 60–61; techniques 102–103,
    125–126, 135–140; *see also*
    embodiment
body work 124–128, 132–133,
    150–153, 214
bonding theory *see* attachment
    parenting; attachment theory
Bowlby John 6, 11, 42, 76

breastfeeding: the breastfeeding
    project 5–8, 124, 157, 159–160,
    209, 220–221; comforting feeding
    191–192; emotional work 139,
    159, 214; as gender performance
    12, 160, 219; health effects 5, 70;
    and hormones 128–129, 135, 219;
    initiation at home 128–140; and the
    law (Switzerland) 60; and liminality
    79, 154–155, 159, 204–205, 216;
    and linear time 63–66, 181–186,
    204–205, 216–220; long–term
    breastfeeding 77–80, 149–158,
    192–196; negotiated 8–11, 209,
    222–223; on-demand 65–66, 174–
    186; and pain 159, 214; productivist
    vs. qualitative approach 61–63, 92;
    relational process *vs.* milk transfer
    65, 72–73, 94, 172–173, 204–205,
    217; responsive feeding 65, 163–164,
    205, 217; scheduled feeding 64–65,
    162; and sexuality 154–155, 219–
    220; support 135–140; as team work
    (partner's involvment) 141–142,
    147–149, 189; *see also* body work
breastfeeding promotion policies:
    individual choice paradigm 57–58,
    209; in Switzerland 5, 8, 59–60,
    149–150
breast milk (as protection) 116, 201
breast pump 60, 150–153
breasts (sexualisation of) 77–78,
    155–156, 195–196, 219
Butler Judith 11–12, 160

caesarean section birth 77, 90, 157–158
childbirth: hospitalisation of 36–37;
    natural childbirth movement 39–41,
    81, 140, 174–175

child-centred approach 10, 69, 163, 196–197, 206, 214–215
choice: health choices as moral choices 8, 120, 159–160; the informed choice ideal 210, 222; logic of choice *vs.* logic of care 102, 222
cloth diapers 201; *see also* Elimination Communication
co-sleeping *see* bed-sharing

dads *see* fathers
Davis Elizabeth 79, 114, 120
Davis-Floyd Robbie E. 3, 45, 46, 79, 86, 92, 114, 120, 204
development (child): and breastfeeding 192, 205–206, 211, 214, 216; psycho-developmental theories 77, 164, 185, 197
Dick-Read Grantly 39, 81–82, 140, 176
Dykes Fiona 3, 7, 44–45, 55, 60–65, 126, 216–217

elimination communication 197–201, 214–215; and breastfeeding 199
embodiment 124–125; embodied parenting 5–7, 13, 162–163, 189, 206, 213–214; interembodiment (between babies and parents) 74–75, 213–215
ethnographic approach 2, 23–24; interviews 29–31; participant-observation 21–23; participants 31–35, 41–43, 210–211; reflexivity 18–19, 23–29
evidence-based medicine 46, 85

Faircloth Charlotte 69, 75, 78, 143, 163, 192, 201, 203–206, 216
Fassin Didier 8, 25, 52, 211
fathers: and attachment parenting 143, 146; and breastfeeding 141–142, 147–149, 173–174, 217–219; and holistic care 140–146
feminism: and attachment parenting 11–12; and breastfeeding 57–58
formula feeding: in combination with breastfeeding 55–56, 221; and growth curve 86; history of formula industry (history of) 54–56; regulation 56–57; stigmatisation of (by parents) 106, 115–116
Foucault Michel 10, 52

gender: and breastfeeding 217–220; and holistic care 11–12, 142–146; transgression (parental roles) 149, 160
Giddens Anthony 69, 71, 131, 137, 158, 203–204, 211
Gottlieb Alma 7, 72–73, 167, 215

holistic care: accessibility 210; and attachment parenting 34–35, 214–215; and the biomedical model 3–4, 9, 40, 211–212; and breastfeeding 91, 120, 149–150, 221; characteristics 21–23, 31–32, 46–47, 210, 221; and child conception 7, 181, 215; and complementary medicines 34, 42, 137, 170, 212; and continuity of care 2, 33–34, 45–46, 130–131, 166–167, 221; definition 1–2, 3, 9; and heterocentrism 32–33; the holistic care script 6, 35–36, 208; and hospital protocols 87, 92, 93, 120; and normative injunctions 115, 131, 159, 166–167, 203, 204, 211, 222; and risk management 10, 82–83, 95, 97, 99–104, 120, 211, 212; stigmatization of 2, 18–20, 23; and time 43–45, 184, 204, 217
home birth: safety of 1–2; in Switzerland 1–2; *see also* childbirth
hormones *see* breastfeeding, hormones
hospital: and iatrogenic risks (*vs.* home birth) 90, 212; and infant feeding 3, 63, 86, 91, 126, 163–164; *see also* holistic care, and hospital protocols

infant weighing *see* weight (of the baby)
intensive mothering 58, 66–70, 74, 214; and breastfeeding 68–70, 76; and holistic care 10, 82–83; and maternal availability 174–175, 204, 205, 214

Jordan Brigitte 35, 45, 46, 63

Kahn Robbie Pfeufer 66
Katz Rothman Barbara 46–47, 86, 92
Kukla Rebecca 51–53, 75, 77, 81

lactation (management) 131–132, 137, 144, 149–153, 214
La Leche League 60, 104

Lee Ellie 63, 69–70, 72, 77, 163
Lock Margaret 124–125, 213
Lupton Deborah 59, 74–75, 118, 155

Maher Vanessa 63, 125
Martin Emily 43–44, 47, 60–61
maternity leave 4, 183–184, 201, 216
Memmi Dominique 7, 8, 159–160, 206, 211, 213
midwives: gendered approach of 11–12, 142–146, 218–219; independent midwives 3, 41–43; midwifery model of care 46; as newborns' interpreters 166–167; *see also* holistic care
Moscucci Ornella 37, 81
motherhood: embodied motherhood 5–8, 69, 213–214; intensification of 9, 50, 68–70; scientific motherhood 66–68
Murphy Elizabeth 59, 68, 71

natural childbirth *see* childbirth, natural
nature: breastfeeding as natural 10–11, 128–129; *vs.* culture 81–82; natural motherhood 35, 80–82; *see also* childbirth, natural
negotiated breastfeeding *see* breastfeeding, negotiated
neoliberalism: and "civilised babies" 64–65, 171, 178, 181; and definition of the individual 79–80, 204, 206; and risk management 70–71, 211

Odent Michel 10, 40–41, 77, 178
out-of-hospital birth *see* home birth

paediatricians 107–114; and breastfeeding 109–110; collaboration with independent midwives 107–109, 120–121; and diversification 115–116; emergence of paediatrics 52–54; and vaccines 109
Palmer Gabrielle 54–55
paternity leave 4, 147, 208–209, 219
pumping milk *see* breast pump

risk: customized risk management model 85–87, 115–120, 212–213; emotional risk management 118–121; and infant feeding 71–72, 211–213; "parental determinism" 71–72,

159–160; parenting as managing risks 9–10, 71–72, 121, 159–160; parents' negotiations with health professionals 99–102, 104–107, 118–119; *see also* holistic care, and risk management
Rose Nikolas 71, 206, 214–215
Rousseau Jean-Jacques 51–52, 82

Sachs Magda 96, 102–103, 154–155, 214
Scheper-Hughes Nancy 164–165, 171, 204, 213, 215
Schmied Virginia 59, 70, 155, 217
Sears William & Martha 6, 35, 42
sexuality: and breastfeeding *see* breastfeeding, and sexuality; and post-partum bodies 154–155, 220; resuming sexuality (after giving birth) 154–155, 195–196
sleep (and breastfeeding) 181–182, 189, 195; *see also* bed-sharing
Stearns Cindy A. 124, 126, 152, 156
St. John Gloria 3, 45, 204
Switzerland: breastfeeding data 5; breastfeeding promotion *see* breastfeeding promotion policies, in Switzerland; family policies 4–5, 208; gender system 4–5, 219; healthcare system 1–2, 20–21; and heteronormativity 4–5, 32–33, 210–211; history of breastfeeding 51–57; hospitalisation of childbirth 36–37; midwifery in 3–4, 36–39, 41–43, 108; and race 33, 210

temporalities 43–45, 65–68, 181–186, 216–217
Tomori Cecilia 64, 85–86, 125–126, 143–144, 146, 148, 187

vaccine: breastfeeding as "natural vaccine" 116, 121, 213; hesitancy 108–109, 115–117
voluntary simplicity 34, 36, 205

weaning (from the breast): and full term breastfeeding 192–194; as negotiation between mother and child 193–196
weight (of the baby): emotional weighing 96–99; and evaluation of breastfeeding success 61–63;

and hospital protocols 86, 93; test weighing 113; weighing as symbol of midwifery care 113–114, 121; weighing practices (midwives) 93–96

Wolf Joan B. 61, 69, 80

World Health Organisation: guidelines on breastfeeding (parents' sucription to) 6, 124; guidelines on breastfeeding 5

Young Iris 11, 127–128, 156

For Product Safety Concerns and Information please contact our EU
representative GPSR@taylorandfrancis.com
Taylor & Francis Verlag GmbH, Kaufingerstraße 24, 80331 München, Germany